# Pre-Clinical PROSTHODONTICS

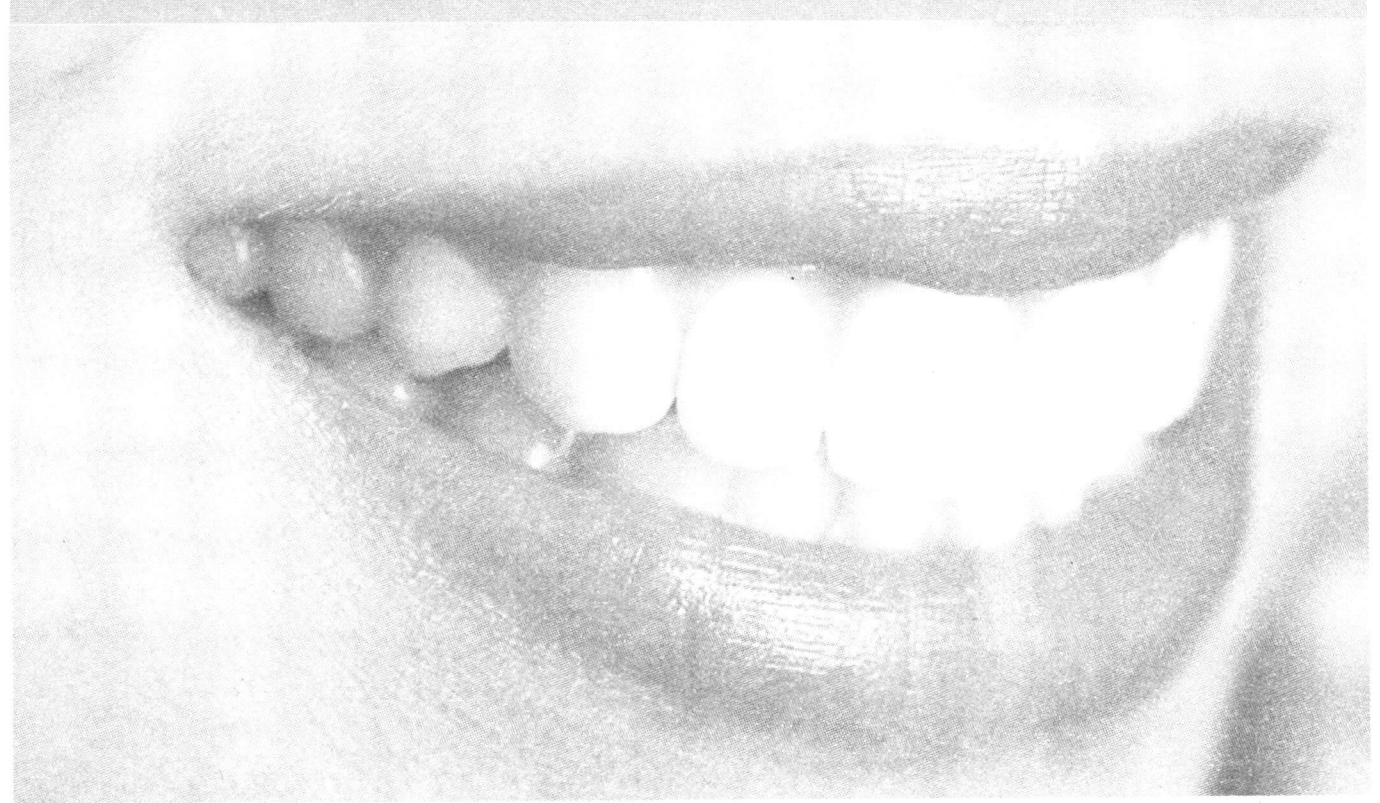

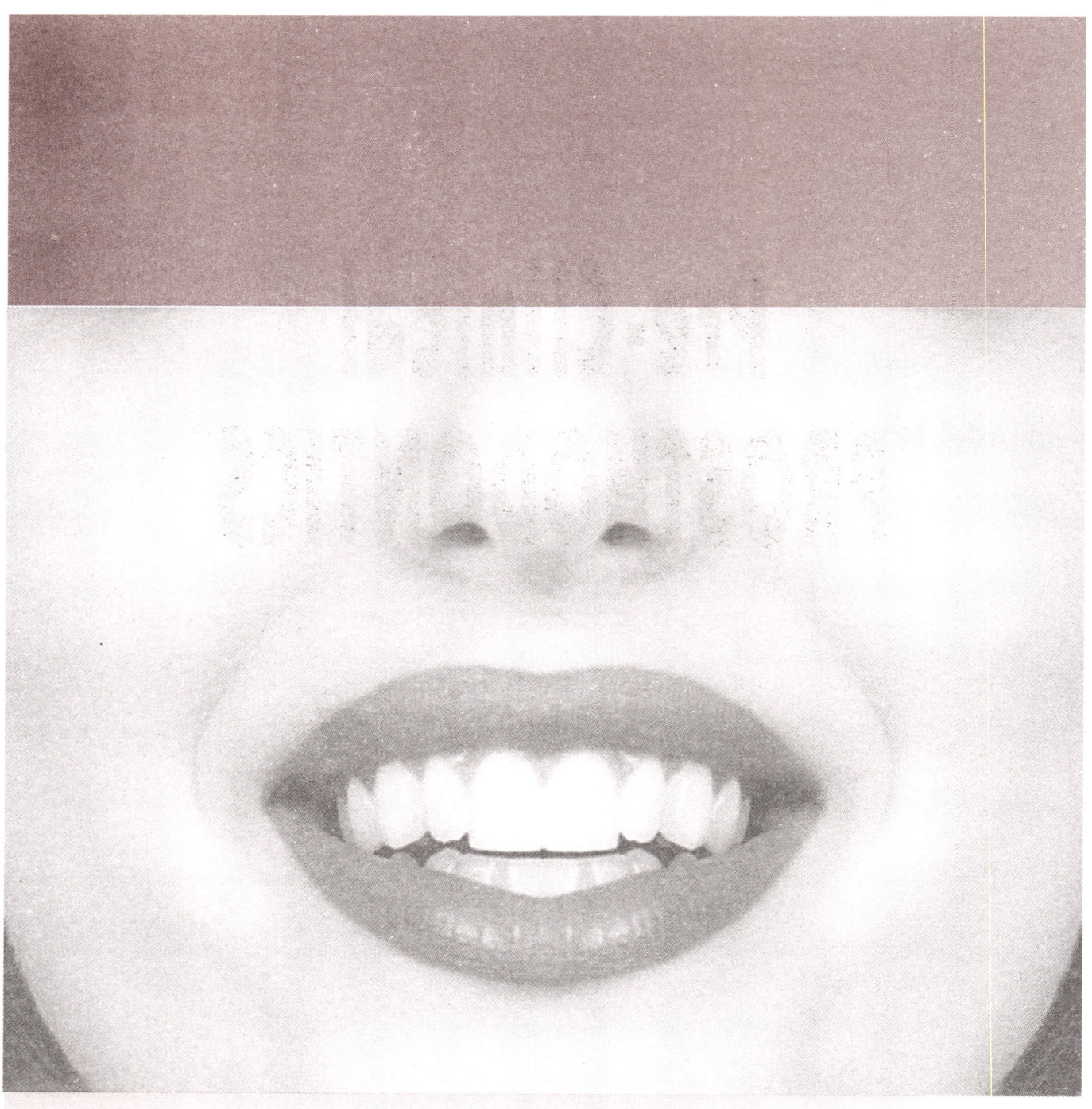

Other CBS books by the same authors:
- Pre-Clinical Operative Dentistry and Endodontics
- Notes on Operative Dentistry and Endodontics, 2/e

# Pre-Clinical PROSTHODONTICS

### Narendranatha Reddy P.
### Vanitha N.

Bangalore

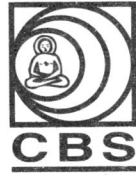

**CBS PUBLISHERS & DISTRIBUTORS PVT. LTD.**
NEW DELHI • BENGALURU • CHENNAI • KOCHI • MUMBAI • PUNE

ISBN : 978-81-239-1767-2

First Edition: 2009
Reprint: 2011, 2015

Copyright © 2009 Authors & Publisher

All rights reserved. No part of this book may be reproduced or transmitted in any form or by any means, electronic or mechanical, including photocopying, recording, or any information storage and retrieval system without permission, in writing, from the authors.

*Published by:*
Satish Kumar Jain for CBS Publishers & Distributors Pvt. Ltd.,
CBS Plaza, 4819/XI Prahlad Street, 24 Ansari Road,
Daryaganj, New Delhi – 110002, India
delhi@cbspd.com, cbspubs@airtelmail.in • www.cbspd.com
Ph.: 23289259, 23266861, 23266867 • Fax: 011-23243014

*Branches:*
- *Bengaluru:* Seema House, 2975, 17th Cross, K.R. Road,
  Bansankari 2nd Stage, Bengaluru - 560070
  Ph: +91-80-26771678/79 • Fax: +91-80-26771680
  E-mail: cbsbng@gmail.com, bangalore@cbspd.com
- *Chennai:* 20, West Park Road, Shenoy Nagar, Chennai - 600030
  Ph: +91-44-26260666, 26208620 • Fax: +91-44-42032115
  E-mail: chennai@cbspd.com
- *Kochi:* 36/14, Kalluvilakam, Lissie Hospital Road, Kochi - 682018
  Ph: +91-484-4059061-65 • Fax: +91-484-4059065
  E-mail: cochin@cbspd.com
- *Mumbai:* 83-C, Dr. E. Moses Road, Worli, Mumbai - 400018
  Ph: +91-9833017933 • E-mail: mumbai@cbspd.com
- *Pune:* Bhuruk Prestige, Sr. No. 52/12/2+1+3/2,
  Narhe, Haveli (Near Katraj-Dehu Road Bypass), Pune - 411041
  Ph: +91-20-64704058/59, 32342277 • E-mail: pune@cbspd.com

*Printed at :*
SDR Printers Pvt. Ltd., Delhi

# Preface

The aim of the authors was to bring out a book on the pre-clinical prosthodontics which should be copious with the requirements of the first and second BDS students. Unfortunately, no book is available on this subject and it is a known fact that the students need to study from at least four or five textbooks for this speciality. Most of the students face difficulty in studying and understanding those texts. Therefore, in trying to fill that pitfall, we have come up with the present volume which furnishes the theory part in a simple and logical manner, as well as the practical aspects. Although utmost care has been taken, any bloopers are purely coincidental and are regretted. As this is the first book of its kind, a few lapses are inevitable. Hence, we welcome the constructive suggestions from the readers, students and the teachers for further improvement and will be duly acknowledged.

Narendranatha Reddy P.
Vanitha N.

drpnnreddy@in.com
drvanithan@in.com

***to***
*our beloved friend*
**Dr KSR PRASAD**
*who has given us the real support
and encouragement
during the years that this
incubus was nurtured*

# About the Course

Prosthodontics is a branch of dentistry pertaining to the restoration and maintenance of oral function, comfort, appearance and health of the patient by the restoration of natural teeth and/or the replacement of missing teeth and contiguous oral and maxillofacial tissues with artificial substitutes. Viewing from academic perspective, this is one of the two subjects that will be studied throughout the BDS course from first to the final year, although the theory examination will be given in the last year (the other being Operative Dentistry and Endodontics). The clinical part of the course will commence in third year. To get accustomed to the clinical environment, a laboratory curriculum called **Pre-Clinical Prosthodontics** is designed and followed for the first two years of the BDS programme. Basic principles of prosthodontics will be taught in this course to enable the dental student to accomplish various clinical procedures necessary to treat the edentulous and the partially edentulous patient, as well as the patient requiring fixed restorations. It has only university practical examination (no theory examination) which will be held at the end of the second year. The examination consists of arrangement of teeth in class I relation, waxing, carving, polishing and a viva voce (some universities examination scheme has survey and designing of RPD and crown preparation on mounted teeth too). This course is intended to prepare the student as fully as possible for his/her introduction to clinical prosthetic dentistry. With successful completion of laboratory training, students will be competent to • properly use and maintain applicable materials and equipment, • produce properly contoured casts, • fabricate accurate impression trays, • record bases and occlusion rims neatly, and • articulate and set up complete denture teeth properly with an esthetic waxup along with its processing. They will also have a basic understanding of • edentulous oral anatomy and • accessory complete denture processing techniques such as relining, rebasing and tissue conditioning, etc. A student's admittance into the clinic is an implied departmental trust that he/she possesses the requisite baseline skills necessary to treat patients.

# Acknowledgements

First and foremost, we would like to express our deep gratitude to our beloved friend Dr. Sitha Ram Prasad Kasina for his immense and constant support. Without his help this book would not have seen the light of the day. We are appreciative of Dr. Naveen D, Coordinator, Brihaspathi Academy, Bangalore, for lending his helping hand in the preparation of this work. We also thank our friends Dr. Sashikanth and Dr. Srinivas for their cooperation during this work. We extend our heartfelt thanks to our friend Mr. Babu Prasad, Ushakirana Innovations, Bangalore, for his excellent typesetting and graphic work.

We are obliged to Mr. Satish Kumar Jain, Managing Director, CBS Publishers & Distributors, who came forward to publish this title, and also to Mr. Y.N. Arjuna, Publishing Director, and Mr. Deepak Rao, General Manager (South), of CBS P&D for their cooperation in this project. Last but not least, we are grateful to our parents and family members for their tolerance of our absence and their sustained backup.

Narendranatha Reddy P.
Vanitha N.

# Contents

Preface  v
About the Course  vii

## Section 1
## INTRODUCTION TO PROSTHODONTICS

**Chapter 1**
**PROSTHODONTICS: AN OVERVIEW**  3
Prosthesis  3
Appliance  5
Prosthodontics  5
Glossary  6

**Chapter 2**
**ANATOMICAL AND PHYSIOLOGICAL ASPECTS**  13
Osteology of Head  13
Temporomandibular Joint  17
Mandibular Movements  19
Muscles of Mastication  19
Depressor Muscles  22
Muscles of Facial Expression  22
Modiolus  23
Tongue  24
Oral Mucous Membrane  24
Saliva  25

**Chapter 3**
**THE ORAL CAVITY**  26
Dentulous and Edentulous  26
Anatomic Landmarks  26
Topography of Edentulous Oral Cavity  27
The Face  29
The Oral Cavity  29

**Chapter 4**
**The Teeth**  41
Teeth—Types and Function  41
Tooth Loss  42
Treatment Considerations  42

**Chapter 5**
**PROSTHODONTIC LABORATORY AND ARMAMENTARIUM**  43

**Chapter 6**
**STERILIZATION AND INFECTION CONTROL**  47

**Chapter 7**
**DENTAL CASTS AND MODELS**  52

## Section 2
## COMPLETE DENTURES

**Chapter 1**
**INTRODUCTION** — 57

**Chapter 2**
**FABRICATION OF COMPLETE DENTURE: AN OVERVIEW** — 59

**Chapter 3**
**EXAMINATION, DIAGNOSIS AND TREATMENT PLANNING** — 61

**Chapter 4**
**IMPRESSION MAKING** — 64
Impression  *64*
Impression Trays  *69*
Primary Impressions  *74*
Final Impression Trays  *78*
Impression Border Molding  *89*
Secondary Impressions  *91*
Beading and Boxing of Final Impression  *93*

**Chapter 5**
**RECORD BASES** — 97

**Chapter 6**
**OCCLUSION RIMS** — 108
Occlusion/Record/Bite/Rims/Bite Blocks  *108*

**Chapter 7**
**POSTERIOR PALATAL SEAL AREA** — 113

**Chapter 8**
**JAW RELATIONS/MAXILLOMANDIBULAR RELATIONSHIPS** — 115
Orientation Jaw Relations  *116*
Face Bow  *116*
Vertical Jaw Relations  *119*
Horizontal Jaw Relations  *120*
Methods of Recording Jaw Relations  *123*

**Chapter 9**
**TEETH SELECTION** — 130

**Chapter 10**
**OCCLUSION** — 140

**Chapter 11**
**ARTICULATORS** — 147

**Chapter 12**
**TEETH ARRANGEMENT** — 153

**Chapter 13**
**TRY-IN PROCEDURES** — 164

**Chapter 14**
**WAXING AND CARVING** — 166

**Chapter 15**
**PROCESSING OF DENTURES** — 169

**Chapter 16**
**INSERTION OF FINISHED DENTURE AND PATIENT EDUCATION** — 185

**Chapter 17**
**MISCELLANEOUS** — 187
Relining and Rebasing  *187*
Repair of Denture Bases  *190*
Immediate Denture  *191*
Overdenture  *191*
Single Complete Denture
  Opposing Natural Teeth  *192*

## Section 3
## REMOVABLE PARTIAL DENTURE

**Chapter 1**
**REMOVABLE PARTIAL DENTURE** — 195

## Section 4
## FIXED PARTIAL DENTURE

**Chapter 1**
**FIXED PARTIAL DENTURE** — 207

## Section 5
## PROSTHODONTIC MATERIALS

**Chapter 1**
**PROSTHODONTIC MATERIALS** — 213

Index — 217

# Section 1
# Introduction to Prosthodontics

# Prosthodontics: An Overview

**CHAPTER 1**

Prosthodontic dentistry deals with the substitution or replacement of oral structures. Prosthodontic dentistry can include anything from replacing one missing tooth to constructing a complex—designed device to replace structures of the face such as eyes, ears, or a cleft palate. Prosthodontic treatment is concerned primarily with replacing missing teeth with some type of artificial substitute. Substitutes for natural teeth are called prosthodontic prostheses. Prosthodontic prostheses are either fixed permanently into the patient's mouth or removable.

This chapter presents in brief about the Prosthesis-definition and types, appliance-definition and differentiation with prosthesis, prosthodontics-definition, scope and objectives and branches, and lastly glossary of important terms.

## PROSTHESIS

- The term *'Prosthesis'* has got varied meanings. It may be defined as *"an artificial replacement of an absent part of the human body"* or *"a therapeutic device to improve or alter function"* or it can also be said as *"a device used to aid in accomplishing a desired surgical result"*.

### TYPES

- Prosthesis is of three types:
  I. Dental prosthesis
  II. Maxillofacial prosthesis
  III. Axillary prosthesis

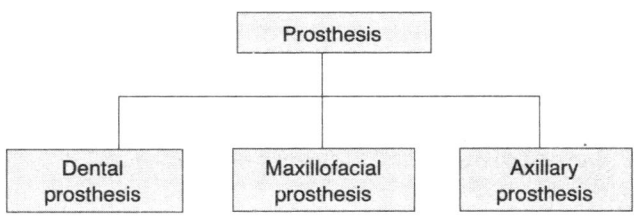

**Fig.1.1.1:** Types of prosthesis

### I. DENTAL PROSTHESIS

- *Dental Prosthesis* can be defined as *"an artificial replacement of one or more teeth (upto entire dentition in either arch) and associated dental/ alveolar structures"*.
- It is subdivided as *"Fixed Dental Prosthesis"* and *"Removable Dental Prosthesis"*.
- Fixed Dental Prosthesis (FDP) is again categorized into three types, i.e.
  i. Cement retained FDP
  ii. Screw retained FDP
  iii. Friction retained FDP

# 4 Pre-Clinical Prosthodontics

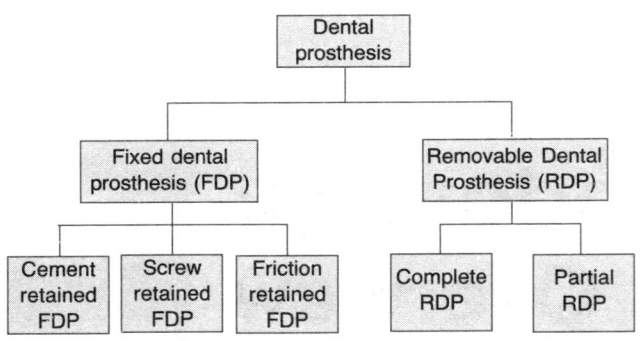

Fig. 1.1.2: Types of dental prosthesis

- Removable dental prosthesis is also catagorized but into two types, i.e.
   i. Complete RDP
   ii. Partial RDP

1. **Fixed Dental Prosthesis**
- FDP can be defined as *"any dental prosthesis that is luted (cemented), screwed or mechanically attached (frictional) or otherwise securely retained to natural teeth, tooth roots and (or dental implant abutments"* (that furnish the primary support for the dental prosthesis).

2. **Removable Dental Prosthesis**
- RDP can be defined as *"any dental prosthesis that replaces some or all teeth in a partially edentulous (without teeth) arch (partial RDP) or edentate/edentulous arch (complete RDP) and that can be removed from the mouth and replaced at will"*.

3. **Partial Removable Dental Prosthesis**
- Also called as *"Removable Partial Denture Prosthesis"*.
- It is defined as *"any prosthesis that replaces some teeth in a partially edentulous arch and that can be removed from the mouth and replaced at will"*.

4. **Complete Removable Dental Prosthesis**
- Also called as *"Removable Complete Denture Prosthesis"*.
- It is defined as *"a removable dental prosthesis that replaces the entire dentition and associated structures of the maxillae or mandible"*.

## II. MAXILLOFACIAL PROSTHESIS (MP)

- It is defined as *"any prosthesis that is used to replace a part or all of any stomatognathic and/or craniofacial structures"*.
- Depending on the source of its retention, it is subdivided in *tissue retained MP, tooth retained MP, implant retained MP, tissue and implant retained MP*.

## III. ANCILLARY PROSTHESIS

- It is a prosthesis, that cannot be categorised as either a dental prosthesis or a maxillofacial prosthesis.
- They are intended for short term or special usage purposes.
- Examples include splints, carriers (fluoride gel, radiation), feeding aids, guides, stents, etc.
- **Prosthodontics** is *"a branch of dentistry pertaining to the diagnosis, treatment planning, rehabilitation and maintenance of the oral function, comfort, appearance and health of patients with clinical conditions associated with missing or deficient teeth and/or maxillofacial tissues using biocompatible substitutes"*. The term *Prosthodontics* has been derived from Latin—*pros*: replacement, *dons*-teeth, *ics*-science.

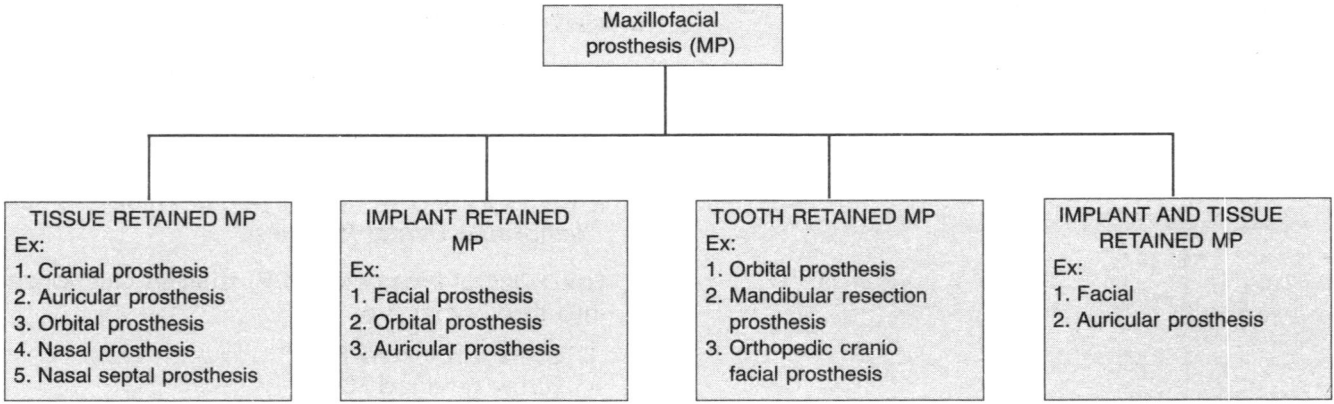

Fig. 1.1.3: Types of maxillofacial prosthesis

## APPLIANCE

- Appliance is defined as "a dental or surgical device designed to perform a therapeutic or corrective function."

## PROSTHODONTICS

- **Prosthodontist** is a specialist in prosthodontics and who has successfully completed an advanced education programme in the speciality of prosthodontics that is accredited (recognised) by the appropriate body. In India, those bodies are the Universities of Health Sciences and which are inturn under the control of Dental council of India (DCI).
- Father of Prosthodontics.

### SCOPE AND OBJECTIVES OF PROSTHODONTICS

- Prosthodontics is pertaining to the restoration and maintenance of oral function, comfort, appearance and health of the patient by the restoration of natural teeth and/or the replacement of missing teeth and contiguous oral and maxillofacial tissues with artificial substitutes.
- The objectives of prosthodontics are:
  1. Preservation of remaining oral structures.
  2. Promotion of health.
  3. Restoration of function and esthetics.

### BRANCHES OF PROSTHODONTICS

- Prosthodontics is broadly categorized into 4 branches, i.e.
  1. Removable Prosthodontics
     - Which is again divided into two sub branches, i.e.
       i. Complete denture prosthondontics.
       ii. Partial denture prosthondontics.
  2. Fixed prosthodontics.
  3. Maxillofacial prosthodontics.
  4. Implant prosthodontics.

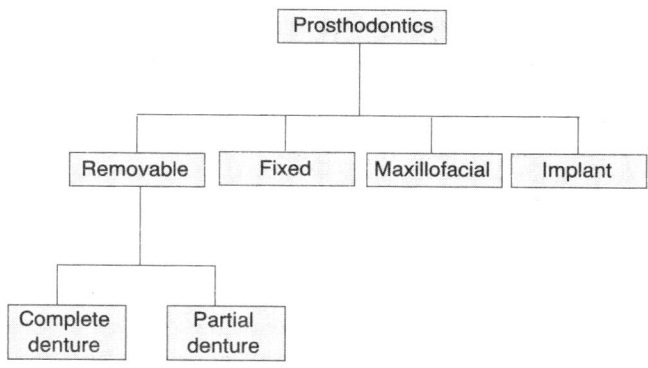

Fig.1.1.4: Branches of prosthodontics

1. **Removable Prosthodontics**
   - The branch of prosthodontics concerned with the replacement of missing teeth and adjacent structures for edentulous or partially edentulous patients by artificial substitutes that can be removed at will.

2. **Complete Denture Prosthodontics**
   - That body of knowledge and skills pertaining to the restoration of the edentulous arch with a removable dental prosthesis.

3. **Removable Partial Denture**
   - Any prosthesis that replaces some teeth in a partially dentate arch, that can be removed from the mouth and replaced at will.
   - It is also called as **partial removable dental prothesis**.

4. **Fixed Prosthodontics**
   - The branch of prosthodontics concerned with the replacement and/or restoration of teeth by artificial substitutes that are not readily removed from the mouth.

5. **Maxillofacial Prosthodontics**
   - The branch of prosthodontics concerned with the restoration and/or replacement of the stomatognathic and craniofacial structures with prosthesis that may or may not be removed on a regular or elective basis.

6. **Implant Prosthodontics**
   - The phase of prosthodontics concerning the replacement of missing teeth and or associated structures by restorations that are attached to dental implants.

# GLOSSARY

*Abutment:* A tooth used to support a removable partial denture or anchor a fixed partial denture.

*Acrylic Resin:* The plastic material widely used in dentistry to make the denture base.

*Alloy:* A combination of two or more metals. Golds for casting, wires, and solders are alloys.

*Alma Gauge:* A precise measuring device for accurate denture construction that pinpoints the vertical and horizontal position of the central incisor teeth relative to the incisive papilla in a two dimensional prescription.

*Alveolar Bone (al veel' ar bone):* The specialized bone structure, which supports the teeth.

*Amalgam:* An alloy of mercury and silver (with other alloying metals) used as a restorative material and for making dies.

*Anneal:* To soften a metal by controlled heating and cooling. Normally done before bending or swaging.

*Anterior Teeth:* Central incisors, lateral incisors, and canines of either upper or lower arch.

*Antero-Posterior:* Extending from the front backward.

*Articulate: (teeth):* To arrange the denture teeth in their proper positions in the trial baseplate. To "set-up" the teeth, (casts); To bring two casts together in occlusion. To mount the upper and lower casts on the articulator.

*Articulation:* (1) The harmonious contact of the opposing teeth in closed position and in lateral and protrusive movements. (2) Junction of two bones which may or may not be movable joint.

*Articulator:* A mechanical instrument that represents the temporomandibular joints and jaws, to which maxillary and mandibular casts may be attached to simulate some or all mandibular movements.

*Artificial Stone:* Gypsum product similar to Plaster of Paris but with much greater density and strength. May be colored to distinguish it from plaster.

*Backing:* A metal support which serves to attach a facing to a prosthesis.

*Balance (in occlusion):* The simultaneous harmonious contacts of tooth surfaces in different parts of the mouth, which act to prevent tipping of the denture.

*Balancing Side:* The side opposite the working side of the dentition or denture.

*Base Metal:* A metal such as copper or iron not classified as a noble metal.

*Baseplate:* A temporary form representing the base of a denture which is used for making jaw relation records and for the arrangement of teeth. STABILIZED B. A baseplate lined with a plastic material to improve its fit and stability.

*Baseplate Wax:* A hard pink wax used for making occlusion rims, waxing dentures, and other dental procedures.

*Bennett Movement:* The lateral shift of the condyle first described by a British dentist.

*Bite Block or Occlusion Rim:* Occluding surfaces fabricated on interim or final denture bases for the purpose of making maxillomandibular relation records and arranging teeth.

*Bonding Agent:* A material used to promote adhesion or cohesion between two different substances, or between a material and natural tooth structures.

*Boxing:* The placing of a retaining wall of wax around an impression to confine the plaster or stone as the cast is poured.

*Bridge (fixed partial denture):* A restoration of one or more missing teeth which cannot be readily removed by the patient or dentist; it is permanently attached to natural teeth or roots which furnish the primary support to the appliance.

*Brilliance or Value:* The amount of whiteness or darkness in a color. The more white a color contains the more brilliant it appears. The more black or grey, the less brilliant it appears.

*Buccal:* Pertaining to the cheek; the surface of the tooth toward the cheek.

*Buccal Frenum:* The string-like tissue, which attaches the cheeks to, the alveolar ridge in the premolar region of each arch.

*Burnish:* The drawing or flattening out of a malleable metal through pressure.

*Cast (noun):* An object formed by pouring a material (usually stone, plaster, or investment) into an impression; also called "model."

*Cast (verb):* To cast a material into a mold (such as inlay, crown, or partial denture).

*Cast Relator (Gothic Arch Relator):* A mechanical device that orients a cast to an articulator using a gothic arch tracing, without reference to anatomic landmarks.

*Cast Study:* A positive likeness of dental structures for the purpose of study and treatment planning.

*Central Bearing*: Application of forces between the maxilla and mandible at a single point that is located at the center of the maxillary and mandibular denture supporting areas. It is used for distributing forces evenly throughout the supporting structures during the registration of maxillomandibular relations and during the correction of occlusal errors.

*Central Bearing Point*: The anatomical center of the upper arch. The critical point that determines the upper cast-to-articulator mounting position. It is located on the median suture line of the upper cast (the vertical line dividing the arch in left and right halves), halfway between the incisive papilla and the foveae palatinae.

*Centric Occlusion*: The relations of opposing tooth surfaces when the jaws are in centric relation. For dentures, this will be the same position as the maximum planned contact and/or intercuspation.

Centric Relation

1. The most posterior relation of the mandible to the maxilla at the established vertical dimension.

2. The relation of the mandible to the maxilla when the condyles are in their most posterior position in the glenoid fossa, from which unstrained lateral movements can be made at the normal occluding vertical dimension for the individual.

*Clasp*: The metal part of a partial denture which partly encircles an abutment tooth and helps to support, stabilize, and retain the denture.

*Class I Arch Form*: Arch form with a shallow palatal vault; generally square or ovoid arch form.

*Class II Arch*: Arch form with a moderate palatal vault; generally square tapering arch form.

*Class III Arch*: Arch form with a deep palatal vault; generally tapering arch form.

*Condyle*: The rounded end of a bone at the articular end of the mandible.

*Connector*: A term used in partial denture prosthesis meaning a bar, which connects two or more parts of the appliance: (a) major connector: the rigid bar which connects the saddles or major parts. (b) minor connector: the bar which connects clasps to frame.

*Coping*: A thin cover or matrix usually made of cast metal or acrylic resin to fit over a prepared tooth. A crown is then constructed over the coping.

*Cross Bite*: A condition in which the ridge of the mandible lies so far outside the maxillary ridge that normal arrangement of teeth is not feasible.

*Crosslinked*: A typing together of acrylic resin molecules chemically to produce a more stable resin.

*Crown*: Artificial: A replacement of the coronal portion of a tooth.

*Curing*: The process by which denture base materials are hardened to the form of a denture in a denture mold.

*Curve of Spee*: Anatomic curvature of the occlusal alignment of teeth beginning at the tip of the lower canine and following the buccal cusps of the natural premolars and molars, continuing to the anterior border of the ramus.

*Curve of Wilson*: The curvature of the cusps of the teeth as projected on the frontal plane; that of the inferior dental arch is concave and that of the superior dental arch is convex.

*Cuspid Line*: The area marked on an occlusion rim noting the desired position of the cuspid (canine) teeth. It may indicate the distal, mesial, or middle of the cuspid, but must be agreed upon by the clinical professional and the dental laboratory. (Source: DENTSPLY Trubyte literature).

*Deciduous Teeth*: The first teeth of childhood which are later replaced by the permanent dentition.

*Dentition*: Natural teeth in the dental arch.

*Dentulous*: Having natural teeth present in the mouth and capable of function.

*Denture*: An artificial substitute for missing natural teeth and adjacent tissues.

*Denture, Complete*: A dental prosthesis which is a substitute for the lost natural dentition and associated structures of the maxilla or mandible.

*Denture, Immediate*: A dental prosthesis constructed before removal of the teeth and inserted at the time of extraction.

*Denture Service*: Those procedures which are involved in the diagnosis, construction, and maintenance of artificial substitutes for missing natural teeth.

*Devesting or Deflasking*: The retrieval of a processed denture from an investing medium.

*Diagnosis*: A scientific evaluation of existing conditions.

*Diagnostic Model*: A life-size reproduction of a part or parts of the oral cavity and/or facial structures for the purpose of study and treatment planning.

*Diastema*: A space between two adjacent teeth in the same dental arch.

*Diatoric*: The retentive hole or channel in a denture tooth that allows denture base material to fill the space, producing a mechanical lock for retention.

*Die*: A positive reproduction of a tooth or preparation, usually in metal or stone.

*Distal*: The side of a tooth farthest away from the median line in the dental arch.

*Edentics*: A program of continuing care for the edentulous patient.

*Edentulous*: Without teeth. It may be a specific area, one arch or the entire mouth.

*Enamel*: The white, compact, and very hard substance that covers and protects the dentin of the crown of the tooth.

*Endodontics*: Deals primarily with the treatment of diseased tooth pulp, and adjacent areas in the jaw.

*Esthetics*

(1) The branch of philosophy dealing with beauty, especially with the components thereof, viz., color, form, and arrangement. (2) The qualities involved in the appearance of a given restoration.

*Extra-Oral*: Outside the mouth.

*Facial*: Pertaining to the face. The surface of the tooth or appliance nearest the lips or cheeks. Used synonymously for the words buccal and labial.

*Face-Bow*: A caliper-like device used to record the relationship between the maxilla and condyles of the mandible and to transfer this relationship to an articulator.

*Festooning*: Carvings in the base material of a denture that simulate the contours of the natural tissues that are being replaced by a denture.

*Finishing*: The procedure where scratches and/or surface defects are removed using grinding instruments.

*Fixed Bridge*: A fixed partial denture. One that is cemented firmly in position.

*Flash*: Denture base acrylic that has seeped onto land area or tooth surfaces during processing.

*Flask*: A frame constructed in sections into which a denture is invested for processing.

*Foramen*: A hole or perforation in the bone.

*Fossa*: A shallow depression of the bone.

*Fovea*: A pit, dimple, or depression.

*Foveae Palatinae*: Two small pits or depressions in the posterior aspect of the palate, one on each side of the midline, at or near the attachment of the soft palate to the hard palate.

*Frenum*: The small band or fold of connective tissue covered with mucous membrane, which attaches the tongue, lips, and cheeks to adjacent structures.

*Gerodontics*: That branch of dentistry, which deals with the dental problems and conditions of the aged.

*Gingiva*: That part of the gum tissue, which immediately surrounds a tooth.

*Glaze*: The final firing of porcelain which imparts a high gloss.

*Hamular Notch*: The palpable notch formed by the junction of the maxilla and the pterygoid hamulus of the sphenoid bone.

*High Lip Line*: The greatest height to which the lip is raised in normal function or during the act of smiling broadly.

*Hue*: A color as seen in the visible spectrum, i.e., red, yellow, blue, etc.

*Immediate Denture*: A dental prosthesis constructed before removal of the teeth and inserted at the time of extraction.

*Impression*: A negative reproduction of a given area.

*Incisive Papilla*: The elevation of soft tissue covering the foramen (opening) of the incisive or nasopalatine canal.

*Index*: A core or mold used to indicate relative positions so that a part may be removed and replaced in exactly the same position as before.

*Inlay*: A restoration (gold, porcelain) made to fit a prepared tooth cavity and then cemented into place.

*Inter-Condylar Distance*: The distance between the rotational centers of two condyles or their analogues.

*Interproximal*: Between adjoining tooth surfaces.

*Intra-Oral*: Within the mouth.

*Invest*: To surround, embed, or envelop in a material to hold the pieces in place during a subsequent operation.

*Investing or Flasking*: The process used to fabricate an exact duplicate of the wax-up by covering it with a suitable investment material in a flask before processing.

*Investment*: A refractory material used to form a mold for casting.

*Labial*: Pertaining to the lip or toward the lip.

*Labial Flange*: The portion of the flange of a denture that occupies the labial vestibule of the mouth.

*Labial Frenum*: The connective tissue "string" which attaches the upper and lower lip to the alveolar ridge at or near the midline.

*Lateral Movement*: Movement of the mandible to the side.

*Lingual*: Pertaining to the tongue or towards the tongue.

*Lingual Bar*: A metal bar (cast or wrought) used to connect the right and left sides of a lower partial denture.

*Low Lip Line*: The lowest position of the lower lip during smiling or voluntary reaction. The lowest position of the upper lip at rest.

*Malocclusion*: Any deviation from a normal occlusion.

*Mandible*: The lower jaw.

*Masking*: An opaque covering used as an undercoat so that metal will not show through plastic or porcelain veneers.

*Master Cast (model)*: The positive reproduction in stone made from an accurate final impression.

*Master Model*: A replica of the tooth surfaces, residual ridge areas, and/or other parts of the dental arch and/or facial structures used to fabricate a dental restoration or prosthesis.

*Mastication*: The process of chewing food for swallowing and digestion.

*Matrix*: The foundation in which something is formed. The space remaining in the flask after a wax denture is eliminated and into which material for the denture is packed.

*Maxilla*: The upper jaw.

*Maximal Intercuspal Position*: The position where maxillary and mandibular teeth have maximal contact and interdigitation. This is the same as centric occlusion-when the jaws are in centric relation.

*Mechanical Retention*: Parts bound together by mechanical means, for example, rough surfaces, undercut areas or diatoric holes.

*Median Line*: An imaginary line running vertically through the center of the face. It is marked on the occlusion rim as a guide to placement of the central incisors.

*Mesial*: Toward the median line. That surface of a tooth towards median line.

*Milling*: The procedure where specific areas are ground or adjusted to achieve a specific fit or interface. Also referred to as selective grinding.

*Milling-In*: The procedure of refining or perfecting the occlusion of teeth by the use of abrasives while the occluding surfaces are rubbed together either on the articulator or in the mouth.

*Model*: Reproduction in plaster or metal of any object, as a tooth, or the dental arch, by pouring the material into an impression taken from the object.

*Mold (Mould)*

(1) A term used to specify the shape and size of a tooth according to a certain system of classification. (2) A form in which an object is cast or formed.

*Mould Chart*: A chart depicting the moulds available in a given line of artificial teeth and listing their dimensions and combinations with appropriate lowers or posteriors.

*Mould Guide*: All mould available in a given line of artificial teeth. Aids in the selection of the most appropriate mould for an individual and permits interchanging of teeth for better esthetics. Non-usable tooth mould guide: teeth contain iron pins for use as selection aid only. Usable tooth mould guide: all moulds in a given line in usable teeth.

*Mounting*: The attachment of casts to the articulator with plaster or stone.

*Mucobuccal Fold*: The line of flexure of the mucous membrane as it passes from the mandible or maxilla to the cheek.

*Mylohyoid Ridge*: An oblique ridge on the lingual surface of the mandible that extends from the level of the roots of the last molar teeth and that serves as a bony attachment for the mylohyoid muscles forming the floor of the mouth.

*Neutral Zone*: The potential space between the lips and cheeks on one side and the tongue on the other; that area or position where the forces between the tongue and cheeks or lips are equal.

*Noble Metal*: A metal not easily oxidized. Example: gold, platinum. Opposite of base metal.

*Obturator*: A prosthesis used to close a congenital or acquired opening in the palate.

*Occlude*: To bring together. To bring the mandibular teeth into contact with the maxillary teeth.

*Occlusal*

(1) Pertaining to the contacting surfaces of opposing occlusal units (teeth or occlusion rims). (2) Pertaining to the masticating surfaces of the posterior teeth.

*Occlusion*: The relationship between the opposing surfaces of upper and lower teeth when they are in contact either in the mouth or on an articulator.

*Occlusion Rim*: Occluding surfaces built on baseplates for the purpose of recording maxillomandibular relationships. Also used as a base for arranging the teeth.

*Oral Surgery*: Deals primarily with the removal of teeth, treatment of jaw fractures, removal of tumors, and correction of malformed facial bones. Other specialties include oral pathology, and public health dentistry.

*Orthodontics*: Deals with prevention and correction of irregularities of the teeth and jaws.

*Overbite*: Vertical overlap of the upper anteriors over lowers.

*Overjet*: Horizontal protrusion of the upper anteriors beyond the lowers.

*Palate*: The roof of the mouth.

*Cleft P.*: An opening in the palate. It may be in the hard or soft palate or both and may be present from birth or caused by surgery, disease, or accident.

*Papilla*: A small nipple shaped elevation.

*Incisive P.*: A rounded projection at the anterior end of the palate. Interdental P.: The triangular pad of gum which fills the space between the necks of the teeth.

*Partial Denture*: A dental prosthesis which restores one or more, but less than all, of the natural teeth and/or associated parts and which is supported by the teeth and/or the mucosa; it may be removable or fixed.

*Pennyweight (DWT)*: 1/20 part of a troy ounce. 24 grains equal 1 dwt.

*Petrolatum*: A petroleum ointment base used as a lubricant in dentistry (examples: Vaseline®, Triad®, and Model Release Agent).

*Periphery*: The outward part of the surface or border. A term frequently used to describe the border of a denture or an impression.

*Phonetics*: The science of sounds used in speech.

*Polishing*: The procedure where tool marks are removed by the use of fine abrasives to achieve a high gloss surface.

*Pontic*: That part of a fixed bridge which is suspended between abutments and which replaces a missing tooth or teeth.

*Posterior Teeth*: Premolars and molars of either jaw.

*Postpalatal Seal Area*: The soft tissue area at or beyond the junction of the hard and soft palate on which pressure, within physiologic limits, can be applied by a denture to aid in its retention.

*Postpalatal Seal*: The seal area at the posterior border of a maxillary prosthesis.

*Post Dam*: The seal at the posterior border of a denture. Preferred term is posterior palatal seal.

*Post Dam or Postpalatal Seal*: The seal area at the posterior border of a maxillary prosthesis.

*Prosthesis*: (Dental) an artificial replacement of one or more teeth and/or associated structures.

*Prosthodontics*: Prosthetic Dentistry; The branch of dental art and science pertaining to restoration of oral function by the replacement of missing teeth and structures by artificial devices.

*Protrusive Bite (Occlusion)*: Contact relation of the upper and lower teeth when the mandible is brought forward with the anteriors edge to edge.

*Proximal Surface*: The surface of a tooth which lies next to another tooth. Nearly always the mesial or distal surface unless the tooth is rotated.

*Pulp*: The connective tissue found in the pulp chamber and canals. It is made up of arteries, veins, nerves, lymph tissue, and connective tissue.

*Pumice*: An abrasive agent used in many polishing procedures.

*Quick Cure Resin (Autopolymer Resin)*: An acrylic resin wherein an activating substance has been added to the monomer which will initiate polymerization or cure without the use of external heat.

*Ramus*: The ascending part of the mandible.

*Rebase*: A process of refitting a denture by replacement of the denture base material on a new case without changing the occlusal relations of the teeth.

*Relief*: The reduction or elimination of pressure from a specific area under a denture base.

*Reline*: To resurface the tissue side of a denture with new base material to make it fit more accurately.

*Removable Partial Denture*: A partial denture which may be removed and replaced by the patient.

*Resorption*: The gradual reduction in volume and size of the alveolar portion of the mandible or maxilla.

*Retainer*

(1) Any type of clasp, attachment, or device used for the fixation or stabilization of prosthesis. (2) A device used by orthodontist to maintain teeth in the desired position after orthodontic treatment.

*Retromolar Pad*: A mass of tissue usually pear-shaped, which is located at the distal termination of the mandibular residual ridge.

*Retrusion*: A backward position of the mandible.

*Ridge*: The remainder of the alveolar process and its soft tissue covering after the teeth are removed. *Center of R.*: The bucco-lingual midline of the residual ridge. *Crest of R.*: The highest continuous surface of the ridge, but not necessarily the center of the ridge. (2) The top of the residual or alveolar ridge.

*Ridge Lap*: The area of an artificial tooth which normally overlaps the alveolar ridge. It corresponds on the inner surface of the tooth approximately to the location of the collar on the facial surface.

*Roentgenogram*: Photograph made with X-rays.

*Rugae*: The irregular ridges found in the anterior region of the upper hard palate. They aid in speech and manipulation

*Saddle (Base)*: The part of a partial denture, upper or lower, which fits on the alveolar ridge and in which the teeth are held.

*Sagittal Plane*: The plane that divides the body vertically into two equal halves.

*Saturation or Chroma*: The relative strength of a hue.

*Scribe*: To write, trace, or mark by making a line or lines with a pointed instrument.

*Separator or Separating Medium*: A coating applied to a surface and serving to prevent a second surface from adhering to the first.

*Set Up*: (noun) A broad term usually denoting a full upper and lower arrangement of teeth in wax. (verb) The act of arranging and positioning artificial teeth in a complete or partial denture.

*Set-Up Wax*: Specially formulated for arranging and articulating artificial teeth, this wax can be "stretched" and moved without breaking, and boils-out cleanly. (Source: DENTSPLY Set-Up Wax directions).

*Shade Guide*: Samples of colors, which are available in manufactured teeth.

*Shade Selection*: The determination of the color (hue, brilliance, saturation) of an artificial tooth or set of teeth for a given patient.

*Shelf Life*: The period of time which a material can be stored without losing its useful properties.

*Sluice Ways*: The escape ways through which food leaves the occlusal portion of the teeth in the process of chewing.

*Spatulate*: To manipulate or mix with a spatula.

*Splint*: An appliance for the fixation of movable, displaced, or fractured parts.

*Sprue*: Wax or metal used to form the aperture or passageway for molten metal to flow into a mold to make a casting; also the metal which later fills the sprue hole.

*Stabilized Baseplate*: A baseplate lined with a plastic material to improve its fit and stability.

*Stippling*: To create depressions in the buccal and labial surface of the denture base to prevent leafy foods from adhering.

*Sulcus*: A groove or depression on the surface of a tooth.

*Surveying*: The procedure of locating and outlining the contour and position of abutment teeth and associated structures on the master cast before designing a removable partial denture. The purpose is to determine the most favorable path of insertion for the partial and to mark survey lines on the teeth to aid in the development of a suitable design for the metal framework.

*Suture Line*: A junction point where the bones of the cranium unite.

*Swage*: To shape metal by hammering or adapting it onto a die.

*Teeth, Anatomic*: Artificial teeth which closely duplicate the form and appearance of natural teeth.

*Teeth, Non-Anatomic*: Teeth whose occlusal surfaces are based on mechanical rather than anatomic forms.

*Teeth, Plastic*: Artificial teeth constructed of synthetic resins.

*Teeth, Porcelain*: Artificial teeth constructed of feldspar, kaolin, and silica.

*Teeth, Tube*: Artificial teeth constructed with a vertical, cylindric aperture extending from the center of the base up into the body of the tooth into which a pin may be placed or cast for the attachment of the tooth to a restoration.

*Teeth, Zero Degree*: Posterior teeth having a flat occlusal surface.

*Template*: A flat or curved plate usually of metal which is used as a guide in arranging artificial teeth.

*Tensile Strength*: Resistance to breakage from a stretching or pulling force.

*Thermal Expansion*: Expansion caused by heat.

*Thermoplastic*: A polymeric material, which can be softened by heat and which, hardens upon cooling.

*Transverse Horizontal Axis*: Also called the hinge axis. An imaginary line around which the mandible may rotate within the sagittal plane. All articulators function within the hinge axis.

*Trauma*: A hurt; a wound; an injury; damage; impairment; external violence producing bodily injury or degeneration.

*Try-In*: A preliminary insertion of a wax-up trial denture, partial denture casting or finished restoration to determine the fit, esthetics, maxillomandibular relations, etc.

*Try-In Selector*: (Shade Selector) A set of 6 upper anterior artificial teeth in each shade available in a given line of teeth to permit visualizing the effect of "staggered" shades by selecting laterals and canines of a shade different from the centrals.

*Tuberosity*: A bulge sometimes found at the posterior end of the maxillary ridge.

*Vacuum Fired*: The baking of porcelain in a vacuum to eliminate trapped air.

*Vault*: The palate or roof of the mouth.

*Veneer*: A thin layer.

*Vertical Dimension*: A vertical measurement of the face between any two arbitrarily selected points which are conveniently located, one above and one below the mouth, usually in the midline.

*Vertical Dimension of Occlusion*: The distance measured between two points when the occluding members are in contact.

*Working Side*: The lateral segment of a denture or dentition towards which the mandible is moved.

# Anatomical and Physiological Aspects

**CHAPTER 2**

Oral cavity is a space that is surrounded by numerous bones and muscles and is constantly influenced by them accordingly. Once a prosthesis is placed in the mouth, it also gets influenced. It is essential to refresh your knowledge about these influential structures on oral cavity for the delivery of better prosthesis

## OSTEOLOGY OF HEAD

- The skull is that portion of the human skeleton which makes up the bony framework of the head. For descriptive purposes, the skull is divided into an upper, dome-shaped, cranial portion; and a lower or facial portion composed of the eye sockets, nasal cavities, and both jaws. The adult skull is composed of 22 bones (8 cranial and 14 facial).

### CRANIAL BONES

- The 8 bones of the cranium are:
    1. Frontal
    2. Parietal (right and left)
    3. Occipital
    4. Temporal (right and left)
    5. Sphenoid
    6. Ethmoid.

### NOTE

- The shape and arrangement of these 8 bones form a bony shell (cranium) that has a central cavity containing the brain. The arched roof of the cranial cavity is called the *Vault* and the floor of the cavity is called the *Base*.

### FACIAL BONES

- There are 14 bones in the facial portion of the skull
    1. Maxilla
    2. Palatine
    3. Zygomatic
    4. Lacrimal
    5. Nasal
    6. Inferior concha
    7. Vomer
    8. Mandible

**NOTE**
- There is only one vomer and one mandible in a skull: the other facial bones are paired.

## CRANIAL AND FACIAL BONES OF PRIMARY INTEREST IN PROSTHETIC DENTISTRY

- Artificial replacements for missing natural teeth (dental prostheses) must be made to fit jaw contours and work in harmony with muscle activity. Therefore, we will discuss only those facial bones which give shape to soft tissues within the mouth, serve as anchorage sites for muscles which move the lower jaw, and give shape to the lower one-half of the face.
- **Cranial Bones of Primary Interest**
  1. Frontal
  2. Parietal
  3. Temporal
  4. Sphenoid
- **Facial Bones of Primary Interest**
  1. Maxilla
  2. Palatine
  3. Zygomatic
  4. Mandible
- Particular features of these bones are important to remember for subsequent reference in this publication and indeed, for the remainder of your professional career.

## FRONTAL BONE

- The frontal bone is a single bone that forms the anterior of the cranial vault, the roof of the eye sockets, and a small portion of the nasal cavity. A temporal line can be found on both lateral surfaces of the frontal bone. The line begins in the region of the eye socket and proceeds posteriorly, often dividing into superior and inferior temporal lines near the posterior border of the frontal bone.

## PARIETAL BONES

- The paired parietal bones are located between the occipital and frontal bones to form the largest portion of the top and sides of the cranium. The parietal bones are marked by two semicircular bony ridges, the superior and inferior temporal lines, which are the posterior continuation of the frontal bone's temporal line. The superior and inferior temporal lines rim the area of origin of the temporal muscle.

## TEMPORAL BONES

- Temporal bones are the paired bones which form a portion of the right and left sides of the skull below the parietal bones. The temporal bones extend down onto the under surface of the cranium and contribute to the formation of the cranial base. Each temporal bone articulates with the parietal above, the sphenoid in front, and the occipital bone behind.
- The significant features of the temporal bone are:
  i. Mastoid process
  ii. Styloid process
  iii. Zygomatic process
  iv. Glenoid fossa
  v. Articular eminence
  vi. Auditory canal or external auditory meatus
- The *convex posterior part* of the temporal bone *(mastoid portion)* is characterized by a rounded, downward projecting mastoid process. The mastoid process presents a roughened exterior surface for attaching several muscles of the neck.
- The *styloid process* is a slender, tapering spur of bone projecting downward from the under surface of the temporal bone. The styloid process has sites of attachment for multiple muscles and ligaments which then go to the mandible, the hyoid bone, the throat, and the tongue.
- The *zygomatic process* is a projection from the approximate center of each temporal bone which extends forward to form a part of the zygomatic arch or cheek bone. This arch or so-called cheek bone is not one continuous bone, but is made up of a number of parts. The zygomatic process of the temporal bone forms the posterior part.
- The *glenoid fossa* is a deep hollow on the under surface of the base of the zygomatic process. The base of the zygomatic process is the place where the process originates from the central mass of the temporal bone.
- The *articular eminence* is a ramp-shaped prominence which extends forward and downward from the anterior boundary of the glenoid fossa.
- The *auditory canal or external auditory meatus* is a hole in the bone found posterior to the glenoid fossa. It leads from the outside surface of the base of the zygomatic process to the inner portions of the ear.

## SPHENOID BONE

- The sphenoid bone resembles a bat with wings extended. It consists of a central portion or body which is situated in the middle of the base of the skull and three pairs of processes: two laterally extended greater wings, two downward projecting pterygoid processes, and two lesser wings. The features of the sphenoid bone we will discuss are:

i. Greater wings
  ii. Spine of the sphenoid
  iii. Pterygoid processes

- *Greater Wings:* A greater wing forms part of the surface contour of the cranium anterior to the temporal bone, and also forms part of the eye socket.

- *Spine of the Sphenoid:* This is just inferior to the lateral, posterior, inferior border of the greater wing of the sphenoid bone. The spine of the sphenoid is the site of attachment of the sphenomandibular ligament.

- *Pterygoid Process:* Extends downward from the junction of the body and greater wing of the sphenoid on the right and left side. The pterygoid process is formed by the union of two bony plates. The depression between the two plates is called the pterygoid fossa. The pterygoid process is a site of origin for the internal and external pterygoid muscles.

## MAXILLA (Plural = Maxillae)

- The maxillae or upper jawbones are paired bones which unite in the midline to give shape to the middle face, form a portion of the floor of the eye socket and lateral wall of the nose, form the anterior two-thirds of the hard palate, and support natural teeth in bony sockets. Each maxilla is irregularly shaped and is made up of a body and these four processes:

  1. Nasal process
  2. Zygomatic process
  3. Alveolar process
  4. Palatine process

- The *nasal process* forms a portion of the lateral wall of the nose. Another name for nasal process is frontal process.

- The *zygomatic process* of the maxilla joins with the zygomatic bone (zygoma) which, in turn, unites with the zygomatic process of the temporal bone to form the zygomatic arch or cheekbone. The term cheekbone, although popular, is incorrect. This so-called single bone is actually made up of the three parts specified.

- The roots of the maxillary teeth are surrounded by the alveolar process. The *alveolar processes* of both maxillae unite to form the maxillary arch. A maxillary tuberosity is found on both of the distal ends of the maxillary arch. Proceeding even further posteriorly, the maxillary tuberosities abruptly rise into deep depressions called the hamular notches. The pterygoid process of the sphenoid bone joins with the posterior aspect of a maxilla to form a hamular notch. The labial portion of the alveolar bone follows the contours of the natural tooth roots; when a root is large and prominent, the labial alveolar bone over the root is raised in comparison to an alveolar area between roots. The labial alveolar bone covering the root of the maxillary cuspid stands out so much that it has a specific name, the cuspid eminence.

- The *palatine processes* of the maxillae join in the midline to form the anterior two-thirds of the hard palate. The midline junction of the right and left palatine processes is called the median palatine suture. An incisive foramen is found in the suture line immediately behind the central incisor teeth. The foramen is an exit hole for nerves and blood vessels which supply palatal tissue.

## PALATINE BONES

- The paired, "L"- shaped palatine bones are located between the maxillae and the sphenoid bone. A palatine bone forms parts of the floor and outer wall of the nasal cavity, the floor of an eye socket, and the hard palate. The horizontal plates of the palatine bones unite in the midline as the posterior continuation of the medial palatine suture. (Read the next sentence slowly and analyze its meaning.) The anterior border of the horizontal plates of the palatine bones join with the posterior border of the palatine processes of the maxillae to form the transverse palatine suture. You should recall that the palatine processes of the maxillae form the anterior two-thirds of the hard palate, and the horizontal plates of the palatine bones make up the remaining posterior one-third.

## ZYGOMATIC BONE (Zygoma, Malar Bone)

- The zygomatic bone is situated laterally to the maxilla. When the zygomatic process of the maxilla, the zygomatic bone, and the zygomatic process of the temporal bone are considered as a unit, the combination is called the zygomatic arch.

## MANDIBLE

- The mandible or lower jaw is the only movable bone of the skull. This bone gives shape to the lower portion of the face, provides sites of attachment for the muscles which make it move, forms the framework for the floor of the mouth, and supports the lower natural teeth. The mandible is connected to the skull by the right and left temporomandibular joints. Within each joint the condyle of the mandible fits into the glenoid fossa on the underside of the temporal bone. In its movements, the condyle also travels onto the temporal bone's articular eminence. The articular eminence projects downward and forward from the anterior border of the glenoid fossa.

- The most prominent features of the mandible are its horizontal body and two vertical projections known as Rami (one projection = ramus). The body is curved, somewhat like a horseshoe; at the posterior limits of the body, the bone turns upward and slightly backward to form the Rami. As the inferior edge of the mandible is traced from anterior to posterior, the sudden transition between the horizontal body and the relatively vertical ramus is known as the mandibular angle (angle of the mandible). Five processes are readily identifiable. The body of the mandible carries the alveolar process which surrounds the root structure of individual teeth; each ramus ends in two processes, and anteriorly positioned coronoid process and the more posterior condyloid process. The deep, "U"- shaped concavity between the two processes is called the mandibular notch. A condyloid process can be divided into a condyle and a neck. The top part of the condyle articulates with the glenoid fossa and articular eminence of the temporal bone to form the temporomandibular joint.

- The important *external surface landmarks* of the mandible are:

  1. *Mental Protuberance:* A roughly triangular prominence occurring in the midline near the inferior border of the mandible (chin point).

  2. *Mental Foramen:* The anterior opening of the mandibular canal. The foramen is usually found between and slightly below the first and second bicuspid root tips. The inferior alveolar nerve passes within the mandibular canal and exits onto the exterior surface of the mandible through the mental foramen to become the mental nerve. Compression of the mental nerve by artificial dental replacements must be avoided. It causes a feeling of pain or numbness.

  3. *External Oblique Ridge (Line):* The external oblique ridge extends at an oblique angle across the external surface of the body of the mandible. This ridge begins at the lower anterior edge of the ramus, continues onto the body, and progressively thins out to end near the mental foramen. The external oblique ridge is most prominent in the molar area and forms a distinct ledge with relation to the base of the alveolar process. This ledge is called the *buccal shelf.*

- The significant *internal surface landmarks* of the mandible are the internal oblique or mylohyoid ridge, genial tubercles, sublingual fossa, mandibular foramen, lingula, and digastric fovea.

  1. *Mylohyoid Ridge:* Located on the internal surface of the mandible, the mylohyoid ridge occupies a position similar to the external oblique ridge on the external surface. The mylohyoid ridge passes forward and downward from the internal aspects of the ramus onto the body of the mandible and fades out near the midline. This ridge serves as the lateral line of origin for the mylohyoid muscle (the mylohyoid muscle forms the major portion of the floor of the mouth).

  2. *Genial Tubercles:* Slightly above the lower border of the mandible in the midline, the bone is elevated to a more or less sharply defined prominence forming the genial tubercles.

  3. *Sublingual Fossa:* A shallow concavity which houses a portion of the sublingual gland, this depression occurs just above the anterior part of the mylohyoid ridge.

  4. *Mandibular Foramen:* The foramen is located in almost the exact center of the inner surface of the mandibular ramus. It opens into the mandibular canal.

  5. *Lingula:* A bony prominence on the anterior border of the mandibular foramen.

  6. *Digastric Fovea:* A depression found on both sides of the midline near the inferior lingual border of the mandible.

## HYOID BONE

- Since dentists and technicians are concerned with sites of anchorage for muscles which move the lower jaw, the hyoid bone which is not a part of the skull must be mentioned. The hyoid is a "U"-shaped bone located anterior to the spinal column between the mandible and the larynx (voice box). There is no joint-like union between the hyoid and any other bone. It is suspended between the mandible above and the clavicle (collar bone) below by suprahyoid (above the hyoid) and infrahyoid (below the hyoid) muscle groups. Some of the suprahyoid muscles act to depress the lower jaw. Those suprahyoid muscles which act to depress the mandible are described below.

# TEMPOROMANDIBULAR JOINT

- Temporomandibular joint (TMJ) is a synovial articulation between the mandible and the cranium, sometimes it is called as craniomandibular joint.
- It is formed by the articulation between the articular tubercle and the anterior part of the mandibular fossa of the temporal bone above and the condylar head of the mandible below.
- As a synovial joint, the TMJ has two unusual features:
  1. Articular surfaces of joint are covered with fibrous tissue instead of hyaline cartilage.
  2. Joint cavity is divided into two joint spaces by an intra-articular disc.
- Surface of the bone that articulates with the opposing bone—is called as articular surface.
- In TMJ between the articular surfaces of temporal bone and mandible are separated by a small space that is called as **joint cavity** or **articular space**.
- In TMJ articular surfaces are
  1. In temporal bone: superior and anterior part of mandibular fossa; posterior of articular eminence/tubercle.
  2. In mandible: superior and anterior part of condylar head.

## ANATOMY

- The TMJ is made up of:
  1. Bones making up the joint.
  2. Articular capsule.
  3. Articular disc.
  4. Synovial membrane.
  5. Ligaments associated with the joint.
  6. Fibrous covering of articular surfaces.
- TMJ is formed by articulation between mandible and temporal bone (part of cranium).
- **Boundaries of TMJ**
  Anteriorly—Posterior wall of articular eminence of temporal bone.
  Posteriorly—Posterior wall of mandibular fossa / glenoid fossa in temporal bone.
  Superiorly—Superior surface of glenoid fossa.
  Inferiorly—Superior surface of condylar head of the mandible.

## 1. BONES MAKING UP THE JOINT

### A. MANDIBULAR FOSSA/GLENOID FOSSA

- Mandibular fossa is an oval depression in the under surface of the temporal bone.
- It lies immediately anterior to the external acoustic meatus.
- It is bounded:
  i. anteriorly by articular eminence / tubercle
  ii. posteriorly by tympanic plate
  iii. laterally by zygomatic process
  iv. medially by sphenoid bone
- Its mediolateral dimension approx. 15 to 20 mm is greater than anteroposterior, in order to accommodate the mandibular condyle.
- It is limited posteriorly (by squamotympanic and petrotympanic fissures); laterally by (root of zygomatic process) and medially (by spine of sphenoid bone).

### B. MANDIBULAR CONDYLE

- Size and shape of mandibular condyle varies considerably.
- When viewed from above, the condyle is roughly ovoidal.
- Anteroposterior dimension (approx. 1 cm) is half of mediolateral dimension.
- Medial aspect is wider than the lateral aspect; and posterior aspect is broader than anterior.
- Long axis of condyle is not at right angles to the ramus, but diverges posteriorly.
- Anterior and superior surfaces of condyle are convex and are called articular surfaces of condyle.
- Articular surface area of condyle is about 200 mm$^2$, which is about half of that of mandibular fossa.
- Posterior surface is broad and flat (which is a non articular surface).
- Articular and non articular surface are separated by a slight ridge.
- Condyle has two parts
  i. **Head of the condyle:** Broad portion of mandibular condyle that has articular and non articular surfaces.
  ii. **Neck of the condyle:** This is the portion of the condyle that unites the broad condylar head to the ramus of the mandible.
  a. Condylar Head:
  b. Condylar Neck:
  – Small depression, pterygoid fovea is present on the anterior part of neck.

### C. ARTICULAR EMINENCE

- It is a bony prominence present in temporal bone anterior to mandibular fossa.

## 2. ARTICULAR CAPSULE

- It is a thin fibrous sac that surrounds the TMJ.
- It does not limit the mandibular movements and is too weak to provide support for the joint.
- It is attached:
  – Superiorly to mandibular fossa.
  – Inferiorly to neck of condyle.

- Anteriorly to articular eminence/tubercle.
- Posteriorly to squamotympanic and petrotympanic fissures.
- Internally it is attached to intra-articular disc and is lined by synovial membrane.
- The collagen fibres of the capsule run predominantly in a vertical direction.
- The capsule is richly innervated.
- The capsule is strengthened laterally by the temporomandibular ligament (lateral ligament).

## 3. ARTICULAR DISC

- Articular disc (meniscus) is interposed between the articular surfaces of mandible and temporal bone.
- It is dense and fibrous.
- When viewed sagittally, upper surface of the disc is concavoconvex from front to back and lower surface is concave.
- The disc is of variable thickness
  - It is thinnest centrally over articular surface of condyle.
  - Anteriorly and posteriorly it is thick, being more thickest posteriorly.
  - Lateral half of disc is thinner than medial half.
- It divides the articular space/joint cavity into two compartments,
  - Upper compartment: temporodiscal—between disc and temporal bone.
  - Lower compartment: condylodiscal—between disc and condyle.
- Articular disc is divided into three portions:
  i. Anterior.
  ii. Intermediate: Thinnest and is in contact with articular surface by condyle.
  iii. Posterior.
- It is connected to:
  Anteriorly—it fuses with articular capsule and fibrous bands connect the disc to anterior margin of articular eminence above and to the anterior margin of condyle below.
  Medially—directly attached to the capsule and medial pole of condyle.
  Laterally—directly attached to the capsule and lateral pole of condyle.
  Posteriorly—it is attached to the capsule by means of bilaminar zone.
- Bilaminar zone/retrodiscal tissue or pad:
  i. It is a thick, loose fibroelastic portion that is continuous with the posterior part of articular disc and attaches it to fibrous capsule.
  ii. It is highly vascular and innervated.
  iii. It has two zones
    - Superior stratum or lamina that attaches. It to posterior wall of glenoid fossa and squamotympanic fissure.
    - Inferior stratum that attaches it to the back of mandibular condyle.
  iv. Superior stratum is more vascular and contains many elastic fibres.
  v. It allows anterior movements of condyle.
- Blood vessels are evident only at the periphery of articular disc, the bulk of it being avascular.
- Some fibres of lateral pterygoid muscle are attached to the anterior border of the disc.

## 4. SYNOVIAL MEMBRANE

- Synovial membrane lines the inner surface of the fibrous capsule and bilaminar zone.
- It does not cover.
  i. articular surfaces of joint.
  ii. articular surfaces of disc.
- It has folds on villi protruding into joint cavity.
- Synovial membrane secretes synovial fluid.
- Synovial fluid:
  - It is a clear, straw-coloured, viscous fluid secreted by synovial membrane.
  - It is found in the articular spaces.
  - It mainly contains proteoglycans.
  - It is formed by diffusion from rich capillary network of the synovial membrane.
  - It lubricates the joint and also provide nutrition to avascular tissues covering condyle and articular eminence and for articular disc.
  - 1 ml of fluid is present in inferior joint cavity and a little more in superior joint cavity.
  - Its hydrostatic pressure is subatmospheric, but is elevated during mastication.

## 5. LIGAMENTS

- TMJ has four ligaments: one principle ligament + three accessory ligaments.

### A. TEMPOROMANDIBULAR LIGAMENT / LATERAL LIGAMENT

- It is the principle ligament of TMJ.
- It strengthens the capsule laterally.
- It takes origin from the lateral surface of articular eminence and inserts into posterior surface of the condyle.
- It provides support to TMJ by restricting distal and inferior movements of mandible and thus resist dislocation during functional movements.

**B. ACCESSORY LIGAMENTS ARE**
  i. Sphenomandibular ligament.
  ii. Stylomandibular ligament.
  iii. Pterygomandibular raphe.

## BLOOD AND NERVE SUPPLY

**Arterial supply:** Branches of maxillary and superficial temporal arteries supply the joint.

**Nerve supply:** Joint tissues are innervated by,
  i. Auriculotemporal nerve (branch of mandibular division of trigeminal nerve).
  ii. Proprioceptor fibres from the joint are carried by masseteric nerves.
- Articular disc is devoid of nerves.

## MOVEMENTS OF TMJ

- Two types of movements seen in TMJ are,
  1. Hinge movement.
  2. Translatory movement.
1. **Hinge movement:**
   - It is a rotational movement about an axis through the heads of the condyles.
   - This movement occurs in lower joint space.
   - It permits opening of the jaws.
2. **Translatory movement:**
   - It occurs in upper joint space.
   - This movement occurs as the disc and the condyles traverse anteriorly along the descending slopes of articular eminence.
   - This movement permits anterior and inferior movement of mandible.
- During opening of mouth, first hinge movement takes place followed by translatory movement.

# MANDIBULAR MOVEMENTS

## OPENING AND CLOSING

- From a position of centric relation, pure hinge movements are possible in opening and closing. In a hinge movement, the condyles rotate within the glenoid fossa. Opening and closing movements, where the measured distance between maxillary and mandibular incisors is greater than 25 mm, result in combined rotation and translation of the condyles. Translation occurs whenever a condyle leaves the glenoid fossa.

## PROTRUSION AND RETRUSION

- Protrusion is when the mandible moves forward and both condyles leave their respective fossae and move down their eminences. The opposite process is called retrusion. Protrusion and retrusion are translatory movements.

## RIGHT AND LEFT LATERAL

- *Working Side:* The side toward which the mandible moves. When the mandible moves laterally, the condyle on the working side stays in its fossa, rotates and moves laterally.
- *Balancing Side:* The side opposite the working side. In a lateral movement, the balancing side condyle leaves the fossa and moves forward down the eminence, and medially.

# MUSCLES OF MASTICATION

- A person's ability to move part of the body depends on a group of specialized cells called the muscle fibers. Muscle fibers have the ability to contract or shorten when stimulated by nerve impulses. A typical muscle consists of a mass of muscle fibers bound together by connective tissue. A muscle can generate varying degrees of power. This variation in power is directly proportional to the number of fibers within the muscle that are contracting at any given time. Muscles can also stretch, but only because a muscle located elsewhere has contracted and forced the extension. The simplest way to express this is that muscles can only pull; they cannot push.
- The two ends of a voluntary muscle usually attach to different bones. In some instances, one end of a muscle may attach in soft tissue such as skin. Some of the very small muscles that give expression to the face have both ends attached to soft tissue. In any case, the muscle attachment site which remains relatively stationary when the muscle contracts is known as the origin. The muscle attachment site having the greater movement during the contraction is called the insertion. A description of the movements which take place as a result of muscle contraction is called the action.
- Two muscle groups are responsible for executing the movements that the mandible is capable of making. They are the muscles of mastication, and the depressor muscles of the mandible. The muscles of mastication enable the lower jaw to make closing, opening, protrusive, and retrusive movements along with movements to the right and left sides. The depressors of the mandible act to open the lower jaw widely, a function which the muscles of mastication cannot perform.
- There are four, paired muscles of mastication:

1. Temporalis
2. Masseter
3. Lateral pterygoid
4. Medial pterygoid

## DEVELOPMENT

- From the mesoderm of the first branchial arch.

## 1. TEMPORALIS

### Origin
- From inferior temporal line, temporal fascia and temporal fossa.

### Insertion
- Inserted to the anterior, posterior borders, tip and medial surface of the coronoid process of the mandible.

### Nerve Supply
- Deep temporal branch of anterior division of mandibular nerve.

### Blood Supply
- Deep temporal branch of maxillary artery and middle temporal artery from superficial temporal artery.

### Actions
1. Elevation of mandible.
2. Posterior fibers—retraction of the protruded mandible.

### Relations
1. *Superficially:* Skin, anterior and superior auricular muscles, temporal fascia, superficial temporal vessels, auriculotemporal nerve, temporal branch of facial nerve, zygomatic temporal nerve, galea aponeurotica, zygomatic arch and masseter.
2. *Deep surface:* Temporal fossa, lateral pterygoid, superficial head of medial pterygoid, buccinator, maxillary artery, deep temporal nerve, buccal nerve and muscle.

### Palpation
- Its contraction may be felt by placing fingers on the side of the head while clenching the teeth.

## 2. MASSETER

- Most superficial muscle among muscles of mastication.
- Quadrilateral muscle.
- Covers lateral surface of the ramus of the mandible.
- It consists of two overlapping heads.
  A. Superficial
  B. Deep

### A. Superficial Head
Origin
- From lower border of anterior 2/3rd of zygomatic arch and adjoining zygomatic process of Maxilla.

Insertion
- Lower and posterior part of the external surface of the ramus of mandible.

### B. Deep Head
Origin
- From the deep surface of the zygomatic arch.

Insertion
- Upper and anterior part of ramus of mandible.

Nerve supply
- Masseteric nerve—a branch of anterior division of mandibular nerve.

Blood Supply
- Masseteric artery—a branch of maxillary artery.

Actions
- *On simultaneous contraction of right and left muscles:*
  Elevation of the mandible to close the mouth and clenches the teeth.
- *On alternate contraction of right and left muscles:*
  Results in a rocking, grinding type of motion that facilitates the breakdown of food.

Relations
1. **Superficially:** Skin, superficial fascia, platysma, risorius, zygomaticus major, parotid gland and duct, branches of facial nerve and transverse facial vessels cross the muscle.
2. **Deep surface:** It overlies the insertion of temporalis and ramus of the mandible; a mass of fat separates it from the buccinator and buccal nerve; masseteric nerve and vessel enter the deep surface; posterior margin is overlapped by parotid gland; anterior margin projects over the buccinator and is crossed below by facial vein.

Palpation
- Outline of the masseter may be traced by palpating the muscle as it contracts while clenching the teeth.

## 3. LATERAL PTERYGOID/PTERYGOID EXTERNUS

- Has two heads—small *superior* and large *inferior*

Origin

1. **Superior Head:** from infratemporal surface and infratemporal crest of the greater wing of sphenoid

2. *Inferior Head:* From lateral surface of the lateral pterygoid plate.

### Insertion
- Fibers run backwards, laterally and converges
- Inserted into pterygoid fovea on the neck of the mandible, articular capsule and disc of TMJ.

### Nerve Supply
- Nerve to lateral pterygoid from anterior division of mandibular nerve.

### Blood Supply
- Maxillary artery

### Actions
1. Depression of mandible when acts alone.
2. Protrusion when acting along with medial pterygoid on both sides at the same time.
3. Side to side/chewing movement when acting along with medial pterygoid on both sides alternatively.

### Relations
1. *Superficial:* Maxillary artery, ramus of the mandible and masseter muscle.
2. *Deep:* Mandibular nerve and its branches, middle meningeal artery, chorda tympani nerve.
3. *Upper Border:* Deep temporal nerves and masseteric nerve.
4. *Lower Border:* Lingual nerve and inferior alveolar nerve.

## 4. MEDIAL PTERYGOID/PTERYGOID INTERNUS
- *Deepest muscle among muscles of mastication.*
- A quadrilateral muscle.
- Has two heads—small *superficial* and large *deep*.

### Origin
#### A. Superficial Head
- Arises from maxillary tuberosity and pyramidal process of palatine bone.

#### B. Deep Head
- Arises from medial surface of lateral pterygoid plate and adjoining part of palatine bone.

### Nerve Supply
- Nerve to medial pterygoid—a branch from the main trunk of mandibular nerve.

### Blood Supply
- Medial pterygoid branch of the maxillary artery.

### Actions
1. Elevation of the mandible.
2. Protrusion when acting along with medial pterygoid on both sides at the same time.
3. Side to side/chewing movement when acting along with medial pterygoid on both sides alternatively.

### Relations
1. *Lateral surface:* Ramus of the mandible, lateral pterygoid, sphenomandibular ligament, maxillary artery, inferior alveolar nerve and vessel, lingual nerve and part of the parotid gland.
2. *Medial surface:* Tensor veli palatini, and is separated from superior constrictor by styloglossus and stylopharyngeus muscle.

## DIGASTRIC
- Located below the inferior border of the mandible.
- Consists of an anterior and a posterior belly connected by an intermediate tendon.

### A. Anterior Belly

### Origin
- From the digastric fossa on the inferior border of the mandible.

### Insertion
- Runs downwards and backwards to the digastric tendon.

### B. Posterior Belly

### Origin
- From the mastoid notch immediately behind the mastoid process of the temporal bone.

### Insertion
- Passes downwards and forwards towards the hyoid bone, where it becomes the digastric tendon.

### Actions
- Depresses and retrudes the mandible.
- Stabilize the position of the hyoid bone.
- Aids in elevation of hyoid during swallowing.

### Nerve Supply
- *Anterior Belly:* Mylohyoid branch of the mandibular division of trigeminal nerve.
- *Posterior Belly:* Digastric branch of facial nerve.

### Blood Supply
- *Anterior Belly:* Facial artery.
- *Posterior Belly:* Posterior auricular and occipital artery.

# DEPRESSOR MUSCLES

- The depressor muscles of the mandible all have the hyoid bone in common as an attachment site. When the hyoid bone is immobilized by a contraction of the muscles below it, the contraction of the depressor muscles located between the hyoid bone and the mandible pulls the mandible downward (open the mouth). The suprahyoid depressors of the mandible are the mylohyoid, geniohyoid, and digastric muscles.

### Mylohyoid Muscle Attachment Sites

- The paired mylohyoid muscles are attached to the mylohyoid lines on the internal surfaces of the mandible, the right and left mylohyoid muscle join in the midline to form the floor of the mouth, and the posterior end of this midline junction attaches to the hyoid bone.

### Geniohyoid Muscle Attachment Sites

- The two geniohyoid muscles are found next to each other, on each side of the midline, directly on top of the mylohyoid muscles. The sites of the attachment are the genial tubercles and the hyoid bone.

# MUSCLES OF FACIAL EXPRESSION

- Eight paired muscles of expression in combination with the single, orbicularis oris muscle control movements of the lips and cheeks. The teeth and alveolar processes of the jaws support this group of muscles against collapse into the oral cavity. When natural teeth are extracted, facial muscle support must be maintained by replacing the missing teeth. A person's appearance can be dramatically affected by the position of the artificial teeth. Inadequate support makes people look older, and excessive support distorts a person's features by making them appear stretched.

- The muscles of facial expression also play an important part in forming the anterior and lateral portions of maxillary and mandibular impression borders. This is because, all of these muscles can alter the depth of vestibular sulci (below) in one way or another. If impression borders are not properly extended and shaped, the muscles act to unseat the dentures.

## ORBICULARIS ORIS

- This ring-like muscle lies within the upper and lower lips and completely surrounds the opening to the mouth. When the orbicularis oris contracts, it causes the lips to close. The orbicularis has no real bony origin. Instead, it is entirely rimmed by the insertions of other muscles of facial expression, most of which do originate on bone. Certain muscles of expression that insert into the orbicularis oris act to draw the corners of the mouth backward, some depress the lower lip, and others elevate the upper lip.

## QUADRATES LABII SUPERIORIS

**Form:** Flat, triangular.
**Position:** Lateral to the nose.

### Origin (by three heads)

1. *Angular:* Frontal process of the maxilla.
2. *Infraorbital:* Inferior margin of the orbit.
3. *Zygomatic:* Anterior surface of the zygomatic bone.

### Insertion

- Fibers of the orbicularis oris beneath the nostrils.

### Action

- Elevates the upper lip, widens the nasal opening, and raises the corner of the nose.

## ZYGOMATICUS

**Form:** Oblong, flat, and cylindrical.
**Position:** Lateral to, and above, angle of mouth.
**Origin:** Zygomatic bone, lateral to quadrates labii superioris muscle.
**Insertion:** Skin at angle of mouth.
**Action:** Draws angle of mouth laterally and upward.

## CANINUS

**Form:** Flat, triangular.
**Position:** In canine fossa of the maxilla, covered by the quadrates labii superioris muscle.
**Origin:** Canine fossa.
**Insertion:** Angle of mouth.
**Action:** Lifts angle of mouth upward, lifts lower lip, and helps to close mouth.

## RISORIUS

**Form:** Flat, triangular.
**Position:** Lateral to angle of mouth.
**Origin:** Tissue over the masseter muscle and parotid gland
**Insertion:** Unites at angle of mouth with triangularis muscle.
**Action:** Draws angle of mouth laterally, causes smile and dimple.

## QUADRATES LABII INFERIORIS

**Form:** Flat, quadrangular.
**Position:** Covers mental foramen.
**Origin:** Lower border of mandible.
**Insertion:** Skin of lower lip.
**Action:** Depresses and inverts lower lip.

## TRIANGULARIS

**Form:** Flat, quadrangular.
**Position:** Covers mental foramen.
**Origin:** Lower border of mandible just beneath mental foramen.
**Insertion:** Angle of mouth.
**Action:** Draws angle of mouth downward.

## MENTALIS

**Form:** Thick, cylindrical, short.
**Position:** On chin, deep to quadrates labii inferioris muscle.
**Origin:** Mandible, deep to quadrates labii inferioris muscle.
**Insertion:** Obliquely downward to skin of chin.
**Action:** Lifts and wrinkles skin of chin.

## BUCCINATOR

- This thin quadrilateral muscle occupies the interval between the maxilla and the mandible in the cheek. It is attached to the outer surfaces of the alveolar processes of maxilla and mandible opposite the molar teeth and to the anterior border of pterygomandibular raphe. The raphe separates the muscle from the superior constrictor of pharynx.
- The fibres converge towards the modiolus with following mode of attachment.
  - Central (pterygomandibular) fibres intersect each other; those from below crosses to the upper part of orbicularis oris and those from above crosses to the lower part.
  - Highest (maxillary) and lowest (mandibular) fibres enter their corresponding lips without decussation.

### Relations

- Posteriorly—covered by buccopharyngeal fascia.
- Superficially—fat separates its posterior part from the ramus of the mandible, masseter and part of temporalis.
- Anteriorly—superficial surface is related to zygomaticus major, risorius, levator and depressor anguli oris and parotid duct.
- The duct pierces it opposite the third upper molar tooth. The duct is crossed by the facial artery, facial vein and branches of the facial and buccal nerves.
- Deep surface—related to buccal glands and mucous membrane of the mouth.

### Nerve supply

- Lower buccal branches of the facial nerve.

### Actions

1. Compresses cheeks against the teeth and gums.
2. During mastication, assists tongue in directing food between the grinding molar teeth.
3. Buccinators expel air from the cheeks between the lips (blowing muscle).

## PTERYGOMANDIBULAR RAPHE

- It extends from the pterygoid hamulus to the posterior end of the mylohyoid line. Medially it can be easily palpated where it is covered by the mucous membrane of the mouth while laterally it is separated from the ramus of the mandible by adipose tissue. It provides attachments to.
- Posteriorly—Superior constrictor of pharynx.
- Anteriorly—Central part of buccinator.

# MODIOLUS

- On each side of the face a number of muscles converge towards a point just lateral to the buccal angle where they interlace to form a compact fibromuscular mass termed as the modiolus.
- In the modiolus the muscles radiate from a central point.
- The muscles lie in different planes and their modiolar stems are spiralized.
- There are nine muscles attached to each modiolus.
- The shape and dimensions of the modiolus varies.

### Structure

- It resembles a blunt cone. The base of the cone (basis moduli) is adherent to the mucosa. It is elliptical and extends vertically about 20 mm above and 20 mm below a horizontal line through the buccal angle and 20 mm laterally from the angle.
- The blunt apex of the cone (apex moduli) is about 4 mm across and about 12 mm lateral to the buccal angle.
- It is divided into basal, central and apical parts.
- Central body has an oblique fibrous cleft which transmits the facial artery.
- The apex of the modiolus is adherent to the panniculus fibrosus. There its free border forms a

crescentic subcutaneous fibroelastic cord that accommodates the various expressions of the modioli, lips, mouth and jaws.

### Modiolar muscles

- Muscles radiate from the modiolus. Some muscles are almost closed and strap-like while others are widely open and their planes vary.
- Most of the muscle stems rotate as they approach the modiolus.
- Peripherally the attachment of the depressor lies in the plane of the body of mandible, whereas at the modiolus it lies in an apicobasal direction. The orbicularis in the free lip lie in a roughly coronal plane, but the stem thickness dorsoventrally and attaches at the modiolus from apex to base.

### Cruciate modiolar muscles

1. Zygomaticus major.
2. Levator anguli oris.
3. Depressor anguli oris.
4. Platysma (pars modiolaris).

- These muscles resemble a compound X.

    Transverse modiolar muscles

    1. Buccinator.
    2. Risorius.
    3. Various parts of orbicularis oris.
    4. Incisivus superior and inferior.

- The attachment of these muscles of the modiolus consists of interdigitation, partly with neighbouring bundles but mainly with antagonists. Most fibres terminate after attachment within the modiolus.

### Modiolar movements

- Mobility of the modioli integrate the activities of cheeks, lips, oral fissure, oral vestibule and jaws.
- These activities include:
    1. Biting.
    2. Chewing.
    3. Drinking.
    4. Sucking.
    5. Swallowing.
    6. Changes in vestibular contents and pressure.
    7. Variations in speech.
    8. Modulation of musical tones.
    9. Production of sounds as in shouting.

## TONGUE

- The tongue is a muscular organ that contains specialized cells for detecting the presence of chemicals in the food we eat. The brain interprets this chemical detection process as taste. The tongue's many different sets of muscles enable it to make the complex movements associated with speaking and with chewing food. The constant motion of the tongue represents a powerful force, and no artificial dental replacement can restrict that motion for long. If a prosthesis is not constructed to work in harmony with the tongue, it will fail. For example, the tongue can maintain a denture in position or throw it out, depending on how the lingual surfaces and borders of the denture are shaped. The tongue is animated by two muscle groups, the intrinsic and extrinsic.

### Intrinsic Muscles

- Intrinsic muscles represent the substance of the tongue. They are responsible for the tongue's ability to change shape.

### Extrinsic Muscles

- Extrinsic muscles originate at sites like the hyoid bone, the styloid process of the temporal bone, and the genial tubercles. The extrinsic muscles proceed from their sites of origin and insert into the tongue's mass. The extrinsic musculature enables the mass of the tongue to move from place to place within the mouth. Intrinsic and extrinsic muscles do not act in isolation from one another. The smooth, precise tongue movements that we take for granted are the result of finely coordinated contractions generated by appropriate muscles in both groups.

## ORAL MUCOUS MEMBRANE

- Body cavities that communicate with the external environment are lined by mucous membrane and that are coated by serous and mucous secretions. Similarly the oral cavity is lined by an uninterrupted mucous membrane that is continuous with the skin near the vermilion border of the lips and with the pharyngeal mucosa in the region of the soft palate.
- In the same way as the skin does, the oral mucosa serves in protecting the underlying tissues / organs and also in receiving, transmitting the stimuli from the environment.
- In an edentulous oral cavity, the mucous membrane helps in supporting the complete denture or it may have contact with it intermittently.
- Structurally, oral mucous membrane resembles the skin in many ways. It is composed of epithelium, connective tissue (lamina propria) and submucosa (may or may not be present). Epithelium is of stratified squamous type, that may be ortho-

keratinized, parakeratinized or non keratinized depending on the location. Lamina propria may attach to the periosteum of the alveolar bone or it may overlay the submucosa (varies in different regions of the oral cavity). Submucosa contains connective tissue of varying thickness and density. Glands, blood vessels, nerves and adipose tissue are present in submucosa. It attaches the mucous membrane to the underlying structures. Whether this attachment is loose or firm depends on the character of the submucosa.
- A thorough knowledge and understanding of the various combinations of epithelium, lamina propria and submucosa is important to best use various areas of the oral cavity for denture support.

## CLASSIFICATION OF ORAL MUCOSA

- Oral mucosa is divided into three categories depending on its function and location. They are,
  1. Lining mucosa
  2. Masticating mucosa
  3. Specialized mucosa

### 1. Lining Mucosa

- Lips, cheeks, vestibular spaces, alveolingual sulcus, soft palate ventral surface of the tongue and unattached gingiva found on the slopes of the residual ridges.
- It usually comes in contact with the denture borders.
- It has a thick, stratified squamous non-keratinized epithelium supported by a thick lamina propria.
- Lamina propria is highly elastic in nature in these areas and hence these tissues are freely movable.

### 2. Masticatory Mucosa

- It covers the hard palate, crests of the residual ridges and residual ridge attached gingiva.
- The epithelium is stratified squamous orthokeratinized or parakeratinized with a thick and dense lamina propria.
- There is no distinct submucosa and the lamina propria blends with the periosteum and thus limits the mobility of the entire mucosa.

### 3. Specialised mucosa
- Covers the dorsal surface of the tongue.
- The mucosa is keratinized and contains specialised papillae.

## SALIVA

- Saliva is a mixture of two types of primary secretions; A serous secretion (thin, watery) for digestion of starches and a mucous secretion (viscid, sticky or adhesive) for lubricative purposes. The quantity of daily secretion normally ranges between 1000 and 1500 mL. Although, it has got varied junctions, the main function is lubrication and protection of the mucosa. Saliva also lubricates the surfaces of a denture, that makes the denture more compatible with movements of the lips, cheeks and tongue.
- Saliva is considered as a major one among the physical factors that contribute to the denture retention. The saliva is involved in the physical forces like adhesion, cohesion, capillary and atmospheric pressure.

### Clinical Significance
- Thin, watery saliva of high surface tension provides good retention.
- Ropy saliva contributes to the poor retention.
- Excessive salivation presents a problem in impression making, so appropriate measures should be taken to overcome the same.
- Excessive mucous secretions from the palatal glands may distort the impression material in the posterior two thirds of the palate.
- Pathologic conditions that are associated with decreased salivation are atrophy of salivary glands with aging, fibrosis of glands following irradiation therapy, poliomyelitis, diabetes mellitus, diabetes insipidus, diarrhoea by bacteria and vitamin A deficiency, etc.
- Pathologic condition that are associated with increased salivation are digestive tract irritants and painful oral lesions, etc.

# CHAPTER 3: The Oral Cavity

To construct a prosthesis, the dentist should have a thorough understanding of the anatomical land marks of the face and oral cavity. This chapter is designed to identify the surface anatomy of the face, edentulous mouth and denture bearing areas. By the end of this chapter, student should be able to recognize and identify the surface anatomy of the edentulous mouth; identify the negative likeness of anatomical fractures presented in an impression; understand the relevance of certain anatomical features to full denture construction.

## DENTULOUS AND EDENTULOUS

- Dentulous is a condition in which natural teeth are present in the mouth (synonym: Dentate).
- Edentulous is a condition of without teeth or lacking teeth. If all the teeth are missing, the condition is *completely edentulous* and if only a few teeth are missing, the condition is called *partially edentulous*.
- Edentulism is the state of being edentulous or without natural teeth.
- Edentics is the art, sciene and technique used in treating edentulous patients.
  Figures 1.3.1 to 1.3.6 gives the parts of the edentulous oral cavity.

## ANATOMIC LANDMARKS

- The knowledge of anatomical landmarks of maxillary and mandibular arches plays a vital role in successful construction of complete dentures.
- Complete dentures function effectively if denture base extends as far as possible without interfering in the health of function of tissues. So, the dentist must fully understand the anatomy of supporting and limiting structures of denture bearing area in order to deliver a successful prosthesis.
- To construct prosthesis, the dentist should have a thorough understanding of the anatomical land marks of the face and oral cavity.
- This chapter is designed to identify the surface anatomy of the face, edentulous mouth and denture bearing areas.
- By the end of this chapter, student should be able to,
  - Recognize and identify the surface anatomy of the edentulous mouth.

# TOPOGRAPHY OF EDENTULOUS ORAL CAVITY

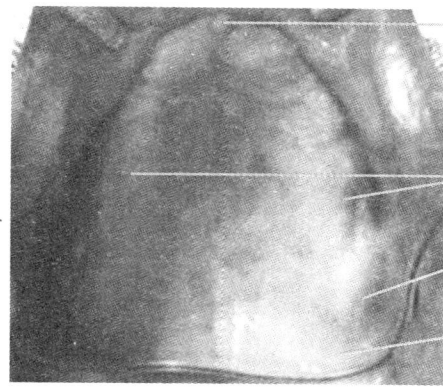
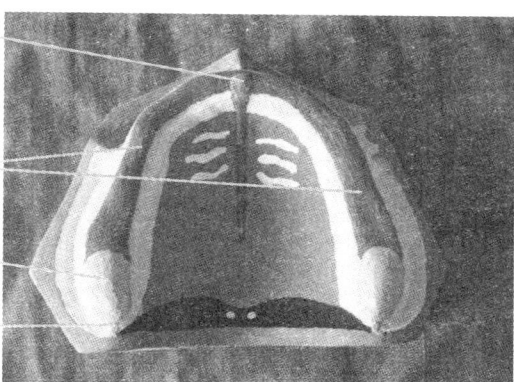

- Incisive papilla
- Residual alveolar ridge
- Maxillary tuberosity
- Hamular notch

Fig. 1.3.1

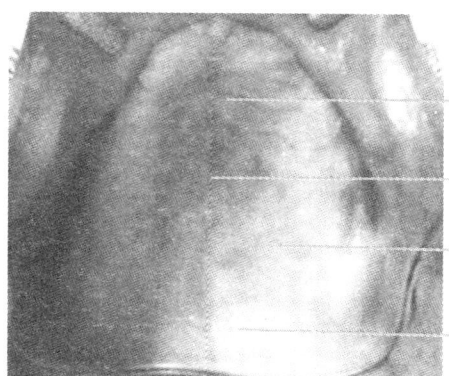
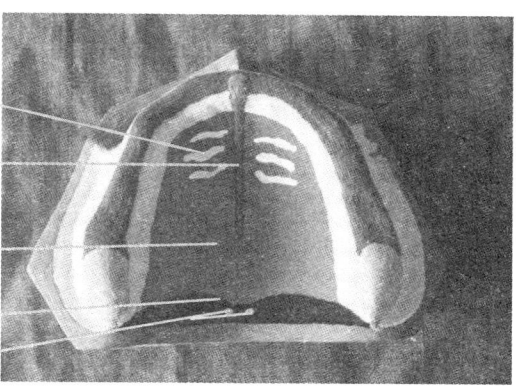

- Rugae area
- Mid palatine raphe
- Hard palate
- Vibrating line
- Fovea palatinae

Fig. 1.3.2

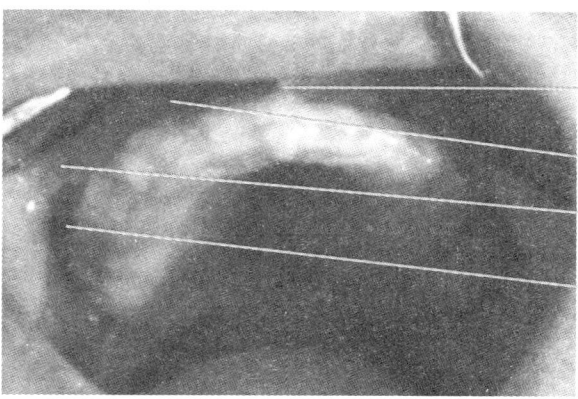
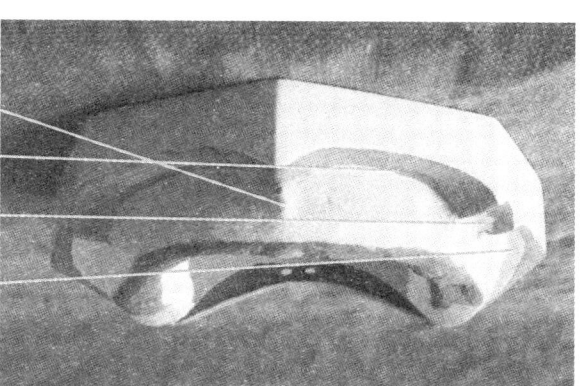

- Labial frenum
- Labial vestibule
- Buccal frenum
- Buccal vestibule

Fig. 1.3.3

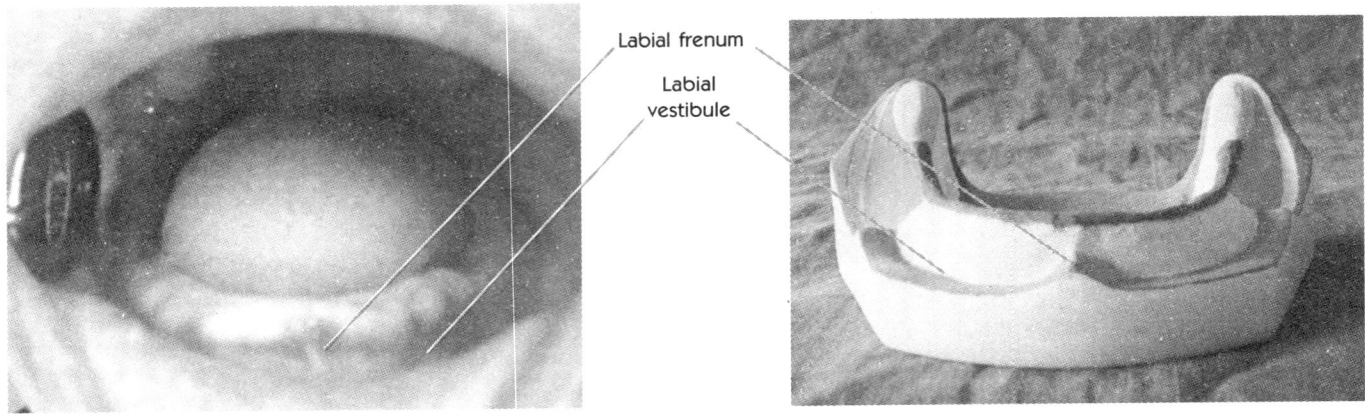

Fig. 1.3.4

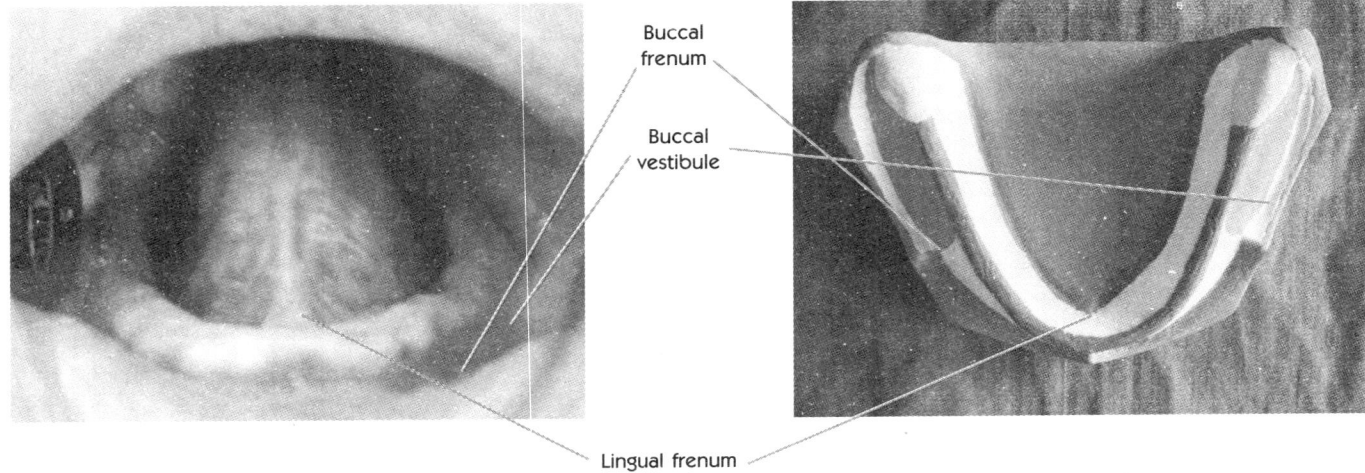

Fig. 1.3.5

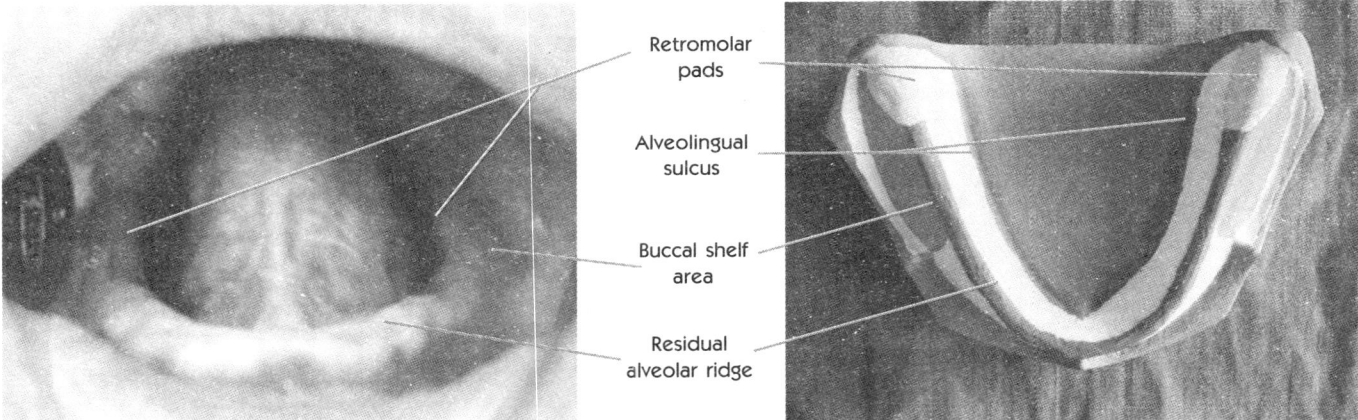

Fig. 1.3.6

- Identify the negative likeness of anatomical features presented in an impression.
- Understand the relevance of certain anatomical features to full denture construction.

## THE FACE

- **Face** is defined as *the part of the head visible in a frontal view that is anterior to the ears and all that lies between the hairline and the chin.*

### REGIONS OF THE FACE

- The face is subdivided into nine regions and are as follows:
  1. Forehead
  2. Temples
  3. External ear
  4. Orbital area
  5. Zygomatic (malar) area
  6. Cheeks
  7. External nose
  8. Mouth and lips
  9. Chin.

### LANDMARKS OF THE FACE

1. *Outer canthus of the eye:* Fold of tissue at the outer corner of the eyelids
2. *Inner canthus of the eye:* Fold of tissue at the inner corner of the eyelids
3. *Ala of the nose:* Wing-like tip on the outer side of each nostril
4. *Philtrum*
5. *Tragus of the ear*
6. *Nasion*
7. *Glabella*
8. *Root of the nose*
9. *Anterior nares*
10. *Labial commissure*
11. *Nasolabial sulcus*
12. *Mental protuberance*
13. *Angle of the mandible*
14. *Zygomatic arch*

### DEFINITION

- A recognizable anatomic structure used as a point of reference—GPT.

### SIGNIFICANCE

- Helps in locating the stress bearing areas, retentives areas, relief areas and limiting structures while impression making.
- Helps in preservation of remaining tissues.
- Helps in construction of complete dentures with good masticatory efficiency, pleasant esthetics and correct phonetics.

## THE ORAL CAVITY

### MAXILLARY ANATOMIC LANDMARKS

- Average available denture bearing area for edentulous maxilla is 24 cms$^2$.

**I. Based on Supporting and Limiting Structures**

  **A. Supporting Structures**
  1. Mucous membrane
  2. Hard palate
  3. Rugae area
  4. Mid palatine raphae
  5. Residual ridge
  6. Incisive papilla
  7. Maxillary tuberosity
  8. Torus palatinus

  **B. Limiting and Peripheral Structures**
  1. Labial frenum
  2. Labial vestibule
  3. Buccal frenum
  4. Buccal vestibule
  5. Hamular notch
  6. Vibrating line
  7. Fovea palatinae

**II. Based on Function**

  **A. Stress Bearing Areas**
  1. Primary
  2. Secondary

  *Primary stress bearing areas:* Horizontal portion of hard palate lateral to midline.
  *Secondary stress bearing areas:* Palatal rugae, crest of alveolar ridge, facial slopes of alveolar ridge, maxillary tuberosity.

  **B. Relief Areas**
  - Mid palatine raphae, torus palatinus, labial frenum, buccal frenum.

### 1. MUCOUS MEMBRANE

**Definition**

- A thin layer of tissue that lines a cavity, envelopes a vessel or part or separates a space or organ—GPT.

**Structure**

- Structure of oral mucous membrane resembles skin in many ways.
- Oral mucous membrane consist of:

A. **Mucosa**
- Epithelium
- Lamina propria (connective tissue).

B. **Submucosa**
- Connective tissue.

A. **Mucosa**

**Classification**
- Oral mucosa is divided into 3 categories depending on its function and location,
  i. Masticatory mucosa
  ii. Lining mucosa
  iii. Specialized mucosa.

i. **Masticatory Mucosa Covers**
- Hard palate.
- Crest of alveolar ridge.
- Residual attached gingiva that is firmly attached to supporting bone.
- Stratified squamous epithelium of masticatory mucosa has well defined keratinized layer.
- It is associated with those parts of oral cavity which are firmly attached to periosteum.

ii. **Lining Mucosa Covers**
- Lips
- Cheeks
- Vestibular spaces
- Alveolingual sulcus
- Soft palate
- Ventral surface of tongue
- Unattached gingiva found on slopes of residual ridges.
- Stratified squamous epithelium of lining mucosa is devoid of keratinized layer.
- It is associated with those parts of oral cavity which are not firmly attached to periosteum.
- These tissues are freely movable because of elastic nature of underlying lamina propria.

iii. **Specialized Mucosa Covers**
- Dorsal surface of tongue.
- This mucosal covering is keratinized and includes specialized papillae on upper surface of tongue.
- In order to support complete dentures, the mucosa should be firmly attached, keratinized or masticatory type.

B. **Submucosa**
- Submucosa is formed by connective tissue and may contain glandular, fat or muscle cells and transmits blood and nerve supply to mucosa.
- It attaches mucous membrane to underlying structures and whether this attachment is loose or firm depends on the character of submucosa.
- In order to support complete dentures, the submucosa should consist of resilient, fibrous connective tissues having average thickness and should be firmly attached.
- In a healthy mouth, submucosa is firmly attached to periosteum of underlying supporting bone and will usually withstand successfully the pressures of the dentures.

**NOTE**
- Mucosa is important from health stand point and submucosa is largely responsible for support that mucous membrane affords a denture because in most instances, sub mucosa makes up bulk of mucous membrane.

2. **HARD PALATE**

**Macroscopic Anatomy**
- The two palatine processes of maxillae and palatine bone form the hard palate and provide support for denture.
- The horizontal portion of hard palate lateral to midline provides primary support area for denture.
- Anterolateral and posterolateral part of hard palate act as secondary retentive areas.

**Microscopic Anatomy**
- Epithelium is normally keratinized.
- Submucosa contains adipose tissue anterolaterally and glandular tissue posterolaterally.

**Clinical Consideration**
- During final impression procedure, posterolateral part should not be compressed as it can interfere with function of glands.

3. **PALATAL RUGAE**

**Definition**
- The irregular fibrous connective tissue ridges located in the anterior third of hard palate—GPT.

**Macroscopic Anatomy**
- These are mucosal folds located in anterior region of palatal mucosa.
- The palatal rugae plays an important role in speech.
- In the area of rugae, the palate is set at angle to the residual ridge and is thinly covered by soft tissue, which resists anterior displacement of dentures. Hence it is considered as **secondary stress bearing area**.

**Microscopic Anatomy**
- It is made up of ketatinized fibrous connective tissue.

### Clinical Consideration
- The rugae area should be recorded without pressure. If the tissue distorts while making the impression, it can rebound and unseat the denture.

### 4. MID PALATAL RAPHAE

#### Definition
- The ridge of mucous membrane that marks the median line of hard palate.

#### Macroscopic Anatomy
- It is the area extending from incisive papilla till the posterior region of hard palate.
- This sutural joint is formed by median fusion of two maxillary processes and two horizontal plates of palatine bone.
- Function of sutural joint is growth and sometimes there will be overgrowth of sutural joint resulting in torus palatinus.

#### Microscopic Anatomy
- Epithelium is normally keratinized.
- Submucosa is extremely thin and practically in contact with underlying bone. Hence soft tissue covering the mid palatine raphae is non resilient and should be relieved.

#### Clinical Consideration
- During final impression procedure mid palatine raphae is relieved to avoid trauma from denture base and to prevent rocking of dentures over centre of palate when vertical forces are applied to the teeth.

### 5. RESIDUAL RIDGE

#### Definition
- It is defined as "the portion of the residual bone and its soft tissue covering that remains after the removal of teeth"—GPT.

#### Macroscopic Anatomy
- The resorption following extraction of teeth is rapid at first, but it continues at a reduced rate throughout life.
- If the teeth have been out for many years, the residual ridge may become small and crest of ridge may lack smooth, cortical bony surface under the mucosa.
- Unlike palate, crest of alveolar ridge undergoes resorption and hence considered as the secondary supporting area, rather than a primary supporting area.
- The inclined facial surfaces of maxillary ridge provides little support and is also considered as secondary supporting area.

#### Microscopic Anatomy
- Crest of residual ridge:
  i. Mucosa is formed by stratified squamous epithelium which is thickly keratinized and firmly attached to underlying bone.
  ii. Submucosa of residual ridge is devoid of fat and glandular cells and is characterised by dense collagenous fibers that are contiguous with lamina propria.
- Slopes of residual ridge:
  i. Mucosa is formed by stratified squamous epithelium which is non keratinized or para keratinized.
  ii. Submucosa contains loose connective tissue and elastic fibers. Hence this loosely attached tissue will not withstand the forces of mastication.

#### Clinical Consideration
- Less stress is placed on loosely attached and movable tissues during making of final impression because the final impression material in that region is close to escape ways.

### 6. INCISIVE PAPILLA

#### Definition
- The elevation of soft tissue covering the foramen of the incisive and nasopalatine canal—GPT.

#### Macroscopic Anatomy
- It is situated on a line immediately behind and between the central incisors about 8–10 mm posterior to central incisors.
- Biometric guide which gives information about location of maxillary canines. A perpendicular drawn posterior to centre of incisive papilla to sagittal plane passes through canines.
- Its location varies in edentulous mouth. It lies nearer to crest of ridge as resorption progresses. Thus the location of incisive papilla gives an indication as to the amount of resorption that has taken place.

#### Microscopic Anatomy
- It is a pad of fibrous connective tissue overlying the orifice of nasopalatine canal.
- It covers the incisive foramen through which the nasopalatine nerves and vessels pass.

#### Clinical Consideration
- During final impression procedure care should be taken not to compress incisive papilla. It is a relief area. If not relieved, the denture will compress the blood vessels and nerves causes necrosis of distributing areas and parasthesia of anterior palate respectively.

## 7. MAXILLARY TUBEROSITY

### Definition
- The most distal portion of the maxillary alveolar ridge—GPT.

### Macroscopic Anatomy
- It is usually a bulbous extension of residual alveolar ridge in the second and third molar region, terminating in hamular notch.
- The tuberosity region can hang down abnormally low when maxillary posterior teeth supra erupt due to early loss and non replacement of lost opposing mandibular posterior teeth.
- It is considered as **secondary stress bearing area** as it is least likely to resorb.

### Clinical Consideration
- An over hanging tuberosity may interfere with location of occlusal plane and reduces space available. It has to be surgically reduced.
- Soft tissue tuberosity should be excised on both sides if present. But bony tuberosity if present should be retained on one side so that it can be used for retention of denture, etc., if patient is right side chewer we should retain that sided tuberosity.
- Teeth are not set on the maxillary tuberosity region.

## 8. TORUS PALATINUS

### Definition
- Torus is defined as a smooth rounded anatomical protuberance—GPT.

### Macroscopic Anatomy
- It is a hard bony enlargement that occurs in midline of hard palate and is found in 20% of the population.

### Microscopic Anatomy
- Mucous membrane covering the torus palatinus is very thin and is easily traumatized by denture unless relief is provided.

### Clinical Consideration
- The relief of torus palatinus should conform exactly to the shape of torus because an extensive relief will reduce the support area of denture.

## 9. LABIAL FRENUM

### Definition
- Frenum is defined as a connecting fold of membrane serving to support or retain a part—GPT.

### Macroscopic Anatomy
- It is a fibrous band covered by mucous membrane that extends from the mucous lining of mucous membrane of lip to or toward the crest of residual alveolar ridge in a fan shaped fashion.
- It contains no muscle and has no action of its own.
- It inserts in a vertical direction.
- The frenum may be narrow or broad.
- Its a relief area.

### Clinical Consideration
- During final impression procedure sufficient relief should be given, if not denture impinges on frenum and results in pain and dislodgement of denture.
- During impression procedure lip should be stretched horizontally outwards for proper recording of frenum.
- The labial notch in the labial flange of denture must be just wide enough and just deep enough to allow for frenum to pass through it without manipulation of lip.
- Frenectomy is indicated in cases where frenum lies close to the crest of alveolar ridge and affects the denture seal and retention.

## 10. LABIAL VESTIBULE

### Definition
- The portion of the oral cavity that is bounded on one side by the teeth, gingiva and alveolar ridge (in the edentulous mouth, the residual ridge) and on the other by the lips anterior to the buccal frenula—GPT.

### Macroscopic Anatomy
- The labial vestibule is divided into a left and right labial vestibule by labial frenum. Labial vestibule area extends on both sides from labial frenum to buccal frenum.
- It accomodates labial flange of denture and provides valve seal.
- The reflections of mucous membrane superiorly determines the height and thickness of labial flange depends on degree of alveolar resorption.

### Microscopic Anatomy
- Mucous of vestibular spaces is described as lining mucosa which is devoid of keratinized layer and is freely movable with tissues to which it is attached because of elastic nature of lamina propria.
- Submucosal layer is thick and contains large amount of loose areolar tissue and elastic fibers.

### Muscles of Importance
- Orbicularis oris is the main muscle of lip which forms the outer surface of labial vestibule.
- The fibres of orbicularis oris muscle pass horizontally through lips anastomose with fibers of buccinator muscle.

- Tone of orbicularis oris muscle depends on support it receives from labial flange and position of teeth.
- Orbicularis oris muscle has only an indirect effect on the extent of impression and denture base as its fibers run in a horizontal direction.

### Clinical Consideration
- Labial flange affects the appearance of patient. If the flange is too thick, the lips bulge out and if too thin the lips loose support and look unsupported.
- For effective border contact between denture and tissue, vestibule should be completely filled with impression material.

## 11. BUCCAL FRENUM

### Definition
- Frenum is defined as a connecting fold of membrane serving to support or retain a part—GPT.

### Macroscopic Anatomy
- Buccal frenum extends from buccal mucous membrane reflection area to or towards slope at crest of residual ridge.
- It forms the dividing line between labial and buccal vestibules.
- It can be single, double or broad and fan-shaped.
- Relief area. Its reflection is an anteroposterior direction.

### Muscles of Importance
- **Levator anguli oris** attaches beneath frenum and hence influenced by other muscles of facial expression.
- **Orbicularis oris** muscle pulls the buccal frenum forwards.
- **Buccinator muscle** pulls the buccal frenum backwards.

### Clinical Consideration
- During final impression procedure buccal frenum should be given sufficient relief and manipulated to mimic its function during chewing, smiling, etc. If not recorded in function results in dislodgement of denture during function.
- Frenectomy may be necessary if frenum is attached close to chest of alveolar ridge.

## 12. BUCCAL VESTIBULE

### Definition
- The portion of the oral cavity that is bounded on one side by teeth, gingiva and alveolar ridge (in the edentulous mouth, the residual ridge) and on the lateral side by the cheek posteior to the buccal frenula—GPT.

### Macroscopic Anatomy
- It extends from buccal frenum to the hamular notch. It is bound externally by cheek and internally by the residual ridge.
- The size of buccal vestibule varies with the contraction of buccinator muscle, position of mandible and amount of bone lost from maxilla.
- This space is usually higher than any other part of the border.
- When the mandible opens or moves to opposite side the width of buccal vestibule is reduced.

### Microscopic Anatomy
- The mucous membrane lining the buccal vestibule is similar to that lining the labial vestibule.

### Muscles of Importance
1. Buccinator muscle
2. Masseter muscle

The size of buccal vestibule varies with contraction buccinator and masseter muscles.

### Clinical Consideration
- The extent of buccal vestibule can be deceiving because the coronoid process obscures it when the mouth is opened wide. So, it should be examined when the mouth is nearly closed as possible.
- The coronoid process affects buccal flange as mandible moves forward, from side to side or opened wide. So, the distal end of buccal flange of denture should be adjusted in such a way that there is no interference to coronoid process during mouth opening. If distal end of buccal flange is too thick the coronoid process can dislodge the dentures.
- To effectively record the buccal vestibule the mouth should be half way closed because wide opening of mouth narrows the space and does not allow proper contouring of sulcus because the coronoid process of mandible comes closer to the sulcus.

## 13. HAMULAR NOTCH (PTERYGOMAXILLARY NOTCH)

### Definition
- The palpable notch formed by the junction of maxilla and the pterygoid hamulus of the sphenoid bone.

### Macroscopic Anatomy
- It forms the distal limit of buccal vestibule and is situated between the maxillary tuberosity and hamulus of medial pterygoid plate.

- The pterygomandibular ligament attaches to the hamulus.
- Hamular notch is a narrow cleft of loose connective tissue approximately 2 mm in extent antero posteriorly.
- Pterygomandibular raph extends from hamulus to top inside back corner of retromolar pad in mandible.

### Microscopic Anatomy

- The mucous membrane of hamulus notch consists of thick submucosa made up of loose areolar tissue.
- Loose areolar tissue present in the centre of deep part of humular notch can be displaced by posterior palatal border of denture to achieve pterygomaxillary seal.

### Clinical Consideration

- Dentures should not be over extended beyond hamular notch because, when mouth is opened wide, the pterygomandibular raphae is pulled forward resulting in trauma of mucous membrane covering the raphe and also dislodgement of dentures.
- Hamular notch is located by using T - burnisher.
- If the dentures is not extended till hamular notch and border is located anteriorly near maxillary tuberosity, denture will not have any retentive properties because of absence of pterygomaxillary seal.

## 14. VIBRATING LINE

### Definition

- An imaginary line across the posterior part of the palate marking the division between the movable and immovable tissues of the soft palate. This can be identified when the movable tissues are functioning.

### Macroscopic Anatomy

- Vibrating line is an imaginary line drawn across the palate that marks the begining of motion in soft palate when an individual says "ah".
- This is not a straight line from hamular notch to hamular notch but follows the contour of the distal border of the palatal bone. At the mid line it usually passess about 2 mm is front of the fovea palatinae.
- Vibrating line is always present on the soft palate. It is not the junction of hard and soft palate.
- It is not a well defined line and should be described as an area.
- Some authors consider the presence of 2 vibrating lines:
  - Anterior vibrating line
  - Posterior vibrating line

- *Anterior vibrating line:* It is an imaginary line present at the junction between immovable tissues over the hard palate and slightly movable tissues of the soft palate.
- It can be located by,
  i. Asking the patient to perform the valsalva maneuver (The patient is asked to close nostrils firmly and gently blow through the nose).
  ii. Asking the patient to say "ah" in short vigorous bursts.
- **Anterior vibrating line** takes the shape of cuspid's bow.
- **Posterior vibrating line:**
  - It is an imaginary line present at the junction of soft palate that shows limited movement and the soft palate that shows marked movement.
  - It also represented the junction between aponeurosis of tensor veli palatini muscle and muscular portion of soft palate.
  - It is recorded by asking the patient to say "ah" in short but normal nonvigorous fashion.
  - Posterior vibrating line is usually a straight line.

### Microscopic Anatomy

- The submucosa in the region of vibrating line contains glandular tissue. But, as the soft palate does not rest directly on bone, the tissue for a few millimeters on either side of vibrating line can be repositioned in the impression to improve posterior palatal seal.

### Clinical Consideration

- The distal end of denture should extend at least to the vibrating line. In most cases it should end 1 to 2 mm posterior to the vibrating line to improve the posterior palatal seal.

## 15. FOVEA PALATINAE

### Definition

- Two small pits or depressions in the posterior aspect of the palate, one on each side of the mid line, at or near the attachment of the soft palate to the hard palate.

### Macroscopic Anatomy

- Fovea palatina are usually two in number located one on each side of midline and slightly posterior to junction of hard and soft palates.

### Microscopic Anatomy

- Fovea palatina are formed by coalescence of several mucous gland ducts.

### Clinical Consideration

- The denture can extend 1 to 2 mm beyond fovea palatine. The secretion of mucous glands spreads as a thin film and aids in retention of denture.

- Fovea palatina should be uncovered in patients with thick ropy saliva because the thick saliva flowing between the tissue and denture can increase the hydrostatic pressure and displace the denture.

## INTERPRETATION OF MAXILLARY ANATOMIC LANDMARKS IN FINAL IMPRESSION

1. Labial frenum appears as labial notch.
2. Labial vestibule forms labial flange.
3. Buccal frenum appears as buccal notch.
4. Buccal vestibule forms buccal flange.
5. Mucous membrane reflections in labial and buccal vestibules makes the impression to turn out towards lips and cheeks. These reflections are smooth.
6. Residual alveolar ridge forms the alveolar groove.
7. Maxillary tuberosity produces a depression at the distal end of alveolar groove.
8. Hamular notch appears as anteroposterior groove distal to maxillary tuberosity region, when extreme mouth opening is allowed in making impression.
9. If patient is asked to open wide, protrude and do lateral movements during final impression, the distobuccal flange in distobuccal vestibule will be contoured by the anterior border of coronoid process.
10. Incisive papilla appear as small round depression in the anterior region.
11. Mid palatine raphae appear as irregular groove (central groove) in the middle of the vault anteroposteriorly.
12. Rugae area appear as small grooves radiating laterally from central groove.
13. Fovea palatina appear as two small raised dots in the impression on either side of mid line posteriorly.
14. At junction of hard and soft palates impression appear smooth. But due to influence of active palatal glands at this region surface will be irregular and (but not smooth) glandular secretions will adhere to impression material.

## MANDIBULAR ANATOMIC LANDMARKS

- Average denture bearing area for edentulous mandible is 14 cm$^2$.

I. **Based on Supporting and Limiting Structures**

A. **Supporting Structures**
  1. Residual alveolar ridge
  2. Buccal shelf area
  3. Mental foramen area
  4. Mylohyoid ridge
  5. Genial tubercles
  6. Torus mandibularis

B. **Limiting or Peripheral Structures**
  1. Labial frenum
  2. Labial vestibule
  3. Buccal frenum
  4. Buccal vestibule
  5. Lingual frenum
  6. Mylohyoid muscle
  7. Retromylohyoid fossa
  8. Sublingual gland region
  9. Alveolingual sulcus
  10. Retromolar pads

II. **Based on Function**

A. **Stress Bearing Areas**
  1. Primary
  2. Secondary

*Primary stress bearing areas:* Buccal shelf area
*Secondary stress bearing areas:* Slopes of residual alveolar ridge.

B. **Relief Areas**
  1. Crest of residual alveolar ridge
  2. Labial frenum
  3. Buccal frenum
  4. Lingual frenum
  5. Mental frenum area
  6. Genial tubercles
  7. Torus mandibularis

### 1. RESIDUAL ALVEOLAR RIDGE

**Definition**

- Refer maxillary anatomic landmarks.

**Macroscopic Anatomy**

- Because of the direction and inclination of teeth and alveolar process, the maxillae resorb upward and inward to become progressively smaller and mandible resorb downwards and outwards to become progressively wider recording to its edentulous age. Hence many edentulous patients appear prognathic.
- Many edentulous mandibles become extremely flat with a concave denture bearing surface, allowing the attaching structures especially on lingual side of ridge to fall over on to the ridge surface.

**Microscopic Anatomy**

- Crest of residual alveolar ridge is covered by a keratinized layer and is firmly attached by its submucosa to the periosteum of mandible in healthy mouths. In some people submucosa is loosely attached to bone and soft tissues are quite movable. But the underlying bone is cancellous. Hence considered as.

- The slopes of residual ridge have thin plate of cortical bone. But slopes are steep and at an acute angle to occlusal forces. Hence it is considered as secondary stress bearing area.

**Clinical Consideration**
- When soft tissues over residual alveolar ridge are movable, it must be registered in its resting position in the final impression.

## 2. BUCCAL SHELF AREA

**Macroscopic Anatomy**
- The area between the mandibular buccal frenum and the anterior edge of masseter muscle is called as buccal shelf area.
- Boundaries of buccal shelf area
  Anteriorly—Buccal frenum
  Posteriorly—Retromolar pad
  Medially—Crest of residual ridge
  Laterally—External oblique ridge
- The width of bony foundation in buccal shelf area increases with resorption due to the fact that width of inferior border of mandible is greater than the width at alveolar process.
- Buccal shelf area is considered as primary stress bearing area for lower denture because.
  1. Bone of buccal shelf area is covered by a layer of dense and smooth cortical bone.
  2. Buccal shelf area lies at right angles to vertical occulsal forces.

**Microscopic Anatomy**
- Mucous membrane covering buccal shelf area is more loosely attached and less keratinized than mucous membrane covering crest of lower residual ridge.
- It contains thicker submucosal layer.

**Muscles of Importance**
- The inferior part of buccinator muscle is attached to buccal shelf area but fibers run in anterior posterior direction, so does not interfere with the function of dentures.

**Clinical Consideration**
- It is advisable to extend the impression beyond external oblique ridge.

## 3. MENTAL FORAMEN AREA

**Anatomy**
- It usually lies between first and second premolar region.
- When the ridge is extremely resorbed, mental foramen will come to lie closer to crest of alveolar ridge.
- Pressure on mental nerve which passes through mental foramen can causes numbness of lower lip. Hence relief should be provided in mental foramen area.

## 4. MYLOHYOID RIDGE

**Definition**
- An oblique ridge on the lingual surface of mandible that extends from level of roots of the last molar teeth and that serves as a bony attachment for the mylohyoid muscles forming the floor of mouth—GPT.

**Anatomy**
- It is a bony ridge found on the lingual aspect of mandible which starts from last molar tooth at level of roots and slopes downward and forwards.
- Anteriorly it lies close to inferior border of mandible and posteriorly it often lies flush with superior surface of residual ridge after resorption.

**Clinical Consideration**
- A thin and sharp mylohyoid ridge can irritate the soft tissues on denture placement. So, it may be corrected surgically (or) relief must be given.

## 5. GENIAL TUBERCLES

**Definition**
- Mental spines; rounded elevations (usually two pairs) clustered around the mid line on the lingual surface of the lower portion of the mandibular symphysis. These tubercles serve as attachments for the genioglossus and geniohyoid muscles.

**Macroscopic Anatomy**
- Usually seen below the crest of ridge on the lingual surface of lower portion of mandibular symphysis.
- In severely resorbed ridges genial tubercles become prominent may lie on crest of residual ridge and hence it should be relieved.

**Microscopic Anatomy**
- Mucosa covering the genial tubercles is thin and tightly adherent to underlying bone.

**Clinical Consideration**
- Failure to relieve genial tubercles results in ulceration of soft tissues present over genial tuberctes.

## 6. TORUS MANDIBULARIS

**Definition**
- Torus is defined as a smooth rounded anatomical protuberance.

## Macroscopic Anatomy
- It is commonly located bilaterally and lingually near the first and second premolars, midway between soft tissues of floor of mouth and crest of the ridge.
- In edentulous patients with considerable resorption, the superior border of torus may be located in flush with chest of residual ridge.

## Microscopic Anatomy
- Torus mandibularis is covered by an extremely thin layer of mucous membrane.

## Clinical Consideration
- Small tori if present and not interfering with denture seal, should be relieved.
- Large tori which interfere with denture seal should be removed surgically.

## 7. LABIAL FRENUM

### Definition
- Refer maxillary anatomic landmarks.

### Macroscopic Anatomy
- It extends from mucous lining of mucous membrane of lower lips to or towards the crest of residual alveolar ridge on labial surface of mandible.
- Its a relief area because unlike maxillary frenum or bicularisoris muscle attaches mandibular labial frenum and hence it is quite sensitive and active.

### Microscopic Anatomy
- Mandibular labial frenum is a fold of mucous membrane and contains a band of fibrous connective tissue which is histologically similar to maxillary labial frenum.

### Muscles of Importance
- It is influenced by incisivus and orbicularis oris muscle which is attached to labial frenum.

### Clinical Consideration
- During final impression procedure the labial frenum should be relieved in such a way that it maintains the peripheral seal without causing soreness.
- During final impression procedure lip has to be reflected anteriorly and horizontally.

## 8. LABIAL VESTIBULE

### Definition
- Refer maxillary anatomic landmarks.

### Macroscopic Anatomy
- Labial vestibule extends from labial frenum to buccal frenum.
- Boundaries

   Anteriorly—Labial frenum
   Posteriorly—Buccal frenum
   Laterally—Labial mucosa
   Medially—Residual alveolar ridge

### Microscopic Anatomy
- The epithelium is thin and non keratinized and submucosa is formed of loosely arranged connective tissue fibers mixed with elastic fibres and muscle fibres.

### Muscles of Importance
- Fibres of orbicularis muscle, incisivius and mentalis muscles are inserted fairly close to crest of ridge and influence the extent of denture flange in this area.

### Clinical Consideration
- When the mouth is opened wide, the orbicularis oris muscle gets stretched and narrows the sulcus. This would displace the mandibular dentures if flange is unnecessarily thick. Hence, labial flange of dentures and impressions should always be narrowest in anterior labial region to prevent dislodgment of dentures when patient opens his mouth wide.

## 9. BUCCAL FRENUM

### Definition
- Refer maxillary anatomic landmarks.

### Macroscopic Anatomy
- It extends from buccal mucous membrane reflection to or towards the slope or crest of residual ridge in the region just distal to cuspid eminence.
- It may be single or double, blood U—shaped or sharp V-shaped.
- The reflection is in anteroposterior direction.

### Microscopic Anatomy
- It is a fold of mucous membrane containing thick fibrous connective tissue.

### Muscles of Importance
- Depressor anguli oris underlines the buccal frenum.

### Clinical Consideration
- Mandibular buccal frenum should be relieved during final impression procedure to avoid dislodgment of dentures.

## 10. BUCCAL VESTIBULE

### Definition
- Refer maxillary anatomic landmarks.

### Macroscopic Anatomy
- The buccal vestibule extends from buccal frenum to the outside back corner of the retromolar pad.
- Boundaries
  Anteriorly—Buccal frenum
  Posteriorly—Outside back corner of retromolar pad
  Laterally—Buccal mucosa
  Medially—Residual alveolar ridge

### Muscles of Importance
1. Buccinator muscle
2. Masseter muscles.
   - The extent of buccal vestibule is influenced by buccinator muscle which runs from modiolus to pterygomandibular raphe posteriorly and has its lower fibers attached to buccal shelf and external oblique ridge. Fibers of buccinator muscle run parallel to the base and hence does not displace the dentures.
   - Masseter muscle contracts under heavy closing pressures and pushes inward against the buccinator muscle to produce a masseteric notch in the distobuccal area of denture base. Masseteric notch in distobuccal area of denture base accomodates mesial border of masseter muscle.

### Clinical Consideration
- The buccal flange may extend to external oblique ridge, upon it or even over it, depending on location of the mucobuccal fold.
- Distobuccal border at the end of buccal vestibule, must converge rapidly to avoid displacement by contracting masseter muscle.
- The impression is always widest in this region.

### 11. LINGUAL FRENUM
- It is the fold of mucous membrane that joins the lingual alveolar mucosa of mandible to tongue anteriorly.
- It can be observed when tip of tongue is elevated. It is active and extremely resistant.

### Muscles of Importance
- Lingual frenum overlies the genioglossus muscle, which takes origin from superior genial spine on the mandible.

### Clinical Consideration
- Lingual frenum should be registered in function because at rest the height of its attachment is deceptive. In function it often comes close to crest of ridge, although it lies much lower at rest.
- Failure to relieve lingual frenum leads to soreness and dislodgement of dentures.

### 12. MYLOHYOID MUSCLE
- Floor of mouth is formed by mylohyoid muscle, which arises from whole length of mylohyoid ridge.
- In the anterior region muscle lies deep to sublingual gland and other structures and does not affect border of denture in this region.
- In the posterior region at the molar area mylohyoid muscle affects lingual impression border in swallowing and in moving the tongue.
- During swallowing, the mylohoid muscle contracts, raising the floor of mouth.
- Lingual flange of denture should not be extended under the mylohyoid ridge, as it will interfere with action of mylohyoid muscle on contraction and displaces denture causing soreness.
- The lingual flange must be made parallel to mylohyoid muscle when it is contracted to prevent displacement of denture.
- If the lingual border stops above mylohyoid ridge, vertical forces will cause soreness and border seal will be easily broken.
- If the lingual flange of lower denture is properly shaped and extended, it will provide border seal and guide the tongue to rest on top of the flange.
- There should be space between lingual flange and mucous membrane when mylohyoid muscle is relaxed contact occurs only when tongue is raised or thrust out.

### 13. RETROMYLOHYOID FOSSA
- It is the area present posterior to mylohyoid muscle.
- As the lingual flange moves into retromylohyoid fossa, it ceases to be influenced by action of mylohyoid muscle and so can move back toward body of mandible producing typical S curve of lingual flange.
- Boundaries of retromylohyoid foosa.
  Anteriorly—Retromylohyoid curtain.
  Posterolaterally—Superior constrictor of pharynx.
  Posteromedially—Palatoglossus and lateral surface of tongue.
  Inferiorly—Submandibular gland.
- Retromylohyoid curtain is a wall of mucous membrane which limits distolingual part of denture flange and is formed.
  Anteriorly by—lingual tuberosity.
  Posteriorly by—superior constrictor muscle.
  Laterally by—mandible and pterygomandibular rophe.
  Inferiorly by—mylohyoid muscle.
- Protrusion of tongue causes retromylohyoid curtain to move forward so this area is carefully moulded to avoid displacement and soreness.

- Medial pterygoid muscle lies posterior to superior constrictor muscle and contraction of medial pterygoid muscle causes bulge in retromylohyoid curtain in the same way as contraction of masseter muscle can cause a bulge in buccinator muscle.

**NOTE**
- Mandibular impression in the lingual aspect is most difficult to accomplish, because the muscles of floor of mouth and tongue do not resist over extension immediately and easily displacable. But over a period of time the over extension causes sorenss, difficulty in swallowing and dislodgement of dentures.

## 14. SUBLINGUAL GLAND REGION

- Sublingual gland rests above the mylohyoid muscle in the premolar region.
- When the floor of mouth is raised, the gland comes close to crest of ridge. Thus even though mylohyoid muscle has low attachment in anterior region a long flange height is not possible.

### Clinical Consideration
- Sublingual gland may be pushed down and laterally out of position by resistant impression material. This should be avoided by shaping anterior part of lingual flange of tray to slope inward toward the tongue and making the final impression with a low viscosity impression material.

**NOTE**
- The anterior portion of lingual flange is commonly called the sublingual crescent area. It is a part of floor of mouth covering sublingual gland, over extension of denture in this area causes burning sensation.

## 15. ALVEOLINGUAL SULCUS

- It is the space between residual ridge and tongue which extends from lingual frenum to retro mylohyoid curtain.
- It is considered in 3 regions.
  1. Anterior region
  2. Middle region
  3. Posterior region

### Anterior Region
- It extends from lingual frenum to premylohyoid fossa (where mylohyoid ridge curves above level of sulcus).
- Lingual border of impression in this anterior region should make contact with mucous membrane floor of mouth when tip of tongue touches upper incisors.
- Lingual flange will be shorter anteriorly than posteriorly. At the premylohyoid fossa, the flange becomes larger as it extends below level of mylohyoid ridge.

### Middle Region
- It extends from premylohyoid fossa to distal end of mylohyoid ridge.
- Middle region is shallowest part of alveolingual sulcus because of the prominence of mylohyoid ridge and action of mylohyoid muscle.
- Lingual flange in this region is made to slope medially towards the tongue because.
  1. It allows tongue to rest on top of lingual flange and aids in stabilizing lower denture on residual ridge.
  2. It provides space for floor of mouth to be raised during function without displacing the lower denture.
  3. It maintains peripheral seal during function.

### Posterior Region
- It extends from the end of mylohyoid ridge to the retromylohyoid curtain.
- Lingual flange in posterior region passes into retro mylohyoid fossa and as it is not influenced by mylohyoid muscle, flange can turn laterally toward the ramus to fill fossa and complete the typical 'S' form of correctly shaped lingual flange of lower denture. This is also called as lateral throat form.

## 16. RETROMOLAR PAD

### Definition
- A mass of tissue comprised of non keratinized mucosa located posterior to the retromolar papilla and overlying loose glandular connective tissue. This freely movable area should be differentiated from the pear shaped pad—GPT.

### Macroscopic Anatomy
- Sicher described retromolar pad as a triangular soft elevation of mucosa that lies distal to third molar.
- **Boundaries** of retromolar pad.
  Posteriorly by—Tendons of temporalis.
  Laterally by—Buccinator.
  Medially by—Pterygomandibular raphe and superior constrictor.
- Contents of retromolar pad.
  1. Glandular tissue
  2. Loose areolar connective tissue
  3. Lower margin of pterygomandibular raphe
  4. Fibres of buccinator
  5. Fibres of superior constrictor muscle
  6. Fibres from temporal tendon.

## Microscopic Anatomy
- Its mucosa is composed of thin, non keratinized epithelium and loose areolar tissue.
- Its submucosa contains glandular tissue and other fibers of muscles.

## Clinical Consideration
- It forms the posterior seal of mandibular denture.
- Muscles present in this region limits the extent of denture and prevents placement of extra pressure on distal part of retromolar pad during impression making. Hence, denture base should extend approximately one half to 2/3rds over the retro molar pad.

## NOTE
- Retromolar papilla is a small pear shaped area just anterior to retromolar pad and distal to third molar. It is a triangular soft pad of keratinized tissue which remains fused to scar after the loss of third molar. It is firmly attached and easily distinguishable from retromolar pad which is readily displaced.

## INTERPRETATION OF MANDIBULAR ANATOMIC LANDMARKS IN FINAL IMPRESSION

1. Labial frenum appear as labial notch.
2. Labial vestibule forms labial flange.
3. Buccal frenum appear as buccal notch.
4. Buccal vestibule forms buccal flange.
5. Mucous membrane reflections in vestibule are more active than in maxilla and appear as small lines in impression material.
6. Residual alveolar ridge forms the alveolar groove.
7. External oblique line appears as a slight groove.
8. Buccal shelf area appear as broad, flat area which extends from external oblique line to begining of slope of residual ridge.
9. When patient is asked to close his mouth forcefully against the downward pressure applied by operator while making mandibular impression results in formation of groove (masseteric groove) at the distal buccal area.
10. Retromolar pad appears as pear shaped depression at the distal end of alveolar groove.
11. Retromolar papilla will appear as small pear shaped depression just anterior to retromolar pad.
12. Lingual frenum appear as lingual notch.
13. Alveolingual sulcus forms the lingual flange.
14. Mylohyoid attachment area from bicuspids forms a groove posteriorly.
15. Retromylohyoid fossa forms on eminence.

# The Teeth

**CHAPTER 4**

## TEETH—TYPES AND FUNCTION

- Humans are omnivorous, which means they eat both meat and plants.
- To accommodate this variety in diet, human teeth are designed for cutting, tearing and grinding different types of food.

### TYPES OF TEETH

- The permanent dentition is divided into four types of teeth, i.e. incisors, canines, premolars and molars.
- The primary dentition has incisors, canines and molars. There are no premolars in the primary dentition.

### 1. Incisors

- These are single-rooted teeth with a relatively sharp, thin edge.
- They are located at the front of the mouth and are designed to cut the food without the application of heavy forces.
- The lingual surface (tongue side) is shaped like a shovel to aid in guiding the food into the mouth.

### 2. Canines

- They are also known as "cuspids".
- They are located at the "corner" of the dental arch.
- They are designed for cutting and tearing the food which require the application of force.
- Canines are the *longest teeth* in the human dentition.
- They are also some of the best-anchored and most stable teeth because of their longest root.
- They are usually the last teeth to be lost.
- Because of its sturdy crown, long route and location in the dental arch, it is referred to as the "corner stone" of the dental arch.

---

After loss of the teeth the remaining alveolar bone forms the alveolar ridge which gives support to a denture and is part of the denture-bearing area. It is likely, particularly in the case of the lower denture, that a substantial alveolar ridge contributes significantly to denture security. Following tooth loss, alveolar bone resorbs, the rate being rapid at first but decreasing with time (so determining the rate of denture replacement - frequent at first, later at longer intervals). During extractions, good surgical technique (avoiding fragmentation or even loss of the associated bone) is particularly helpful. Investigators have shown that the rate of loss of alveolar bone obeys a power law, becoming less with time but never ceasing until all alveolar bone has been lost. There are individual variations, however, with some experiencing very little loss, and others rapid alveolar atrophy. In general bone loss is greater in the mandible than the maxilla by a factor of four.

### 3. Premolars

- There are four maxillary and four mandibular premolars.
- Occasionally, the premolars are also referred to as *bicuspids*, which is inaccurate term because it refers to *two* (bi) cusps and some premolars have three cusps. Therefore, the newer term *premolar* is preferred.
- The pointed buccal cusps hold the food while the lingual cusps grind it.
- They also have a broader surface for chewing the food.
- There are no premolars in the primary dentition.

### 4. Molars

- These are much larger than premolars, usually having four or more cusps.
- Their function is to chew or grind up the food.
- Maxillary and mandibular molars differ greatly from each other in shape, size, number of cusps and roots.

## TOOTH LOSS

- Teeth may be lost due to a variety of reasons; i.e. some are lost during the course of life and others may be absent congenitally.

### CAUSES FOR TOOTH LOSS

- The following are some of the reasons for tooth loss.
  1. Traumatic injuries, i.e. accidents, sports, violence etc.
  2. Dental caries.
  3. Periodontal diseases.
  4. Cysts and malignancies→destruction of alveolar bone →loosening of teeth→tooth loss.
  5. Radiation therapy often demands extraction of teeth as a precaution.
  6. Iatrogenic extraction—wrong tooth extraction.
  7. Therapeutic extraction for orthodontic treatment.
  8. Congenital absence of teeth.
  9. Failure to erupt.

### SEQUELAE OF TEETH LOSS

- Certain changes will occur definitely when a tooth or teeth are lost. The extent of changes may vary from one to another.
- The following are the changes that can occur due to tooth loss.
  1. Resorption of the alveolar socket where the tooth was.
  2. Tilting of adjacent teeth into the edentulous space
  3. Drifting: Total migration of adjacent teeth into the edentulous space.
  4. *Occlusal discrepancies:* The combination of above changes may lead to occlusal malignant that results in abnormal wearing of teeth and discomfort to the individual.

## TREATMENT CONSIDERATIONS

- There are varieties of choices of treatment for an individual with missing teeth:
  1. Removable fixed partial denture
  2. Complete denture
  3. Over denture
  4. Splints
  5. Implant denture
  6. Maxillofacial prosthesis

# Prosthodontic Laboratory and Armamentarium

**CHAPTER 5**

Prosthodontic laboratory is a separate area of the dental clinic, away from the patient treatment area where the dentist and other clinical staff complete various procedures like pouring impressions, trimming and finishing dental casts and models, preparing custom trays and polishing the provisional restorations, partial or complete dentures and indirect restorations. This chapter gives you enough information in brief about the armamentarium that you will be using during the routine procedures

## LABORATORY RULES AND GUIDE LINES

### Professionalism

- While not a percentage of the actual final grade, proper conduct and good work habits are an extremely influential factor in all aspects of the course of dentistry. Start now and continue to conduct yourselves professionally.

### Working, Safety and Dress Code

1. Wear personal protective equipment when working in the lab.
2. White, long laboratory coats, buttoned, must be worn with name tag at all times.
3. Medium to long hair must be pinned or tied back.
4. Keep all cosmetics away from the area.
5. Casual, neat and clean clothing.
6. No sandals or open-toed shoes.
7. No eating or drinking.
8. Follow the manufacturer's instructions for equipment operation.
9. Report all accidents to the staff immediately.
10. Clean the work area before and after every procedure.

## LABORATORY EQUIPMENT/ARMAMENTARIUM

- The dental laboratory is generally equipped with countertops (for adequate work area), cabinets (for safe storage of materials), wall mounted containers (to store bulk supplies of plaster, dental stone and investment materials) and a variety of equipments.

## I. HEAT SOURCES

- Heat source is often required to heat the wax or other materials.
- It may be from a gas line that has been installed into the laboratory and a rubber hose (tube) will be attached to a Bunsen burner or an alcohol torch.

## 1. BUNSEN BURNER

- The Bunsen burner heats wax-carving instruments, waxes, and modeling compound. It requires a balanced air and gas mixture to produce a clean blue flame. The burner is made of metal and consists of a stand, gas-inlet valve, cylindrical barrel and air collar. It is attached to a gas valve with a non-collapsible hose.
- Inspect the unit and hose daily for loose connections and defects.
- Have the hose replaced when it shows signs of wear.
- When wax or similar material drops into the burner, the burner assembly can be detached easily for boiling out and cleaning.

  **WARNING:** Never leave an unattended burner lit or reach over an open flame, because the flame is almost invisible and can cause serious harm.

## 2. ALCOHOL TORCH

- The alcohol torch is used for smoothing wax surfaces, setting teeth and waxing. Also used with a variety of tasks those require an accurate, controlled pointed flame.
- It draws fuel through a wick from a reservoir near the top of the torch.
- Periodically trim all irregular or burned areas of the wick and check the nozzle tip to ensure that it is free from obstructions.

### CAUTION

- *Never overfill the reservoir or attempt to fill it with the flame.*
- *Do not leave the torch unattended when lit.*
- *Extinguish the torch when not in use by covering the wick with the nozzle holder assembly.*
- Before using an alcohol torch, you should check the fuel level. Many different types of fuels can be used with an alcohol torch. Isopropyl alcohol in a solution containing about 70-percent alcohol and 30-percent distilled water by volume produces a flame of very poor quality. Further, 100 percent isopropyl alcohol tends to smoke badly while burning; this makes it somewhat undesirable as torch fuel. The best choice fuel for the alcohol torch is denatured alcohol (ethanol), which produces a clear blue flame. However, care with the accountability of denatured alcohol must be taken when used and distributed.
- The **Alcohol Blowtorch** is designed to be held and operated in one hand. It has a plunger which, when pushed in, ejects a stream of air to produce a pinpoint flame which is useful in applying heat to small, localized areas of wax, modeling plastic or other material. Either ethyl or methyl alcohol may be used for fuel.

## II. MODEL TRIMMER

- The model trimmer is a machine used to trim and contour casts.
- A cast should present a neat, attractive appearance.
- This electrically operated machine has a 10-inch *abrasive wheel,* a small *work table,* and a *water-dispensing mechanism* to keep the abrasive wheel rinsed clean and clog free.
- Before using the trimmer, ensure the water supply is on.
- Allow the water to run for at least 1 minute after the procedure is complete. This will flush most of the particles from the trimmer drain and help prevent clogging.

### CAUTION

- When operating the trimmer, be sure to keep your fingers away from the wheel. Always wear safety glasses or goggles.
- Using light pressure, press the cast against the trimming wheel. Ensure that the water spray is sufficient to contain the grindings.
- Check the unit for water leaks and the power cord for wear or damage.
- If the unit does not operate correctly, contact the dental equipment repair technician. Clean the trimmer at least quarterly, or more frequently, depending on the amount of usage.

## III. VIBRATOR

- The vibrator is used to remove air from the mix of plaster or stone and to aid in the flow of material when pouring a cast. The vibrator also increases the density of the mix by eliminating air bubbles.
- It has a flat working surface that vibrates the bowl or tray.
- A rheostat control is used to adjust the intensity of the vibration from a gentle agitation to a vigorous shaking.
- To maintain the vibrator, cover the rubber platform and body of the unit with a plastic cover. As a safety precaution, check the power cord and plug for defects before use.

## IV. ARTICULATOR

- The articulator is a device used to reproduce the patient's jaw movements.

- The dental casts made from impressions are mounted onto the articulator.
- This allows the dentist and the laboratory technician to recreate the normal movement of the patient's jaw during the fabrication of the prosthesis. There are several types of articulators. The type of articulator used depends upon the type of prosthesis being fabricated.

## V. BENCH LATHE

- The bench lathe (a machine used for cutting or polishing dental appliances) is used during grinding, finishing, and polishing procedures.
- It has a revolving threaded extension from each end of the motor. Attachments such as an abrasive grinding wheel, rag wheel, burs or stones are placed on these extensions.
- An adapter and/or chuck are required to attach these instruments to the lathe.

### CAUTION

- Always wear protective glasses or goggles when working with the bench lathe.
- Ensure that all chucks and attachments are securely mounted before starting the lathe.

## VI. SPECIALIZED SPATULAS

- Spatula is a flat-bladed instrument used for mixing or spreading materials.
- Spatulas are used in prosthodontics for handling dental waxes and mixing impression materials.

### 1. Mixing Spatula
- It has a 2½ inch flexible blade, which is about 1-inch wide with a rounded end.
- The handle is usually made of wood or plastic.

### 2. Wax Spatula
- The wax spatula is a double-ended instrument
- Commonly used are the #7 and the #31.
- Both spatulas are used to hold small bits of wax over a Bunsen burner flame that delivers liquid wax.

## VII. MIXING BOWL

- The mixing bowl is made of flexible material, either rubber or flexible plastic, and used to mix alginate impression material, plaster and dental stone.
- It comes in small, medium, large, and extra large sizes. All sizes are used in the dental laboratory.

## VIII. COMPOUND HEATER

- The compound heater is an electrically operated water bath used to soften modeling plastic.
- Temperature of water is controlled thermostatically.

## IX. MOLD AND SHADE GUIDES

- Denture teeth and facings are made in a variety of sizes, forms, and shades by many tooth manufacturers.
- Size and form are identified by letter or number as are the shades.
- Mold and shade guides are available for denture teeth and facings as special purchase items.

## X. MILLIMETER GAUGE

- The millimeter (Boley) gauge is a measuring instrument calibrated in tenths of millimeters.
- It is used in prosthodontics for determining tooth dimensions and making other measurements.

## XI. PROSTHODONTIC KNIVES

- Usually, two kinds of knives are used in the prosthodontic treatment room: the compound knife and plaster knife.
- As the names imply, one is used with compound and the other with plaster.

### 1. Compound Knife
- The compound knife has a fairly large plastic handle and a detachable blade.
- Routinely the #25 blade is used to trim impression compound, wax and other materials that require an extremely sharp cutting edge.
- The blade is almost identical to a larger version of the #11 surgical blade.

### 2. Plaster Knife
- The plaster knife is a heavy-duty knife used to trim and chisel gypsum products and impression compound.
- It has a large flat blade at one end with a wide projection shaped like a screwdriver at the other end.
- The handle is made of wood and is riveted in place.

## XII. ROACH CARVER

- The roach carver is a double-ended instrument used to cut, smooth, and carve dental waxes.
- At first glance, it appears to look like a wax spatula.
- A closer look reveals a spear-shaped blade at one end, with a deep-welled, very small spoon at the other end.
- Both ends have very sharp edges.
- The deep-welled end may also be used to carry melted wax.

## XIII. IMPRESSION TRAYS

- Impression trays are carriers for the material used in making impressions of the teeth, alveolar ridges, and adjacent structures.

- They are manufactured in various sizes and shapes to accommodate the size and shape of the arch, the type of impression material to be used, and the impression technique to be followed.
- Impression trays hold the impression material in place while it sets.
- The impression may include a portion of the arch or the entire arch.
- Generally, the impression tray is shaped to match the natural contour of the arch.
- The two basic types of trays are stock and custom trays.
- With either type, the tray used for the mandibular impression differs from the maxillary tray because it allows free tongue movement.

1. **Stock Trays**
   - Stock trays come in many sizes for both the maxillary and mandibular arches.
   - Stock trays may be rim locking or mesh.
   - Both stock trays are available in regular, edentulous, and orthodontic styles.
   - Generally, the size of a tray will be identified on the handle tray.

2. **Custom Trays**
   - Custom trays are made in the dental laboratory from tray acrylic. Since custom trays are made for individual patients, you must have a dental cast of the patient's teeth.

# Sterilization and Infection Control

**CHAPTER 6**

Infection control (IC) is an essential part of dentistry. Potential for disease transmission in the dental lab is well documented. Potential pathogens can be transported to lab via orally soiled impressions, dental prostheses/appliances. Microorganisms can be transferred from contaminated impressions to dental casts. Oral bacteria can remain viable in set gypsum for up to 7 days. This chapter outlines you about the sterilization and infection control both in the clinical area and the lab.

## EXPOSURE

- Lab personnel may be exposed via.
  - Direct contact (through cuts and abrasions).
  - Aerosols created during lab procedures.
    - Inhaled or ingested.
- Patients can be at risk due to potential cross-contamination between dental prostheses/appliances.
- Potential for cross-contamination from dental office to lab and back to dental office.
- Potential infection can be transferred in lab from case to case.
  - By surface contact, handpieces, burs, pumice pans, aerosolization, dust/mist, unwashed hands.

## CROSS-CONTAMINATION

- Passage of microorganisms from one person or inanimate object to another.
  - Aseptic techniques must be implemented to reduce occurrence.
- Dentists and lab should establish IC protocol for incoming and outgoing cases.

## GOALS/ACTIONS

- Strive to make dental lab as safe as possible.
- Minimize potential for disease transmission via.
  - Immunizations.
  - Barrier techniques.
  - Aseptic techniques.
- IC compliance.
  - Adhere to standard precautions (SP).
  - Establish written IC policy.

## STANDARD PRECAUTIONS

- Must be observed in the lab at all times.
- Are used by all lab personnel to prevent cross-contamination by dental items entering lab.

- All patients are treated as if they could transmit a bloodborne pathogen (BBP) disease.
  - Examples include hepatitis B, hepatitis C, and human immunodeficiency virus (HIV).

## REQUIREMENTS

- Lab is responsible to comply and enforce all federal, state, and local regulations that affect its operations and employees.
  - Includes the Occupational Safety and Health Administration's (OSHA) BBP Standard.
- All lab personnel
  - Must be included in exposure determination.
  - Must be offered hepatitis B vaccine.
  - Must be given annual BBP training.

## BASICS OF LABORATORY INCORPORATION

- Need coordination between dental office and lab.
- Use of proper methods/materials for handling and decontaminating soiled incoming items.
- All contaminated incoming items should be cleaned and disinfected before being handled by lab personnel, and before being returned to the patient.
- Is most effective, practical method for preventing cross-contamination.
- Is a series of physical cleaning procedures to reduce organic debris and microorganisms on intraorally soiled dental items.
- Accomplished through step-wise process of mechanical and chemical cleaning and disinfection.
- Results in a product that can safely be handled by lab personnel without need for personal protective equipment (PPE).

## BARRIERS

- Include
  - Handwashing with plain or antimicrobial soap (or an alcohol-based hand rub if hands are not visibly soiled).
- Use of PPE when there is potential for occupational exposure to BBPs.
  - Examples
    - Gloves
    - Mask
    - Protective eyewear, chin length face shield.
    - Protective clothing (i.e. lab coat/jacket).

### Gloves

- Disposable gloves
  - Use when there is potential for direct hand contact with contaminated items.
  - Should be changed and disposed of appropriately after completion of procedure.
  - Hands should be washed before gloving and after removing gloves.
- Utility gloves
  - Should be used when cleaning/disinfecting equipment/surfaces.

### Mask/Protective Eyewear/Clothing

- Must be used when there is potential for splashes, spray, spatter, or aerosols.
  - Examples: when operating lathes, model trimmers, and other rotary equipment.
- Lab coat/jacket should be worn at all times during fabrication process.
  - Change daily
  - Do not wear outside of the lab
  - Launder appropriately.

## CHEMICAL DISINFECTANTS

- Two functions
  - Must be an effective antimicrobial agent.
  - Must not adversely affect dimensional accuracy or surface texture of impression materials and resulting gypsum cast.
- Want to reduce likelihood of ill fitting, non-functional prostheses.
- All employees must be properly trained to handle these materials in accordance with OSHA's hazard communication standard.
- Disinfectant must have an environmental protection agency (EPA) registration number.
- Must have at least intermediate-level of activity.
  - Tuberculocidal, hospital-grade.

### Dental Laboratory

- All disinfection procedures are accomplished prior to delivery to lab.
  - Done in dental operatory or professional work area.
- Recommend a sign and monitor system be implemented stating *"Only Biologically Clean Items Permitted"*.

### Incoming Items

- Rinse under running tap water to remove blood/saliva.
- Disinfect as appropriate.
- Rinse thoroughly with tap water to remove residual disinfectant.

- No single disinfectant is ideal or compatible with all items.
- Annotate the DD Form 2322: *"Disinfected with _____ for _____ minutes"*.

## Outgoing Items

- Clean and disinfect before delivery to patient.
- After disinfection: rinse and place in plastic bag with diluted mouthwash until insertion.
- Do not store in disinfectant before insertion.
- Label the plastic bag: *"This case shipment has been disinfected with _____ for _____ minutes"*.

## IMPRESSIONS

- Many studies have been performed to evaluate effects of various disinfectants on different types of impression materials.
- Research findings have been contradictory.
- No single disinfectant is compatible with all impression materials.
- The least distortion is associated with products having the shortest contact times.
- Many variables can affect impression materials.
  - Composition and concentration of disinfectants
  - Exposure time and compatibility of various disinfectants with specific impression materials.
  - Physical/chemical properties can vary in a given category of material or disinfectant.
- Do an in-office "test run" when using new combinations of impression materials and disinfectants.
- Consult dental materials' manufacturers regarding their compatibility with disinfectants.

### Disinfectants

- Methods.
  - Spraying, dipping, immersing.
- Exposure time should be that recommended by the manufacturer of disinfectant for tuberculocidal disinfection.
- Iodophors, sodium hypochlorite (1:10 concentration), chlorine dioxide, phenols, and other approved products are all acceptable.

### Disinfecting Impressions

- Polyether materials cannot be immersed in disinfectants due to potential for absorption and distortion.
- Immersion disinfectants can only be used once before discarding (except for glutaraldehydes).
- Most reports indicate dimensional stability is not significantly affected by immersion technique.
- Clean and rinse impression in dental operatory.
  - Cleaning efficiency can be improved by gently scrubbing impression with camel's hair brush and antimicrobial detergent.
- Sprinkle dental stone into impression before rinsing to aid in cleaning.
- Cleaning and rinsing.
- Reduces bioburden present.
- Lessens overall microbiologic challenge to disinfectant.
- Spray, dip, or immerse impression in appropriate intermediate- or high-level disinfectant and place in sealed bag.
- Disinfection can be accomplished in the dental operatory or a professional work area depending on facility policy.
- After required contact time, rinse impression and pour-up.

### Spray Technique

- Rinse entire impression/tray under running tap water after removal from oral cavity.
- Trim excess impression material from noncritical areas.
  - Reduces number of microorganisms and organic debris present.
- Place impression in bag and liberally spray the entire impression/tray.
- Seal bag to create "charged atmosphere".
  - Reduces exposure to vapors and liquid.
- Remove from bag at end of exposure time; rinse and pour.
- Once stone has set, remove cast from impression.
- Dispose of impression material and disposable tray (if applicable) in general waste.
- Sterilize reusable tray (if applicable).
- Advantages
  - Uses less disinfectant.
  - Same disinfectant can often be used to disinfect environmental surfaces.
- Disadvantages
  - Probably not as effective as immersion.
  - Can be released into air increasing occupational exposure.

### Dipping/Immersion Technique

- Select disinfectant with short exposure time to minimize distortion and deterioration of surface quality of resulting stone cast.
- Follow same procedures as above except fully immerse or dip impression in disinfectant for recommended exposure time.

## DENTAL CASTS

- Very difficult to disinfect.
- Is preferable to disinfect impression.
- If casts must be disinfected:
  - Place casts on end to facilitate drainage.
  - Spray with iodophor or chlorine product, then rinse.
- Another option
  - Soak casts for 30 minutes in 0.5% concentration of sodium hypochlorite and saturated calcium dihydrate solution (SDS).
  - SDS is produced by placing uncontaminated, set gypsum (i.e. stone) in a container of water.

## ORALLY SOILED PROSTHESES

- Scrub with brush and antimicrobial soap to remove debris and contamination.
  - Can be accomplished in operatory or professional work area.
  - Sterilize brush or store in approved disinfectant.
- Place prosthesis in sealable plastic bag or beaker filled with ultrasonic cleaning solution or calculus remover.
- Place in ultrasonic cleaner for required time as specified by manufacturer of ultrasonic cleaner.
- Place cover on ultrasonic cleaner to reduce spatter potential.
- Remove and rinse under running tap water, dry, and accomplish required work.

## SUB-SURFACE DISINFECTION

- Place prosthesis in sealable plastic bag containing 1:10 dilution of sodium hypochlorite or other intermediate to high-level disinfectant (not glutaraldeyde or phenols).
- Place in ultrasonic cleaner for 10 minutes.

## DENTAL PROSTHESES

- Do not exceed manufacturer's recommended contact time on metal components to minimize corrosion.
  - There is little effect on chrome-cobalt alloy with short-term exposures (10 minutes).
- Do not store in disinfectant before insertion.
- Store in diluted mouthwash until insertion.

## LATHE

- Ways to reduce risk of injury from aerosols, spatter, and macroscopic particles.
  - Use protective eyewear.
  - Ensure plexiglass shield is in position.
  - Activate vacuum.
- Pumice has been shown to pose a potential contamination risk.
  - Via aerosol or direct contact.
- Mix pumice with
  - Clean water, diluted 1:10 bleach, or other appropriate disinfectant.
  - Add tincture of green soap if desired.
- Change pumice daily.
- Machine should be cleaned and disinfected daily.
- No need for separate pans for new and existing prostheses if isolated properly.
- At a minimum clean and disinfect pumice brushes and rag wheels daily. Daily heat sterilization is preferable.

## STERILIZATION

- Heat sterilize all metal and heat-stable instruments that contact oral tissues, contaminated appliances, or potentially contaminated appliances should be heat sterilized after each use.
  - Examples: facebow fork, metal impression trays, burs, polishing points, rag wheels, laboratory knives.

### Impression Trays

- Precleaning removes bioburden and any adherent impression material.
- Ultrasonic cleaning can aid in removing residual set gypsum.
- Chrome-plated or aluminum trays.
  - Clean, package, heat sterilize.
- Single-use trays.
  - Discard after one use.
- Custom acrylic trays.
  - Can be disinfected (by spray or immersion), then rinsed (if to be used for second appointment).

## DISINFECTION

- Prosthodontic items contaminated by handling should be disinfected (by spray or immersion technique based on type of item) after each use.
  - Examples: alcohol torch, facebow, articulator, mixing spatula, mixing bowl, lab knife, shade/mold guide.

### Wax Bites/Rims, Bite Registrations

- Immersion disinfection may cause distortion to some items.
  - Use spray disinfection.
- Heavy-body bite registration materials.
  - Usually not susceptible to distortion and can be disinfected in same manner as an impression of the same material.

## LAB EQUIPMENT

- Follow manufacturer instructions for:
  - Maintenance
  - Cleaning
  - Disinfection
  - Compatibility with disinfectants.

## PERSONAL HYGIENE

- Refrain from the following activities while in the lab where there is potential for occupational exposure:
  - Eating
  - Drinking
  - Smoking
  - Applying cosmetics or lip balm
  - Handling contact lenses.

# CHAPTER 7: Dental Casts and Models

Dental casts and models serve as a main bulk in the prosthodontic procedures as they act as a patient's mouth in their absence. Hence, it is must to know about them in detail. This chapter outlines the definitions, parts of casts, models along with its grading criteria.

## CAST

- A life-size likeness of some desired form. It is formed within or is a material poured into a matrix or impression of the desired form.

## DENTAL CAST

- A positive life size reproduction of a part or parts of the oral cavity.
- They are of varied types, i.e. preliminary cast, final cast, refractory cast and remount cast, etc.

## DENTAL MODEL

- A positive full-scale replica of teeth, soft tissues and restored structures.
- They are also referred to as study casts.
- Because these models show a three-dimensional view of conditions, they prove to be a valuable diagnostic tool.
- Dentist can use these models to study the patient's mouth from angles impossible during the clinical examination.

### Parts of a Model/Cast

- A model consists of two parts:
  1. **Anatomic portion:** It is that portion of the cast/model which represents the respective parts of the oral cavity and is created from the impression.
  2. **Art portion:**
     - It is that portion of the cast/model which forms the base of the cast/model.
     - It has three surfaces, i.e. top, back and heel.
- The ratio of anatomic to the art portion is 3 : 1 (Fig. 1.7.1).

### Pouring Methods

- Three different methods are employed to create the cast or model.
  1. **Double-pour method:** Here, the anatomic portion of the cast is poured first, then a second

# Dental Casts and Models

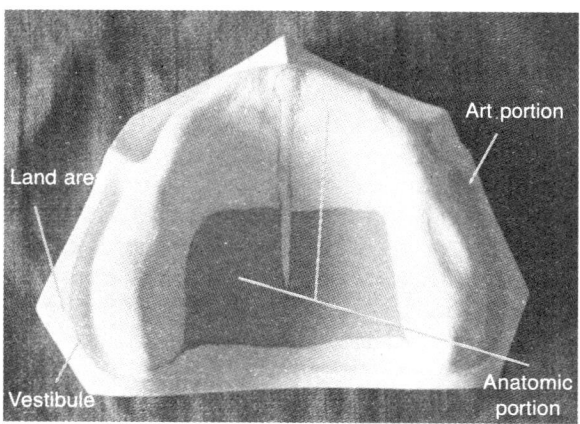

Fig. 1.7.1

mix of plaster or dental stone is used to prepare the art portion. A free-form base can be created by hand or by the use of a rubber mold.

2. **Box and pour method:** Here, the impression is surrounded with a 'box' made of boxing wax. (Details are given in Section-II, Chapter 4).
3. **Inverted-pour method:** This method employs mixing one large mixture of plaster or stone and pouring both portion of the model in a single step.

## Uses

1. Diagnostic purpose.
2. Visual presentation of dental treatment
3. To prepare custom trays, denture bases, etc.
4. To prepare orthodontic appliances.
5. To prepare provisional restorations and mouth guards, etc.

## PRELIMINARY CAST

### Synonyms

1. Primary cast
2. Diagnostic cast
3. Preoperative cast
4. Study cast

### Definition

- A cast formed from a preliminary impression for use in diagnosis or the fabrication of an impression tray (GPT-8)

### Rationale and Objectives

1. For the purpose of study, treatment planning
2. Fabrication of final impression trays

### Equipment and Materials

1. Plaster spatula, vacuum mixer bowl.
2. Buffalo knife.
3. Yellow stone
4. Wax spatulas
5. Vibrator
6. Plastic vacuform sheet on which to pour stone bases for the casts
7. Model trimmer

### CRITERIA FOR GRADING

- Preliminary casts and final impression trays for complete dentures must be evaluated prior to bringing the patient to the clinic for visit 2. Although the preliminary cast and final impression trays are separate steps, we recommended you to show the preliminary cast and final impression tray to one of the faculty at the same time to use your time most efficiently. These are the grading criteria for preliminary casts.

- *Grade A:* Casts are neat, clean, free of voids and/or defects, have sharp detail. Tongue area of mandibular cast trimmed flat and smooth. Casts reflect entire basal support area. The cast base is approximately 10–15 mm thick in thinnest area and is trimmed approximately parallel to the ridge. No impingement of impression tray evident. Cast is labeled with patient name and date. Cast is smoothly trimmed with at least 2–3 mm of vestibule present lateral to the deepest part of the vestibule labially and buccally. Cast edges are beveled and smooth. Land area of the cast is trimmed so no undercut is present. The sides of the cast and the edentulous ridges should be parallel and perpendicular to the base.

- *Grade B:* Minor discrepancies from the above which do not compromise the quality of the clinical treatment. Casts reflect correct extension, but minor, non-critical defects in areas of stone not covered by tray are present. Casts slightly thinner or thicker than ideal. Cast is not smoothly trimmed. Cast is not labeled.

- *Grade C:* Cast extension adequate to make a clinically acceptable tray but marginally so. Full vestibular depth missing in isolated areas. Cheek slightly captured in distobuccal areas of mandibular cast. Tissue surface of cast somewhat unclear and slightly scarred. Land area slightly interferes with correct tray construction. Blockout wax remains on cast. Stone debris left on cast. Cast is not clean and neatly trimmed.

- *Grade E:* Cast prevents construction of clinically acceptable impression tray. Border extension inadequate for correct tray construction. Land areas poorly defined, missing, or so high they prevent proper tray construction. Tongue space not trimmed neatly and/or prevents access to lingual borders. Cast base excessively thick or thin (less than 5 mm or greater than 20 mm).

## SECONDARY CAST

### Synonyms
1. Final cast
2. Master cast
3. Definitive cast.

### Definition
- A replica of the tooth surfaces, residual ridge areas, and/or other parts of the dental arch and/or facial structures used to fabricate a dental restoration or prosthesis (GPT-8).

### Rationale and Objectives
1. Fabrication of denture base.

### Equipment and Materials
1. Plaster spatula, vacuum mixer bowl
2. Buffalo knife.
3. Yellow stone
4. Wax spatulas
5. Vibrator
6. Plastic vacuform sheet on which to pour stone bases for the casts
7. Model trimmer.

### Criteria for Grading
- Master casts and record bases and occlusion rims for complete dentures must be graded through one of the faculty prior to bringing the patient to the clinic for visit 3. Although the master cast and record bases and occlusion rims have separate criteria for grading, we recommend you show them both to one of your faculty at the same time to use your time most efficiently. Step 4, Posterior palatal seal is evaluated after visit 3. These are the grading criteria for the master casts.
- *Grade A:* Base of cast parallel to ridges (mean foundation plane). Cast is 11–13 mm thick in the thinnest areas. Land areas clearly present, are contoured to follow depth of vestibules, beveled at a 30–45 degree angle, and are no more than 2 mm above the depth of the vestibules. Land areas are 3–4 mm wide. Land is 4–6 mm wide on the posterior border of the mandibular cast. Vestibules present and 1–3 mm deep. All areas of denture support present in cast with no obvious over or under extensions. Repositioning indexes present and approximately 10 mm wide and 3–5 mm deep. Tongue area flat and smooth and no more than 3 mm above depth of vestibules. Casts neat and clean with no voids or blebs and non-tissue surfaces smoothed.
- *Grade B:* Minor discrepancies from Grade A which will not compromise the quality of the denture.
- *Grade C:* Master cast is adequate to make a clinically acceptable complete denture, but marginally so. Cast thickness beyond criteria above, less than 11 mm thick. Land areas not smooth, does not follow vestibule, and/or has insufficient width. Vestibule present, but insufficient depth causes a future loss of contour to denture flange. Repositioning indices present, but too deep or shallow. Cast not neat, smooth, and clean. Wax remains in undercuts on cast.
- *Grade E:* Master cast prevents clinically acceptable complete denture treatment. Master cast is broken and/or glued in place

### KEYING THE MASTER CASTS
- Objective: To groove the master casts so that they can be returned to the articulator in the same position after processing or any time. With a sharp plaster knife or a Fast-Cut wheel, make four "V-shaped" cuts as shown in the sketch. The cuts are about 3 mm deep and 5 mm wide.
- Before mounting the casts, soak them in tap water for a few minutes and lubricate the grooves with vaseline. 'This will facilitate separating the casts from the mounngs and will also preserve the grooves so remounts are more accurate (Fig. 1.7.2).

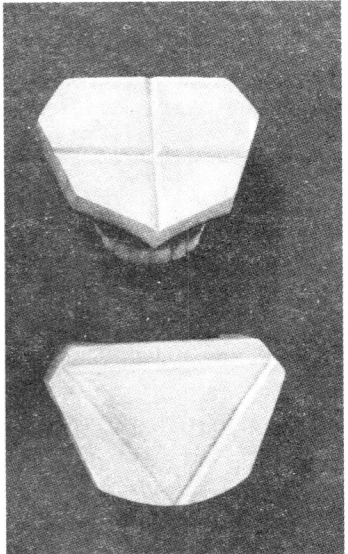

Fig. 1.7.2

- **Note:** 'This is a keying method and not the splint-cast technique as used in occlusion. The long grooves are needed in case the laboratory technician must trim the casts for flasking.

# Section 2
# Complete Dentures

# Introduction

**CHAPTER 1**

## DEFINITION

**Complete Denture:** A removable dental prosthesis that replaces the entire dentition and associated structures of the maxillae or mandible; called a complete removable dental prosthesis.

## SURFACES/PARTS

- A complete denture replaces lost teeth and alveolar bone.
- *From the point of view of function,* however, a complete denture has three surfaces, **occlusal, polished and fitting** – the buccal and lingual surfaces of the teeth being part of the polished surface (Fig. 2.1.1).
- Each of these surfaces has a different function and each surface must be shaped accordingly.
- The occlusal surface is that part which carries out the function of mastication and is designed to operate in contact with the opposing occlusal surface. For foods that are relatively easily crushed,

A *complete denture* (CD) is a type of removable prosthesis designed to replace all of the natural teeth in an arch and associated structures of the maxilla or mandible. However, a CD denture does not usually replace third molars. The CD consists of an acrylic base and porcelain or acrylic artificial teeth. The base is designed to fit over the alveolar ridge, and is composed of the saddle and gingival area. Sometimes, patients need a set of CDs; one for each arch. If a CD is constructed for insertion immediately following the surgical removal of all remaining teeth, it is considered an *immediate complete denture*. Before a conventional prosthesis is fabricated, the extraction sites must be completely healed. Therefore, immediate dentures are often considered temporary or interim prostheses. The immediate denture also functions as a psychological aid to the patient, who will never have to be completely without teeth. Immediate dentures usually require relines 3 to 12 months after initial insertion. This is because of the dramatic reduction in the ridge size during the healing process. This section describes about the steps involved in the fabrication of complete denture along with its relining, rebasing and repair.

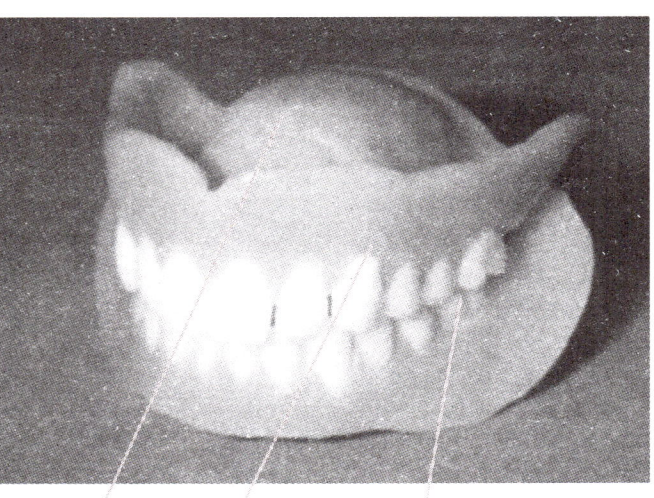

Fitting    Polished    Occlusal surfaces

**Fig. 2.1.1:** Surfaces/parts of complete denture

the degree of comminution of food particles will be proportional to the area of the contacting occlusal surfaces. This surface also has a role to play in stabilising the dentures, and is shaped to promote occlusal balance. Where balance has not been achieved, occlusal interferences can occur. These may be in the intercuspal position or in lateral excursions, and are a common source of lower denture insecurity. To ensure occlusal balance, it is common to carry out a check record which will remove the discrepancies which occur as a result of errors during the recording of the jaw relations and the processing of the denture.
- The polished surface primarily subserves the function of appearance. It consists of the buccal, labial and lingual surfaces of the teeth and the buccal and lingual surfaces of the base. It is designed to achieve good appearance, but must also have a shape which facilitates smooth functioning of the muscles in contact with it. To ensure good appearance and minimal friction with the surrounding tissues it is highly polished. Generally, the polished surfaces are designed to present an overall concave surface to the surrounding musculature in order to enhance stability, but may deviate from this ideal if the demand for the teeth to remain in the neutral zone warrants it.
- The fitting surface is that part in contact with the supporting denture bearing area and is recorded during the stages of primary and working impressions. The denture is designed to conform to the anatomy of the alveolar ridges sufficiently well to permit the force of 'retention' to operate.

## COMPONENTS (Fig. 2.1.2)

1. Denture base
2. Flange
3. Artificial Teeth

## INDICATIONS

1. Extensive bone loss and periodontal disease.
2. Lack of motivation or ability to maintain teeth.
3. Gross decay or abscesses.
4. Edentulous patient.
5. Patient refused partial dentures.
6. Lack of financial resources for alternative treatments.
7. The patient is edentulous.
8. The remaining teeth cannot be saved.
9. The remaining teeth cannot support a removable partial denture, and no acceptable alternatives are available.

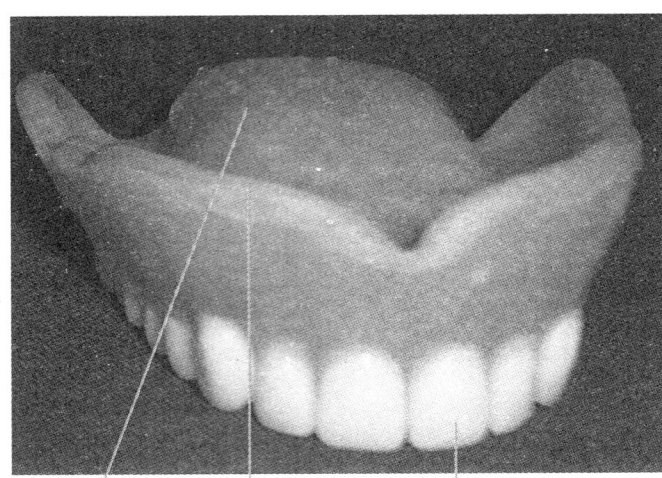

**Fig. 2.1.2:** Components of complete denture

10. The patient refuses alternative treatment recommendations.

## CONTRAINDICATIONS

1. Another acceptable alternative is available.
2. Physical or mental illness affects the patient's ability to cooperate during the fabrication of the denture and to accept or wear the denture.
3. The patient is hypersensitive to denture materials.
4. The patient is not interested in replacing missing teeth.

## ADVANTAGES

Dentures can help patients in a number of ways:

1. **Mastication:** Chewing ability is improved by replacing edentulous areas with denture teeth.
2. **Aesthetics:** The presence of teeth provides a natural facial appearance, and wearing a denture to replace missing teeth provides support for the lips and cheeks and corrects the collapsed appearance that occurs after losing teeth.
3. **Phonetics:** By replacing missing teeth, especially the anteriors, patients are better able to speak by improving pronunciation of those words containing sibilants or fricatives.

## DISADVANTAGES

1. Excess salivation
2. Gagging
3. Retention.

# Fabrication of Complete Denture: An Overview

**CHAPTER 2**

Fabrication of a CD involves one to six appointments. Each appointment will be linked with a corresponding laboratory work (most of the times).

It starts with a complete oral and systemic examination of the patient and ends with the insertion of new denture and its subsequent examination.

The following table provides you synopsis about the steps involved in the CD fabrication.

This chapter gives an overlook about the fabrication of complete denture in a nutshell. This helps the students in better understanding of the steps involved in the fabrication

| CLINICAL SESSIONS | LABORATORY SESSIONS |
|---|---|
| **SESSION I: Preliminary Impressions** ||
| Preliminary impressions are made using plastic dentate stock trays and irreversible hydrocolloid (alginate) impression material. The stock trays are modified with utility rope wax to simulate edentulous stock impression trays.<br>1. Impressions are made with irreversible hydrocolloid impression material. Ideally, there should be fullness to the borders of the impression, no voids present in the impression, no exposure of the impression tray through the impression. | 1. Pour preliminary casts.<br>2. Fabrication of custom impression trays |
| **SESSION II: Final Impressions** ||
| 1. Evaluate/adjust custom trays.<br>2. Border mold custom trays.<br>3. Once the tray has been border molded, the final impression is made with a low viscosity impression material – either low viscosity VPS or low viscosity polysulfide impression material. | 1. Developing master casts<br>2. Construction of stabilized, hard record bases and occlusal rims |
| **SESSION III: Maxillomandibular relations** ||
| The student will use stabilized record bases with baseplate wax occlusion rims. The sequencing of procedures for MMR that is taught in the pre-clinical course is as follows:<br>1. Contour the maxillary occlusion rim for proper lip and cheek support.<br>2. Adjust the mandibular occlusion rim to the VDO.<br>3. Register centric relation<br>4. Take face bow transfer.<br>5. Select teeth. | 1. Mounting of master casts on a semi-adjustable articulator using the face bow transfer and CR registration<br>2. Arrangement of teeth |
| **SESSION IV: Clinical try-in of the trial dentures** ||
| The student and the instructor should perform verification of the esthetics, the phonetics, the vertical dimension of occlusion and the centric relation occlusion. Any minor discrepancies in the orientation of the teeth should be corrected during this session.<br>1. Check CR.<br>2. Check VDO.<br>3. Adjust posterior guidance of articulator / re-evaluate occlusion.<br>4. Carve posterior palatal seal. | 1. Sealing of the trial dentures<br>2. Investing<br>3. Processing<br>4. Equilibration<br>5. Polishing. |
| **SESSION V: Denture Insertion** ||
| Delivery of the complete dentures should involve the following steps:<br>1. Check for areas of overextension and over compression<br>2. Evaluate the labial, buccal and lingual notches to ensure no impingement of the frena.<br>3. Perform a clinical remount.<br>4. Give home-care instructions.<br>5. Confirm time of the first post-insertion appointment on the following day. The student should have scheduled a 24-hour post-insertion appointment at the same time the delivery appointment was scheduled. This post-insertion appointment should be followed by a second post-insertion appointment, scheduled within one week from the delivery appointment. | — |

# Examination, Diagnosis and Treatment Planning

**CHAPTER 3**

The aim of the assessment is to collect, record and evaluate information about the patient. To avoid errors the information is written down in standard format. First the patient's personal details are entered, followed by the complaint, the history of the complaint, the medical history, the dental history, and then the findings resulting from the clinical examination. Subsequently a provisional diagnosis is made and then, following any special tests (usually radiographs) required to resolve doubt, a definitive diagnosis is made and a treatment plan drawn up. The assessment procedure for edentulous patients conforms broadly to that for dentate patients but with differences of emphasis in three major respects: 1. The likely complaints about dentures are limited to pain, looseness, functional disorders, nausea, fracture and poor appearance. 2. An extra area in the mouth must be inspected viz. the denture itself. 3. The average patient is elderly and more likely to have problems of health, mobility and communication.

## INITIAL APPOINTMENT

- Get to know your patient
- Personally, experiences, expectations
- Past medical history
- Past dental history
- Oral examination
- Treatment plan
- Financial agreement—cost / risk / benefit.

## RECORDS

*Very important*
- medical history
- dental history

*Helps determine*
- diagnosis
- prognosis
- fee.

## OBSERVATIONS AFFECTING DIAGNOSIS

### Age

- **Young:** More adaptable, esthetics very important, good health, high tolerance levels.
- **Middle:** Be more aware of psychological and physiological changes.
- **Advanced:** Less tolerant of change, reduced coordination, communication may be more difficult, soft and hard tissue changes, drug regimen.

### Gender

- **Female:** May be more demanding than males.
- **Males:** Indifferent towards appearance and place more emphasis on comfort and function.

### General Health

- May or may not correlate with patients age.
- Observe patients posture and entrance into clinics.
- Communication/listening.

- Friendly questioning usually stimulates patient to readily volunteer information.
- Consultation with physician.

Medical History

- Medical condition.
- Diabetic, psychological state, hypertension, heart problems, allergies, chronic diseases.
- Medications.
- Anti-depressants, anti-anxiety, anti inflammatory, diuretics, antihypertensive, vasodilator.

Extraoral Examination

- View overall facial appearance
- Lip support
- Lip thickness
- Lip length
- Lip fullness
- Facial profile and tone
- Vertical face length

## LIP SUPPORT

- If tissues around the mouth are wrinkled and the rest of the face is not, improvement may be made to decrease the wrinkles.
- If the lips appear collapsed the anterior teeth may be set to far lingually.

## LIP THICKNESS

- Thin lips will not tolerate much change in labio lingual tooth position.
- Any slight change will make changes in the appearance of the lip.
- Thick lips will give the dentist more leeway in tooth position and arch form before changes are noted.

## LIP LENGTH

- Short upper lip will expose all of the maxillary teeth and labial flange of the denture base.
- Pay special attention to tooth size, shape and shade along with the denture base shade.

## LIP FULLNESS

- Directly related to the support it gets from the teeth and mucosa/denture base.
- Do not confuse this with lip thickness which involves the intrinsic structures of the lip.

## FACIAL PROFILE AND CONTOUR

- Gives an indication of the relative jaw size and vertical jaw relations.

- Convex profile maxilla is larger than the mandible. (occlusion that is characteristic of a Class II).
- Concave profile maxilla is smaller than the mandible (occlusion that is characteristic of a Class III).

## TONE OF FACIAL TISSUES

- Age and health affect intrinsic structures of facial tissues.
- Poor tone indicates limitations on what can be done (we are not plastic surgeons).
- Facial tissues can only be supported to their original position.

## VERTICAL FACE LENGTH

- Directly related to the vertical height of the dentures.
- Decreased vertical dimension—lower facial height will not be adequate, difficult to function, soft tissue problems.
- Increased vertical dimension—lower facial height will be extensive, difficult to function, soft tissue problems.

ORAL EXAMINATION

## ELECTRONIC

- MRI, radiographic (CAT, imaging).

## VISUAL

- Eyes, magnification, photography.

## PALPATORY

- Sense of structure (not radiopaque).

## RADIOGRAPHIC EXAMINATION

- Should always be done prior to Tx.

INTRAORAL EXAMINATION

- Pathoses
- Maxillary and mandibular arches
- Oral tissues
- Saliva.

EXAM FORM

- Previous denture experience
- Oral exam
- Radiographic
- Esthetics
- Prognosis
- Fee estimate.

## PREVIOUS DENTURE EXPERIENCE

- Length of time patient has been edentulous?
- How old are current dentures?
- What is the patient's chief complaint?
- This will help you determine if you can help the patient, how successful you will be, and your fee for the service.
- Evaluation
- Esthetics
- Vertical dimension
- Mandibular tissue coverage
- Maxillary tissue coverage
- Retention
- Stability.

## INTRAORAL EXAMINATION

- Oral tissues.
- Mucosa, tongue, soft/hard palate, cheeks, floor of mouth, throat.
- Abrasion, ulcerations, tori, cuts, malignancies, hyperplasia, epulis fissuratum, papillary hyperplasia, lichen planus, leukoplakia.
- Mucosal health is determined by its color, pink.
- Must be healthy prior to impressioning procedures.
- Uniform layer of soft tissue over bone which is firm but resilient.
- Well defined tuberosities and hamular notches, low frenum attachments.
- Broad U-shaped arches are ideal.
- Ideal palatal vault form is of medium depth with well defined rugae.
- Normal tongue size.
- Saliva of moderate flow and serous content is ideal.
- Ideal muscle tone and coordination.
- Free flowing jaw movements.
- Lack of pathological TMJ dysfunction.
- Lack of severe gag reflex.

## TREATMENT PLANNING

- After obtaining all information pertaining to your initial examination, a treatment plan is devised.
- Is treatment indicated considering the patients present medical and/or psychological health?
- Will treatment improve or maintain health?
- Do you as the dentist feel comfortable with the patient and the proposed treatment?
- Discuss with the patient the length of time to complete the procedures and any unforeseen difficulties that may arise.
- Also cost of treatment and **expected outcome.**

# 4 Impression Making

Impressions are a three-dimensional record of patient's dentition and anatomy of the alveolar process. Almost all prosthodontic treatment requires preliminary impressions be taken so that a dental cast can be made and used by the dentist as a diagnostic tool and to fabricate various prosthodontic appliances

## IMPRESSION

### DEFINITION

"An impression is defined as an imprint or negative likeness of the teeth, of the edentulous areas where the teeth have been removed or of both, made in a plastic material that becomes relatively hard or set while in contact with these tissues. Impressions may be made of full complements of teeth of areas where some teeth have been removed or in mouths from which all teeth have been removed"—GPT.

"A complete denture impression is a negative registration of the entire denture bearing, stabilizing and border seal areas present in the edentulous mouth"—GPT.

### RATIONALE/OBJECTIVES

The five primary objectives of complete denture impression as stated by Carl . O. Boucher in 1944 are:
1. Preservation of remaining alveolar ridges
2. Support
3. Stability
4. Retention
5. Esthetics.

### Preservation of Remaining Alveolar Ridges

M. M. Devan stated that "it is more important to preserve what already exists than to replace what is missing". So, this rule is followed in impression making to minimize the soft tissue abuse and bone resorption by:
a. Covering as much of the supporting areas as possible.
b. Using pressure within the physiologic limits of the tissue.

### SUPPORT

Denture support is the resistance to vertical forces of mastication and to occlusal or other forces applied in

a direction toward the basal seat. It is provided by the maxillary and mandibular bones and their covering of mucosal tissue.
- The areas of denture support are divided into primary, secondary and slight.
- Primary supporting areas of edentulous ridge.
  a. Maxillary      – Posterior ridges
                    – Flat areas of the palate
  b. Mandibular     – Buccal shelf
                    – Posterior ridges
                    – Pear shaped pad
- Secondary supporting areas of edentulous ridge:
  a. Maxillary      – Anterior ridge
                    – All ridge slopes
  b. Mandibular     – Anterior ridge
                    – All ridge slopes
- Slight supporting areas of edentulous ridge: All the vestibular areas.
- It is necessary to enhance the available support by utilizing maximum coverage of all usable ridge-bearing areas. This must be accomplished without interference of routine movements or normal functions of the stomatognathic system. Maximum coverage provides the "snowshoe" effect, which distributes applied forces over as wide an area as possible (Fig. 2.4.1).

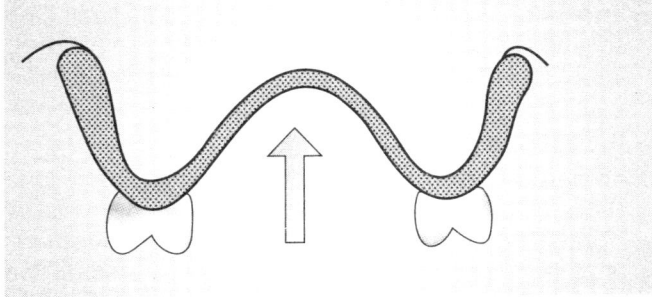

Fig. 2.4.1

### Stability

- Denture stability is the resistance of a denture to movement on its tissue foundation, especially to lateral (horizontal) forces as opposed to vertical displacement (Fig. 2.4.2).

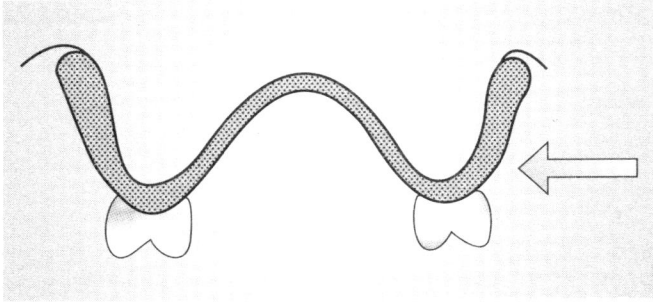

Fig. 2.4.2

- These lateral (horizontal) forces are caused during functions of chewing, talking, singing, whistling, kissing, etc.
- The requirements for a denture to be stable are:
  a. good retention.
  b. non interfering occlusion.
  c. proper tooth arrangement.
  d. proper form and contour of the polished surfaces.
  e. proper orientation of occlusal plane.
  f. good control and co-ordination of patients musculature.
- Boucher stated that stability required the maximum use of all bony foundations where the tissues are firmly and closely attached to the bone.
- Samuel Friedman in 1957 stated that stability is developed in the impression technique through more intimate contact of labial and buccal flanges with the labial and buccal slopes of the ridges.

### Retention

- Denture retention is the resistance in the movement of a denture away from its tissue foundation especially in a vertical direction. In other words, retention of a denture is its resistance to removal in a direction opposite to that of its insertion (Fig. 2.4.3).

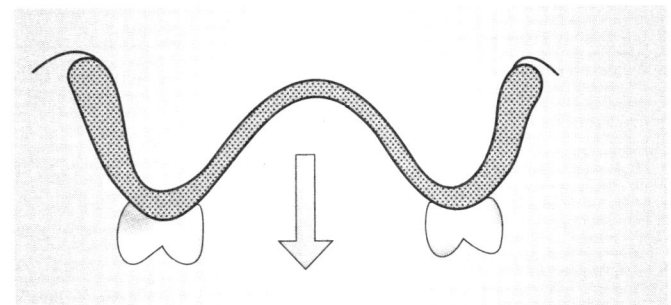

Fig. 2.4.3

- The factors responsible for denture retention are
  a. Adhesion
  b. Cohesion
  c. Interfacial surface tension
  d. Mechanical locking into undercuts
  e. Peripheral seal
  f. Atmospheric pressure
  g. Oral and facial musculature
    a. **Adhesion** is the physical attraction of unlike molecules. It acts when saliva sticks to the denture base and to the mucous membrane of the basal seat. The quality of the adhesion

depends on the close adaptation of the denture, the size of the denture bearing area and the type of saliva. The most adhesive saliva is thin but contains some mucous components. In patients suffering from xerostomia, an artificial saliva such as orex can be given to aid in providing adhesion and thereby retention of denture.

b. Cohesion is the physical attraction between like molecules. In order to be effective, the salivary layer should be thin. It is the attraction of molecules of saliva to each other.

c. Surface tension is the property of liquids in which the exposed surface tends to contract to the smallest possible area, as in the spherical formation of drops, this is a phenomenon attributed to attractive forces or cohesion, between the molecules of the liquid.

d. Mechanical locking into undercuts must be handled correctly because its use can result in abraded and sore areas. Mechanical locking can be an asset only if proper internal relief is done with the use of a disclosing paste and a suitable path of insertion and removal is employed, which is demonstrated and taught to the patient.

e. Peripheral seal is positive contact of the entire perimeter of the denture base to the resilient tissues that outline the basal seat. This includes the posterior palatal seal as well as all labial, buccal and lingual vestibules. Peripheral seal increases retention.

f. Atmospheric pressure resists any dislodging forces of the denture. Atmospheric pressure is provided by the weight of the atmosphere (14.7 lb/sq inch) and the retentive force is directly proportional to the area covered by the denture base. Synder et al have shown that a reduction in atmospheric pressure concomitantly reduces the amount of retention.

g. Oral and facial musculature can significantly contribute to retention but only if the polished surfaces of the denture are correctly shaped and the teeth are correctly positioned.

Relation between stability, support and retention (Fig. 2.4.4)

## Esthetics

- Esthetics in impression making refers to the development of labial and buccal borders so that

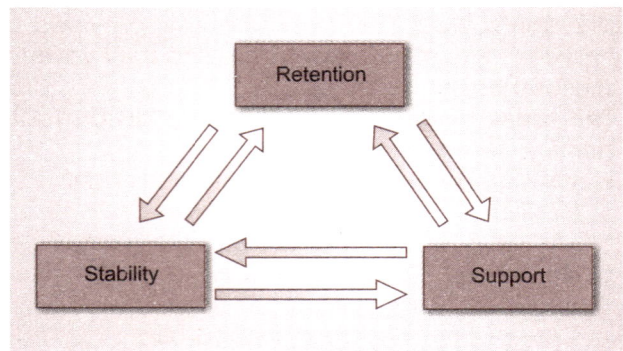

**Fig. 2.4.4:** Relation between stability, support and retention

they are not only retentive but also support the lips and cheeks properly. Border thickness should be varied with the needs of each patient in accordance with the extent of residual ridge loss.

## REQUIREMENTS

Basic requirements of impression making are:

a. Knowledge of oral anatomy: The dentist must know all the anatomical landmarks associated with the making of impressions and must also know how these landmarks function and how they relate to various parts of the impression.

b. Knowledge of basic and reliable technique: One should have thorough knowledge of accepted impression techniques and also should be familiar with alternative techniques when unusual conditions are present.

c. Knowledge and understanding of materials: One should have thorough knowledge of each and every dental material used for the fabrication of dentures. Abuse of materials can seriously affect the characteristics of the materials and can lead to potential problems or failures.

d. Skill: Impression making is a skill which should be mastered by being in constant touch with the subject and applying them in practice.

e. Patient management: It is impossible to make acceptable impressions if the patient is not cooperative. So, patient education and firm management are more important in making of acceptable impressions.

## TYPES

a. Based on the purpose of the impression:
  - Diagnostic impression.
  - Primary impression.
  - Secondary impression.
b. Based on the theories of impression making:
  - Mucostatic or passive impression.

- Mucocompressive or functional impression.
- Selective pressure impression.

c. Based on the position of mouth while making the impression:
   - Open mouth impression.
   - Closed mouth impression.

d. Based on the type of tray used for making the impression:
   - Stock tray impression.
   - Custom tray impression (special tray).

e. Based on method of manipulation for border molding:
   - Hand manipulation.
   - Functional movements.

## Materials used

*Classification of Dental Impression Materials (Table 2.4.1)*

| Table 2.4.1: By application of mechanical properties | | |
|---|---|---|
| By setting mechanism | Rigid/Inelastic (edentulous ridge) | Elastic (tooth form) |
| Chemical reaction (irreversible) | Impression plaster Zinc oxide-eugenol | Alginate hydrocolloid polysulfides Condensation silicones Addition silicones Polyethers |
| Temperature changes (Reversible) | Impression compound Impression wax | Agar hydrocolloid |

## IMPRESSION PLASTER

*Advantages*

- Accurate reproduction of tissue details.
- Tissue distortion will be minimum.
- Easy manipulation.
- Quick flow of material.

*Disadvantages*

- Plaster impressions may break because of brittleness during removal from oral cavity.
- Untidy to handle.
- Cannot be removed from undercuts.
- Saliva washes the material and distorts the surface when mandibular impression is made.

## ZINC OXIDE EUGENAL IMPRESSION PASTE

*Advantages*

- Do not displace soft tissues because of low viscosity.
- Records surface details accurately.
- Material is not washed out by saliva while making madibular impressions.
- Ease of beading and boxing.

*Disadvantages*

- It does not absorb secretions from palate, hence secretions are profuse.
- It is difficult to control at border and may distort on removing from undercuts.
- It is bitter in taste and has objectionable odour.
- It adheres to skin.

## Impression Compound

*Advantages*

- Impression surface is correctable.
- It can be re-used in the same patient.
- Impression can be reinserted in the mouth for evaluation of fit.
- It can be beaded and boxed for fabrication of casts.

*Disadvantages*

- Over heating results in brittle and grainy impression surface.
- It compresses the tissues while impression making.

## Alginate

*Advantages*

- Accurate reproduction of undercuts. So, mostly used for dentulous impressions.
- Easy to manipulate.
- Relatively inexpensive when compared to elastomeric impression materials.
- It causes little discomfort to the patient.

*Disadvantages*

- Surface details not accurately recorded when compared to elastomeric impression materials.
- Distortion takes place due to syneresis and imbibition.

## Agar

*Advantages*

- Most accurately records surface details.
- Accurate reproduction of undercuts.
- When agar impression material is handled correctly, the dies from different impressions are interchangable.

*Disadvantages*

- Equipment is quite expensive.
- Manipulation is quite difficult.
- Distortion takes place during gelation.

**Polysulfides**

*Advantages*

- High tear resistance.
- Long working time.
- Long shelf life.
- Less hydrophobic.

*Disadvantages*

- Odour offends patients.
- Messy and stains clothes.
- Potential for significant distortion.
- Second pour is less accurate.

**CONDENSATION SILICONES**

*Advantages*

- Better elastic properties on removal.
- Less distortion on removal.
- Adequate tear strength.
- Pleasant odour and no staining.
- Adequate tear strength.

*Disadvantages*

- Poor dimensional stability.
- Potential for significant distortion.
- Poor to adequate shelf life.

**Addition Silicones**

*Advantages*

- Extremely high accuracy.
- Shorter setting time.
- Dimensionally stable even after 1 week.
- Less distortion on removal.
- Easy to mix.

*Disadvantages*

- Hydrogen gas evolution.
- More expensive, especially with automatic mixing device.

**Polyethers**

*Advantages*

- Adequate tear strength.
- Less distortion on removal.
- Fast working and setting times.
- Long shelf life.
- Good dimensional stability.

*Disadvantages*

- Stiffness requires blocking undercuts.
- Bad taste.
- Slightly more expensive.

**PRINCIPLES OF IMPRESSION MAKING**

1. The tissues of the mouth must be healthy.
2. The impression should extend to include all of the basal seat within the limits of the functions of the supporting and limiting tissues.
3. The border must be in harmony with the anatomical and physiological limitations of the oral structures.
4. A physiological type of border molding procedure should be performed by the dentist or by the patient under the guidance of the dentist.
5. Proper space for the selected impression material should be provided within the impression tray.
6. The impression must be removed from the mouth without damage to the mucous membrane of the residual ridges.
7. A guiding mechanism should be provided for correct positioning of the impression tray in the mouth tray.
8. The tray and the impression material should be made of dimensionally stable materials.
9. The external shape of the impression must be similar to the external form of the complete denture.

**THEORIES OF IMPRESSION MAKING**

- The impression procedures are based on the amount of pressure used to record the impression. Thus various theories evolved during late 19th century and early 20th century based on the pressure applied during impression making.

**A. DEFINITE PRESSURE/MUCOCOMPRESSIVE THEORY**

- It was put forth by Greene brothers.
- According to this theory the tissues of oral cavity are recorded in their functional positions and not in their rest positions. They thought that tissues recorded under functional pressure like mastication provides better support and retention for the denture.

Materials used
- Impression compound.
- Wax and soft liners.

Techniques
- A preliminary impression with impression compound is made.
- A special tray is constructed with its periphery 1/8th inch shorter than denture outline.
- A second impression is made with special tray using impression compound again.

- Bite rims with uniform occlusal surfaces are made.
- Relief areas of impression like median palatal raphe are softened and impression is again inserted in the mouth and held under biting pressure for one to two minutes.
- Border moulding is done by asking the patient to do various cheek and lip movements as in whistling and smiling.
- Posterior palatal seal is obtained by the swallowing movements of the patient, under biting pressure.

Advantages
- Better support and retention during functional movements like mastication.

Disadvantages
- Dentures function well during mastication but will rebound when the tissues come back to their resting state.
- Excess pressure on peripheral tissues results in transient ischaemia and tissue breakdown.
- Excess pressure over alveolar ridges leads to increased bone resorption resulting in loose fitting dentures.

### B. NON PRESSURE / MINIMAL PRESSURE / MUCOSTATIC THEORY

- It was first proposed by Richardson and later popularized by Henry Page in 1946.
- According to this theory, interfacial surface tension was the only way of retaining complete dentures and impression should cover only those areas of denture foundation where the mucosa is firmly attached.
- In this technique the tissues of oral cavity are recorded in their resting position and border moulding is not done.

Materials used
- Impression plaster.
- Alginate.

Techniques
- A preliminary impression with impression compound is made and primary cast is fabricated.
- Two sheets of base plate wax is placed as the spacer to cover the whole primary cast slightly beyond the border line.
- Special tray with acrylic resin is fabricated on the base plate wax and then the tray is perforated.
- Spacer is removed from special tray and an impression is made with special tray using impression plaster or alginate.

Advantages
- Preservation of health of tissues.
- Good stability.

Disadvantages
- Poor retention due to lack of peripheral seal.
- Poor esthetics and support due to short flanges.
- Lack of peripheral seal results in seeping of food beneath the dentures.

### C. SELECTIVE PRESSURE THEORY

- It was put forth by Boucher.
- This theory was based on the principles of both mucocompressive and mucostatic theories. Mucocompressive procedure is used in primary stress bearing areas and mucostatic procedure is used in non stress bearing areas.
- In this technique, the impression is made to extend over as much denture bearing area as possible within the comfort and functional limits of surrounding muscles and tissues.

Materials used
- Zinc oxide eugenol impression paste.

Techniques
- A preliminary impression with impression compound is made and primary cast is fabricated.
- Sheet of base plate wax is placed as the spacer over the non stress bearing areas on the primary cast.
- Special tray is fabricated with less relief in primary stress bearing areas and greater relief and more impression material in non stress bearing areas, such that more pressure is applied over stress bearing areas and less pressure applied over non stress bearing areas.
- Spacer is removed from special tray and tray is perforated. Now impression is made with special tray using zinc oxide eugenol impression paste.

Advantages
- It considers physiologic functions of the tissues.
- It confines forces acting on denture to stress bearing areas.

Disadvantages
- It may not be possible to record tissues with varying pressure.
- Tissues recorded under function may rebound at rest and results in loss of retention.

## IMPRESSION TRAYS

### DEFINITION
- A device that is used to carry, confine and control impression material while making an impression— GPT.

### RATIONALE/OBJECTIVES
- Impression tray must be rigid. Flexible trays cause distortion of the impression.

- It should be dimensionally stable.
- It should provide uniform space for impression material.
- It should be smooth to avoid injury to oral structures.
- It should not distort the tissues in the vestibular areas.
- It should support set impression material when removed from mouth so that a cast can be poured.

## CLASSIFICATION

*I. Based on whether they are prefabricated or individualized (Figs 2.4.5 and 2.4.6)*

1. Prefabricated trays / stock trays:
   a. Perforated trays
   b. Non perforated trays
   c. Rim lock trays
2. Individualized trays / custom trays / special trays:
   a. Close fitting special trays
   b. Loose fitting or spacer special trays

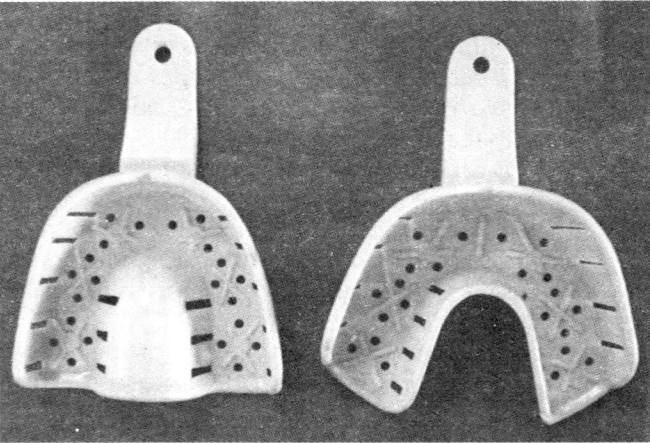

**Fig 2.4.5:** Dentulous plastic perforated trays

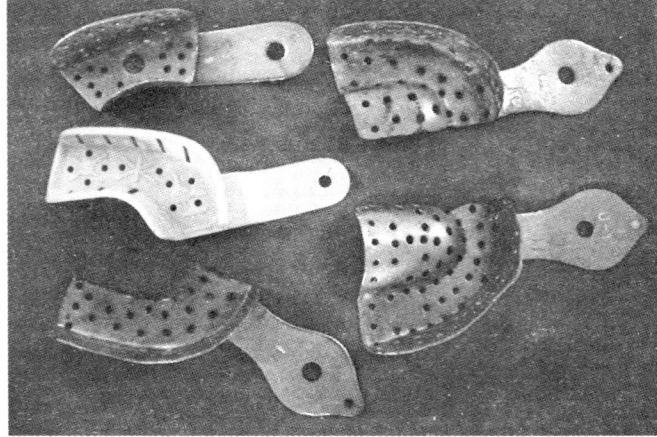

**Fig. 2.4.6:** Dentulous sectional stock trays

*II. Based on use of impression trays:*

1. Dentulous trays
2. Edentulous trays
3. Combination trays

*III. Based on whether it can be reused again or not*

1. Disposable trays
2. Non disposable trays

*IV. Based on material used for fabrication of impression trays*

1. Metallic trays
2. Non metallic trays

### Tray Materials

1. Materials used for fabrication of stock trays:
   A. Metal :
      a. Tin–lead alloy
      b. Stainless steel
   B. Plastic
2. Materials used for fabrication of custom trays
   A. Tray compound
   B. Tray acrylic
   C. Shellac base plate
   D. Vacuum formed thermoplastic resin sheets
   E. Wax
   F. Old dentures

### Advantages

A. Stock trays
   - Rigid and support the set impression material.
   - Dimensionally stable.
   - Tray is smooth, so injury to oral tissues is avoided.
   - Multiple use in several patients.
B. Custom trays
   - Dimensionally accurate impressions can be made.
   - Uniform space available for impression material.
   - Over or under extensions of tray flanges can be avoided.
   - Non stress bearing areas can be relieved with the use of spacer.
C. Tray acrylic special trays
   - Easy to fabricate.
   - Require no special equipment.
   - Sufficient dimensional stability.
   - Can be made thin but reasonably rigid.
   - Modified easily by grinding with an arbor band or an acrylic bur and smoothned or polished readily.
D. Shellac special trays
   - Impression tray can be fabricated very rapidly using thermoplastic shellac base plate.
E. Thermoplastic resin special trays:

- Very minimal amount of time is used in constructing the tray.

**Disadvantages**

A. Stock trays
- Dimensionally accurate impression is difficult to make with stock trays.
- Uniform space is not available for impression material.
- Flanges of stock trays may be over extended or under extended.

B. Custom trays
- Can be used only for individual patient.
- Fabrication of custom tray is time consuming based on the material selected.
- Rigidity is less when compared to metallic stock trays.
- Dimensional stability is less when compared to metallic stock trays.

C. Tray acrylic special trays
- Dimensional stability is less due to polymerization shrinkage.

D. Shellac special trays
- Lack of dimensional stability, especially during application of heat when border moulding the tray with impression compound.
- Brittle material, so chances of breakage while impression making and fabrication of cast.

E. Thermoplastic resin special trays
- Specialized equipment required.
- Expensive due to the requirement of costly equipment.

**Selection of Trays**

1. Based on type of impression
   a. Diagnostic impression—stock trays
   b. Primary impression—stock trays
   c. Secondary impression—custom trays/special trays
2. Based on complete or partial abscence of teeth
   a. Edentulous impression
      - Non perforated trays
   b. Dentulous impression
      - Perforated trays
      - Non perforated trays with tray adhesive.
3. Based on impression material used
   a. Alginate—perforated trays
   b. Impression compound—Non perforated trays

**Special Trays**

1. Based on the fit of trays on denture bearing area
   A. Close fitting special trays.
   B. Loose fitting special trays or spaced special trays.
2. Based on material used for fabrication of special tray
   A. Acrylic special tray.
   B. Shellac special tray.
   C. Tray compound special tray.
   D. Thermoplastic resin special tray.
   E. Wax special tray.
   F. Use of old dentures as special tray.
   G. Modifying the primary impression made with impression compound as special tray.

Close fitting special trays
- These special trays do not have much space to accomodate for the thickness of the impression material. These type of trays are fabricated when impression materials that form thin sections and have low viscosity are selected for impression making, such as thin consistency zinc oxide eugenol impression paste and light bodied elastomers.

Loose fitting special trays / spaced special trays
- Some impression materials require adequate bulk and hence space should be provided in the special tray for accomodation of the impression material. Spaced special trays are fabricated after adaptation of appropriate thickness of spacer over the primary cast. Impression material such as alginate require spacer of about 3 mm.

Tray compound special trays
- A primary impression made using tray compound can be used as special tray if it is separated from stock tray and modified by scraping. In this case primary cast is not required and final impression is direclty made in the compound tray. This technique is used frequently for the maxillary arch and less frequently for the mandibular arch. It is considered particularly desirable when the patient is not available for numerous appointments.

**Spacer Design (Table 2.4.2)**

- A wax spacer is a layer of wax placed within the impression tray which when removed leaves a space in the impression tray. The location of wax spacer reflects the type of impression technique used.

Table 2.4.2: Recommended spacer thickness to be used when constructing special tray

| Impression material | Spacer thickness |
| --- | --- |
| 1. Alginate | 3.0 mm |
| 2. Impression plaster | 1.5 mm |
| 3. Elastomeric impression materials | 0.5–1.5 mm (depending on viscosity) |
| 4. Zinc oxide eugenol paste | 0.5 mm |

1. Spacer design for mucocompressive pressure technique
   No spacer is adapted for this technique.
2. Spacer design for mucostatic or minimal pressure technique
   A. Maxilla—Full coverage spacer with tissue stops in canine and molar region (Figs 2.4.7 and 2.4.8).
   B. **Mandible—Full coverage spacer with tissue stops in canine region anteriorly. The buccal shelf area acts as posterior tissue stop (Figs** 2.4.9 and 2.4.10).
3. Spacer design for selective pressure technique
   A. Maxilla
      a. Shallow vault—'I' shaped.
      b. Anterior flabby tissue—'T' shaped.
      c. Deep palatal vault—Dumbell shaped/pot shaped.
      d. Relief areas—Incisive papilla, mid palatine raphe (Fig. 2.4.11).
   B. Mandible—Spacer only on the crest of the ridge.
      – Relief areas in mandible crest of the alveolar ridge (Figs 2.4.12 to 2.4.14).
   C. Material used
      – Modelling wax and non asbestos casting liner are most commonly used materials for spacer.
      – Impression compound can be used as spacer if special tray has to be fabricated with shellac base plate.
   D. Thickness
      – The spacer should be about 2 mm thick.
4. Spacer design for anterior flabby tissues
   Double spacer is adapted on the anterior flabby tissue region over the primary cast (Fig. 2.4.15)

## Tissue Stops

- Spacer should be cut out in 2–4 places to form windows in the spacer so that part of the special tray extends into the cut out of the spacer or windows. This extended part of special tray is called as the stopper (tissue stop).
- The location of stopper is not very critical, usually 4 stoppers are placed, two on the canine region on either side and two in the molar region.
- The dimensions of stopper can be a square of 2 mm or rectangle of 2 by 4 mm (2 mm mesiodistally and 4 mm bucco lingually) (Figs 2.4.16 and 2.4.17).

## Uses

- Tissue stops ensure uniform thickness of about 2–3 mm of impression material.
- Tissue stops help in stabilizing the special tray during impression making.
- Tissues stops can be produced by several ways:

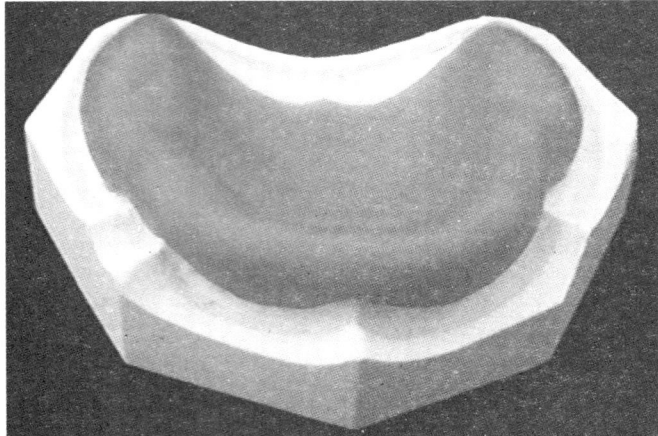

**Fig. 2.4.7:** Maxilla—front view showing the spacer design for mucostatic pressure technique

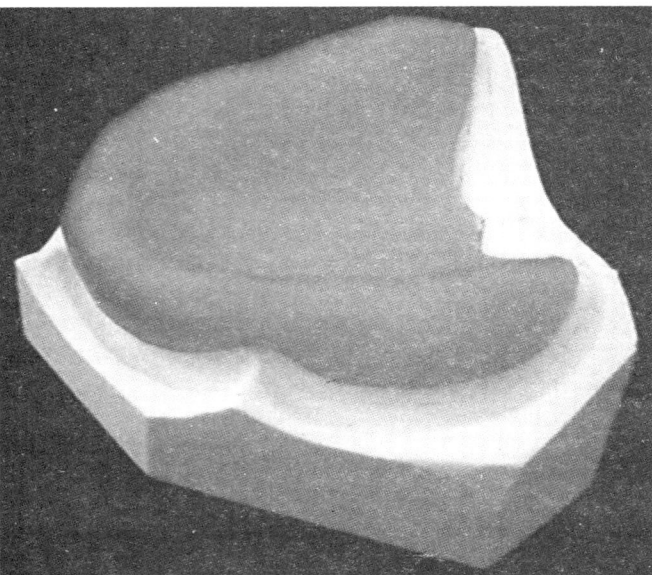

**Fig. 2.4.8:** Maxilla—side view showing the spacer design for mucostatic pressure technique

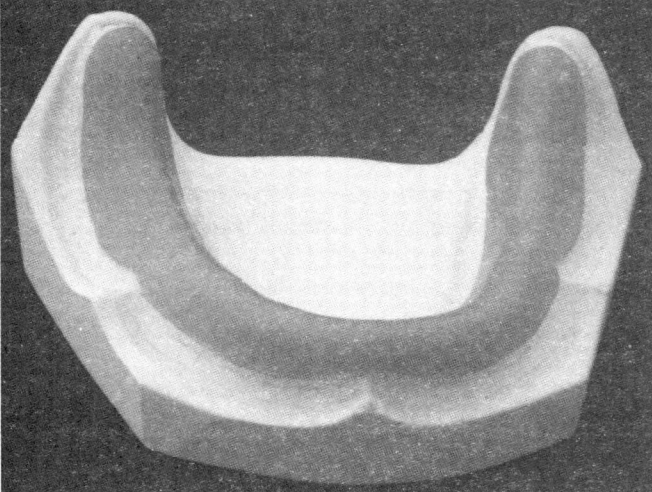

**Fig. 2.4.9:** Mandible—front view showing the spacer design for mucostatic pressure technique

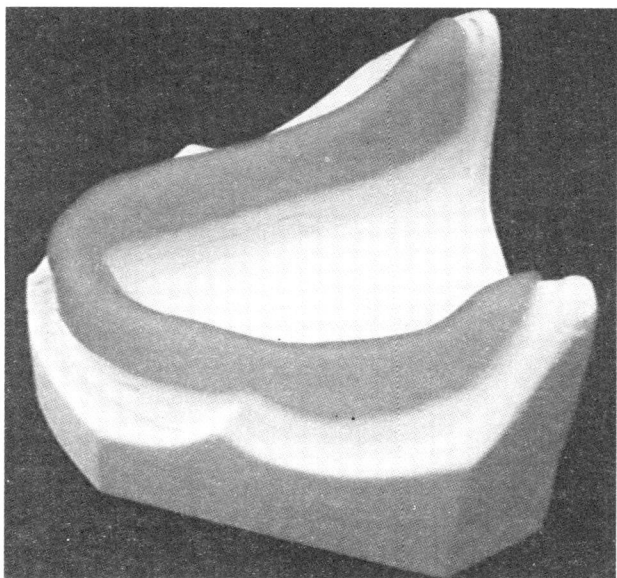

**Fig. 2.4.10:** Mandible—side view showing the spacer design for mucostatic pressure technique

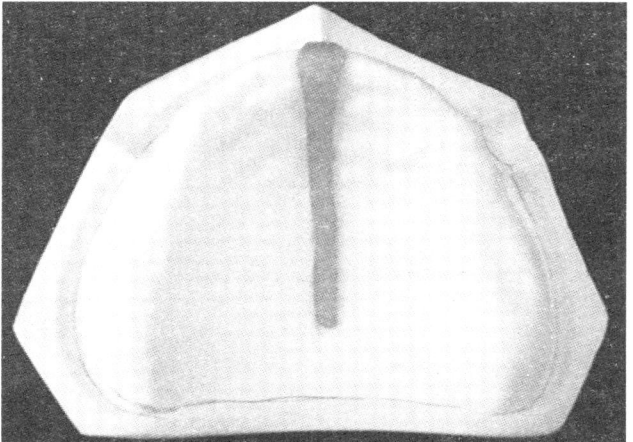

**Fig. 2.4.11:** Spacer design on maxilla for selective pressure technique

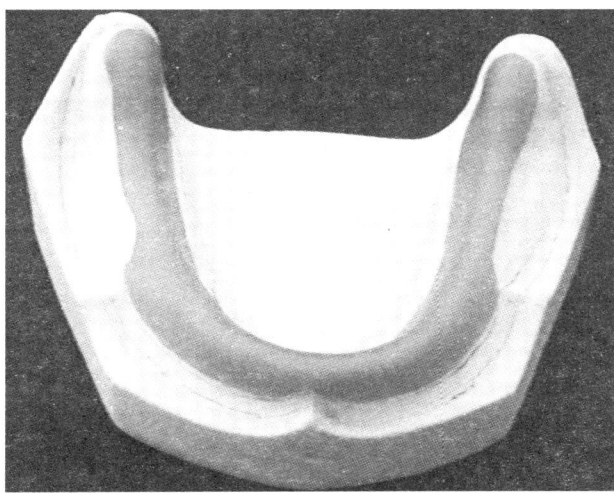

**Fig. 2.4.12:** Spacer design on mandible for selective pressure technique—front view

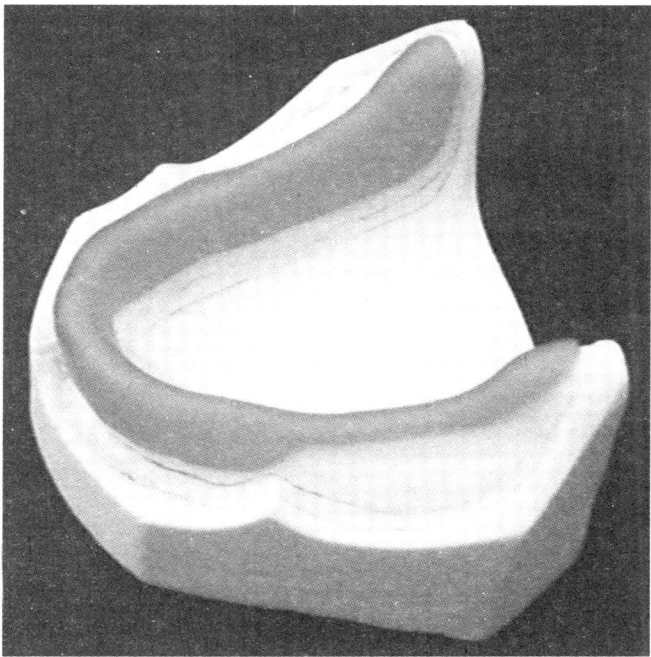

**Fig. 2.4.13:** Spacer design on mandible for selective pressure technique—side view

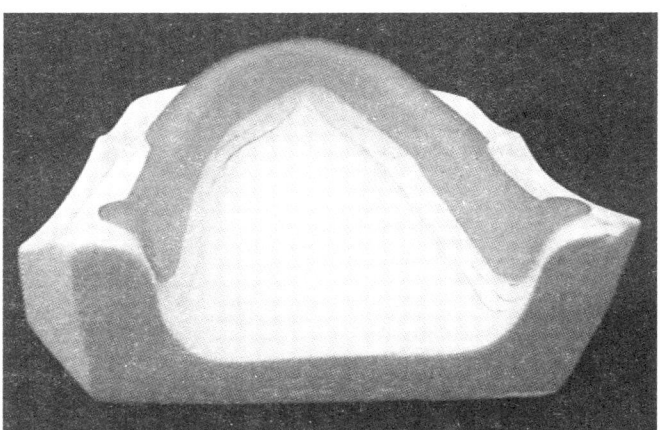

**Fig. 2.4.14:** Spacer design on mandible for selective pressure technique—lingual view

1. During construction of an acrylic tray in the laboratory
   - Windows are cut in the wax spacer at appropriate places on the primary cast used to fabricate special tray when acrylic dough flows into these windows, tissue stops are produced. This method produces accurate tissue stops and saves chair side time.
2. At the chairside in the mouth
   - Tracing compound is applied to the tray and tempered in warm water to avoid burning of the mucosa. The tray is then placed in the mouth to mould the tracing compound to the ridge tissues

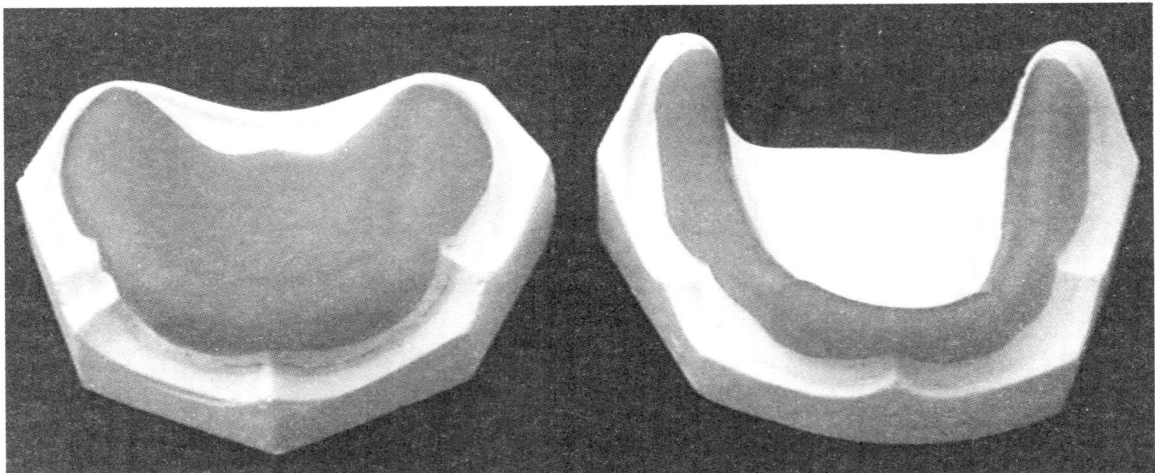

Fig. 2.4.15: Double spacer design on maxilla and mandible for anterior flabby tissues

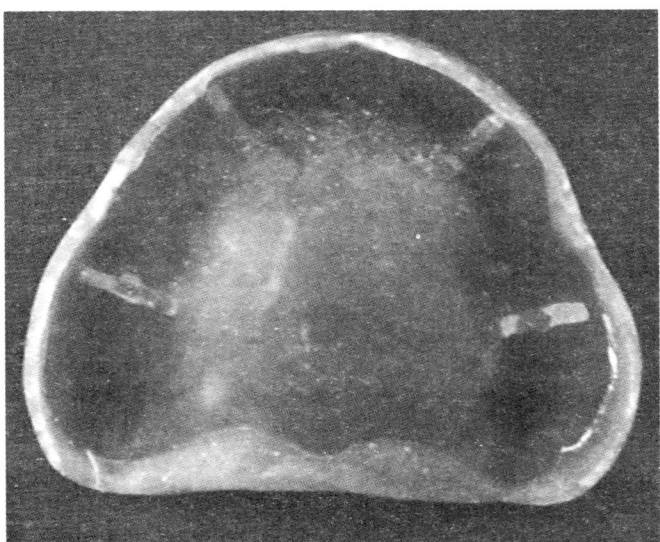

Fig. 2.4.16: Tissue stops in maxillary special tray

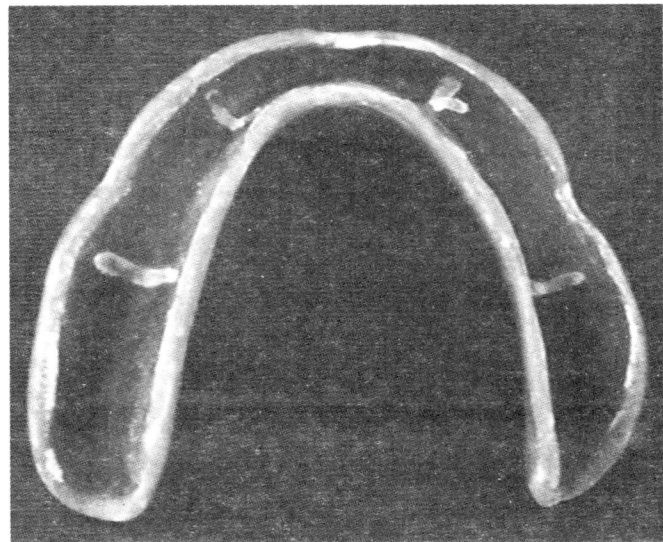

Fig. 2.4.17: Tissue stops in mandibular special tray

creating the required space between the tray and mucosa.
3. At the chair side on the cast
   - Tracing compound is applied to the tray and the tray is then placed on the dampened cast. This technique has advantage of checking visually whether the tray is centred correctly on the ridge while the stops are being formed.

## PRIMARY IMPRESSIONS

### SYNONYMS

- Primary impressions
- Preliminary impressions
- Diagnostic impressions

### DEFINITION

"A negative likeness made for the purpose of diagnosis, treatment planning or the fabrication of a tray" – GPT.

### RATIONALE/OBJECTIVES

1. Preliminary impression is as important as final impression. It is important that preliminary impression is as accurate as possible. An accurate preliminary impression helps to control the accuracy of the remaining impression procedures.
2. Preliminary impression should record all areas to be covered by the impression surface of the denture and the adjacent landmarks with an impression material that is accurate and incorporates the minimum of tissue displacement.

3. The peripheral borders of preliminary impression should be accurate in both height and width for the special tray to be properly extended.
4. The maxillary impression should include the hamular notches, fovea palatina, entire buccal vestibule, frenum attachments, palate and entire labial vestibule.
5. The mandibular impression should include the retromolar pads, the buccal shelf areas, the external oblique ridge, frenum attachments, sublingual space, retromylohyoid space, the posterior mucous membrane floor of the mouth to include and be below the mylohyoid line and the entire labial and buccal vestibules.
6. The completed preliminary impression must closely resemble the eventual denture base.

## INSTRUMENTS AND MATERIALS (Fig. 2.4.18)

A. For preliminary impressions made with alginate.
　1. Impression trays—perforated
　2. Utility wax
　3. X-ray time clock
　4. Irreversible hydrocolloid (alginate)
　5. Water at 70°F
　6. Water measurer
　7. Thermometer
　8. Trimming knife
　9. Napkin and mirror
　10. Rubber bowl
　11. Curved spatula

B. For preliminary impressions made with impression compound.
　1. Stock impression trays—non perforated.
　2. Thermostatically controlled water bath, containing compound.
　3. Rubber bowl.
　4. Alcohol torch.
　5. Bunsen burner and matches.
　6. Mouthwash.
　7. Napkin and mirror.
　8. Trimming knife.
　9. Wax knife.
　10. Large pair of scissors.
　11. Patients bib and chain.

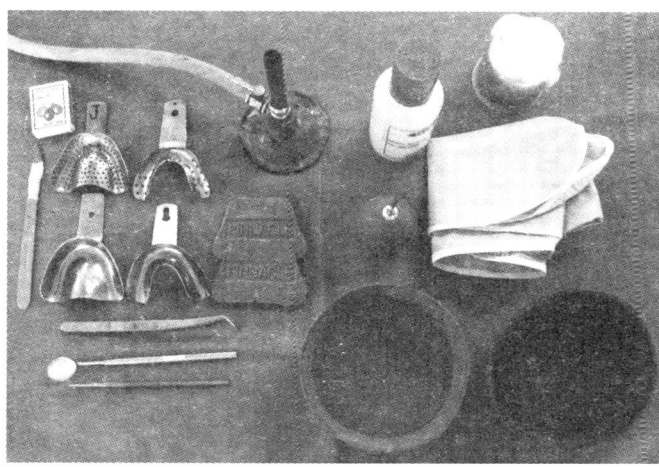

**Fig. 2.4.18**

### Preparation

- Choose the correct impression material and impression technique suitable for particular patient.
- Arrange all the instruments and materials required for the impression procedure. Make sure that sterilization procedures are followed at each and every level.
- Seating the patient: Patient should be seated up right in a comfortable position with the occiput resting firmly in the head rest. Gravity influences the position of the tissues and since dentures are, in most instances, constructed for patients who will use them while in an upright position, the tissues should be recorded in the impression at this position.
- The dentist should instruct the patients about the procedures, prior to impression making and ensure them of the ease of the procedures so that they will work with and not against the dentist.
- Before making the preliminary impression it is advisable to practice placing the tray in position. The patient is asked to perform the various movements required of him by the dentist inorder to mould the impression. This practice is done with the tray in the mouth.

### Selection of Impression Trays

- "The journey of a thousand miles begins with one step", Jao Tsu said. The begining of a good impression starts with the selection of correct impression tray. Good impressions can be made from properly selected trays with relative ease. Poor tray requires tray adjustments at the chair that are time consuming and messy and result in an inferior impression.

- If the impression material to be used is alginate then perforated tray is selected and if it is impression compound non perforated tray is selected.
- The tray is selected according to the size of the arches. It should cover the entire denture bearing area and extend upto the reflection of the mucosa.
- The tray that is approximately 5 mm larger than the outside surface of the residual ridge is selected.
- In maxilla, the tray must include both the hamular notches and vibrating line posteriorly.
- In mandible, the tray must cover the retromolar pads posteriorly.
- For making alginate impressions, the under extension of the tray can be corrected by the addition of impression compound or pink wax to the deficient flange, while over extension can be corrected, if the tray is plastic, by trimming back the flange with a bur.

## MAKING IMPRESSION

### A. Using Alginate

Mandibular arch: The lower impression is usually taken first as it is easier for the patient to tolerate than the upper.

- Select the appropriate tray according to size of the arch and refine its posterior borders with utility wax to carry the impression material to place.
- Instruct the patient to rinse his mouth vigorously with cold water and then to hold some additional cold water in his mouth until the impression is ready to be made. Ask the patient to either expectorate or swallow the water before impression is made. Rinsing with cold water dilutes and minimizes saliva build up and also cools the tissues so that alginate that is manually placed does not set too quickly when it contacts the tissue.
- Mix the alginate according to manufacturers instructions and load the tray from the side slightly over level full.
- Insert the loaded tray with operator sitting or standing infront of the patient, with patient's mouth slightly above the operator's elbow.
- The lower impression tray should be rotated into the mouth, with the cheek retracted by the operator's finger.
- Instruct the patient to lift his tongue up and out, while he is doing this, seat the impression tray posteriorly into retromylohyoid area. Next, instruct patient to relax his tongue in a protruded position. Continue to seat the tray anteriorly using anterior flange of stock tray as guide. Express the material around buccal and labial borders by lifting the cheeks and lip to mimic functional movements in these areas.
- Lift the buccal fat pad over the distobuccal corner of the stock tray. Instruct patient to close his mouth with his tongue in a relaxed forward position, stopping before contact is made between the maxilla and the tray. Hold impression lightly in place for two minutes with no movement.
- Remove the impression with one quick, controlled sharp jerk movement. Inspect the impression for its acceptability.

Maxillary arch

- If the sulci buccal to the maxillary tuberosities are deep, air may be trapped as the loaded tray is inserted. So, ask the patient to open his mouth and prepack the material into both of the retrozygomatic areas opposite the tuberosities place alginate material in the remaining right and left labial and buccal vestibules. Place additional material to cover palate.
- Place loaded impression tray in patients mouth, from a position behind the patient. Place the anterior metal flange of the tray so that it is in the proper border position. Use the handle of tray as a guide for midline.
- Exert bilateral pressure to cause the alginate to flow and record the shape of the tissues. Continue to seat the tray evenly while using fingers to mould the cheeks and lips to form the periphery.
- Hold the impression tray lightly in place for two minutes without any movement. Lift the lip away from the tray and remove the impression with one quick, controlled sharp jerk movement.
- Inspect the completed impression for acceptability.

### B. Using Impression Compound

Mandibular arch

- Soften the impression compound in water bath at temperature of 55°C to 70°C. Knead the compound with fingers by folding the material inwards from the periphery to the centre. Kneading helps to produce a smooth, crease-free surface on one side of compound and also improves flow and maintains uniform consistency of material.

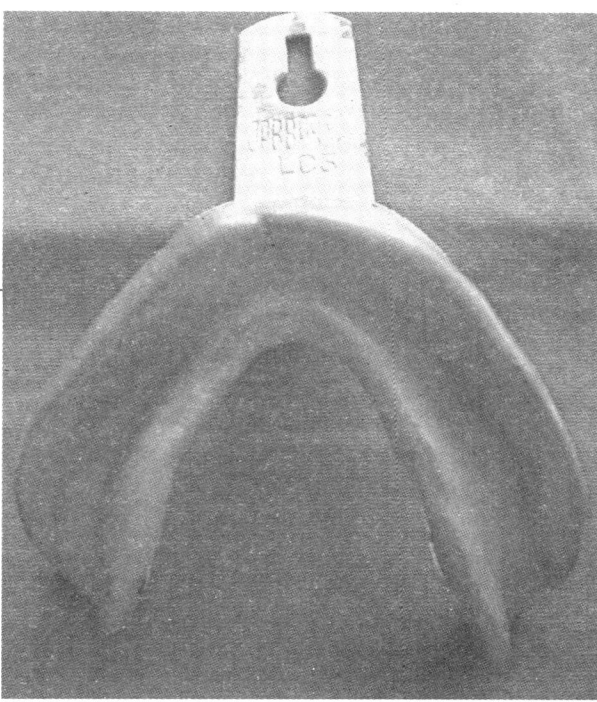

Fig. 2.4.19: Mandibular impression made with impression compound

- The kneaded impression compound is placed in the selected tray so that the smooth side will be towards the tissues and is then moulded with fingers to the approximate shape of the ridge. The surface of the compound can be lightly flamed to improve its flow, tempered in warm water and coated with petroleum jelly.
- The loaded tray is then seated firmly in patients mouth and procedures carried out as described for aliginate preliminary impression. But, as the impression compound is more viscous than alginate, moulding the borders should be carried out with vigour to prevent over extension of the impression.
- When the impression has hardened, remove from mouth and check for deficiencies and over extensions. Do any corrections by trimming excess material or adding excess compound and resoften the surface of impression before reseating in the mouth.
- Once a satisfactory impression has been made, it must be hardened by placing in cold water (Fig. 2.4.19)

Maxillary arch

- Soften the impression compound, knead it and obtain the size and shape of a golf ball.
- Place the golf ball sized portion of this compound into the centre of selected tray and mould it with finger to the shape of the ridge and palate.
- The remaining procedures are as described for the lower compound impression (Fig. 2.4.20).

## IMPRESSION EVALUATION

- The completed impression should be observed next to the patients mouth and the junction of the attached and unattached mucosal tissue visually identified on the border of the impression.
- The completed impression should include the entire denture bearing area.
- The surface of the completed impression should be smooth and show evidence of having been moulded by the tissues.
- The border areas should be rounded and include impressions of the frenal attachments.
- Impression should be repeated or modified if errors are seen in impression like over extension, under extension, incomplete impressions, large voids, seperation of impression from tray during removal, etc.

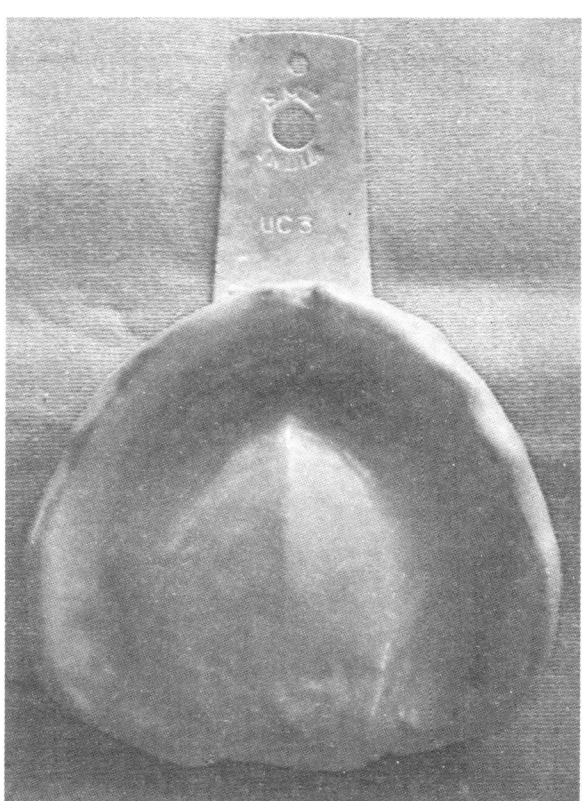

Fig. 2.4.20: Maxillary impression made with impression compound

# FINAL IMPRESSION TRAYS

## DEFINITION

- A device that is used to carry, confine and control impression material while making a final impression.

## RATIONALE/OBJECTIVES

1. The tray should be rigid but not overly thick.
2. It should retain its shape throughout the construction and pouring of the impression.
3. The method of construction should be simple enough so that an acceptable impression tray can be made in a minimal amount of time at a reasonable cost.
4. It should be possible to trim or thin the tray readily with a bur, mounted stone, scissors or an arbor band.
5. The tray should be smooth because sharp edges may injure oral tissues.

## EQUIPMENTS AND MATERIALS

1. Preliminary cast
2. Indelible pencil
3. Base plate wax
4. Separating medium
5. Autopolymerizing acrylic resin polymer and monomer
6. Polymer and monomer dispensors
7. Paper cup or suitable container
8. Bard Parker blade
9. Lecron carver
10. Petrolatum
11. Plaster bowl
12. Acrylic burs.

## FABRICATION

### A. Tray Outline

- To make a tray outline one must know how to interpret the anatomic landmarks on the primary cast obtained from preliminary impression.

#### a. Maxillary cast

- With an indelible pencil, draw a line transversely across the posterior border connecting the two hamular notches, with the mid point approximately 2 mm distal to the fovea palatina.
- Draw a line outlining the mucobuccal fold at the point where the buccal reflection leaves the lateral wall of the alveolar ridge. Carry the outline well above the frenal attachments.
- All trays are subject to refinement in the mouth when tissue is displaced by the borders. Displacement should be checked in the patients mouth prior to making the border moulding with green stick compound (Figs 2.4.21 to 2.4.23).

#### b. Mandibular Cast

- With an indelible pencil, draw a line distal to the retromolar pad continue this line buccally in an inferior and anterior direction following the masseter groove to the beginning of the external oblique ridge.
- Progressing anteriorly, follow the oblique ridge to the buccal frenum attachment carry the outline well above the frenum attachment and end at the buccal frenum.

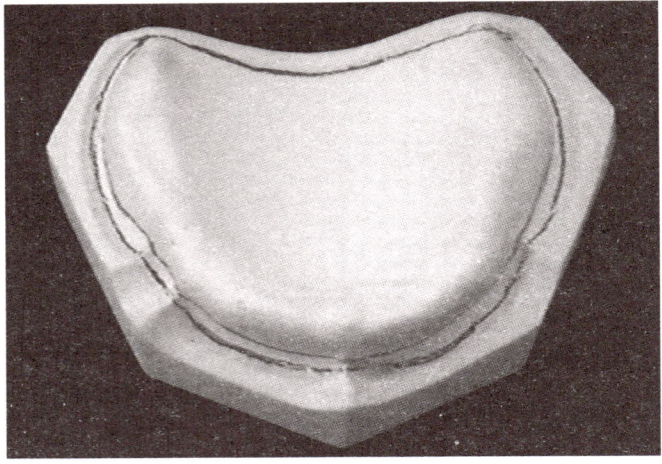

**Fig. 2.4.21:** Maxillary cast—Tray outline, front view (superior line represents tray outline)

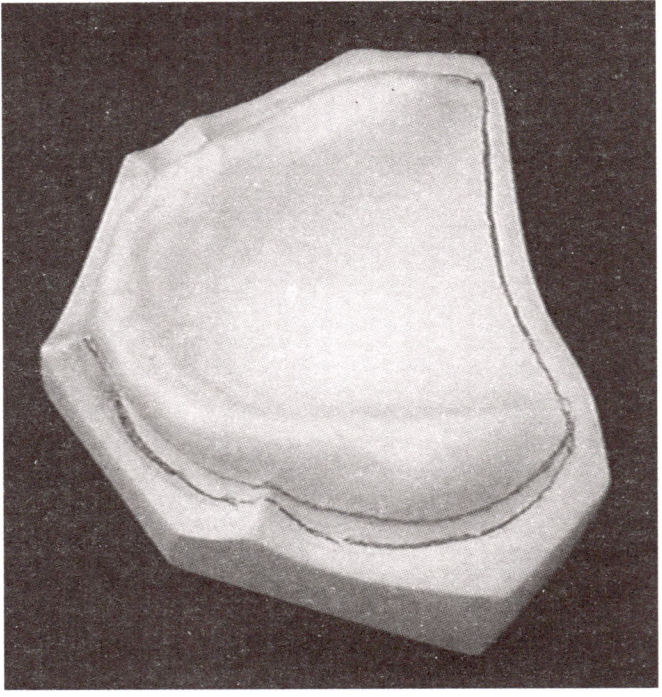

**Fig. 2.4.22:** Maxillary cast—Tray outline, side view (superior line)

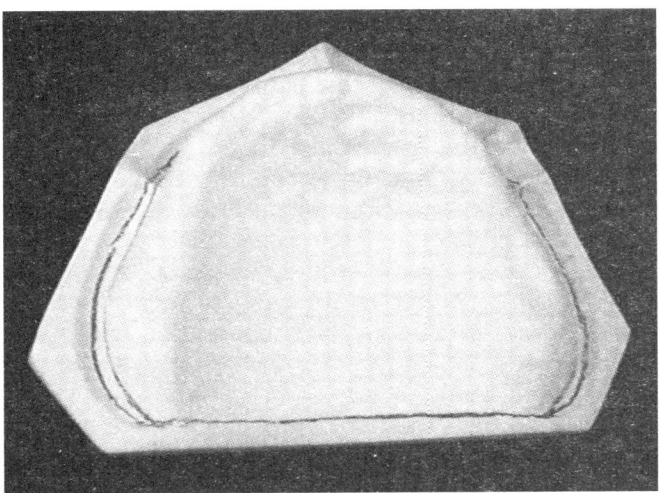

Fig. 2.4.23: Maxillary cast—Tray outline, back view

- Mark the outline similarly on other side also and join these two outlines anteriorly by following the mucobuccal reflection and allowing space for the labial frenum attachment.
- On the lingual side, make a line inferiorly from distal aspect of retromolar pad to lingual tuberosity.
- From lingual tuberosity, extend a line anteriorly and inferiorly to mylohyoid ridge but 2 or 3 mm short of the mucous membrane floor of the mouth reflection to a point opposite the cuspid eminence.
- Mark the outline similarly on the other side of lingual aspect also and join these two outlines anteriorly by following the sublingual mucous membrane reflection and allowing space for the lingual frenum attachment (Figs 2.4.24 to 2.4.26).

### B. Methods

1. Autopolymerizing resin impression trays.
   a. *Sprinkle on method*
      - After making outline of impression tray on cast, block out the severe undercuts with wax and adapt a layer of base plate wax to cast for relief. Trim the relief wax to desired outline.
      - Apply separating medium on the stone cast and over the relief wax.
      - Sprinkle polymer powder on the cast and relief wax and saturate with liquid monomer from an eye dropper, until uniform layer of approximately 2 mm thickness is obtained.
      - The cast should be tilted during shifting to prevent excess resin build up in the palatal region of maxillary casts or in the mucobuccal fold areas of madibular casts.

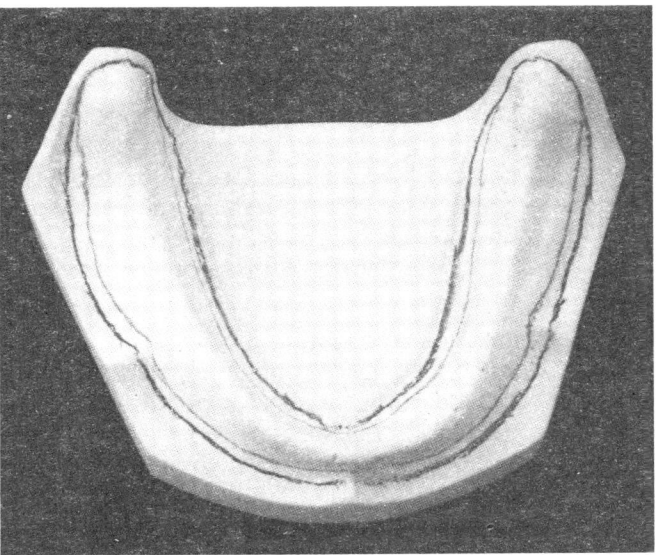

Fig. 2.4.24: Mandibular cast—Tray outline, front view (superior line represents tray out line)

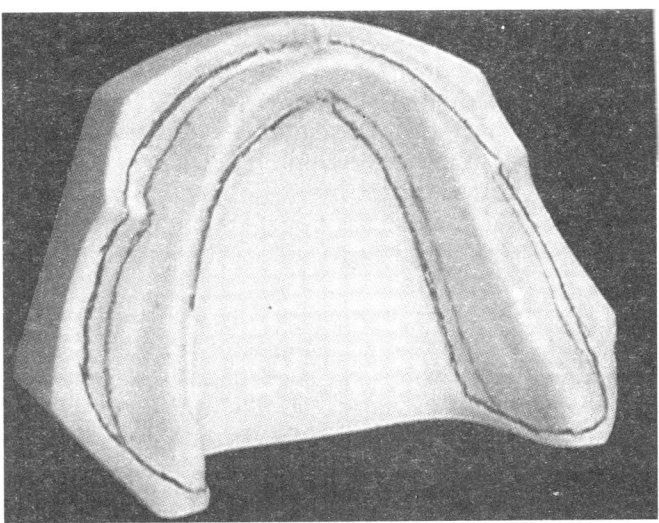

Fig. 2.4.25: Mandibular cast—Tray outline, front view

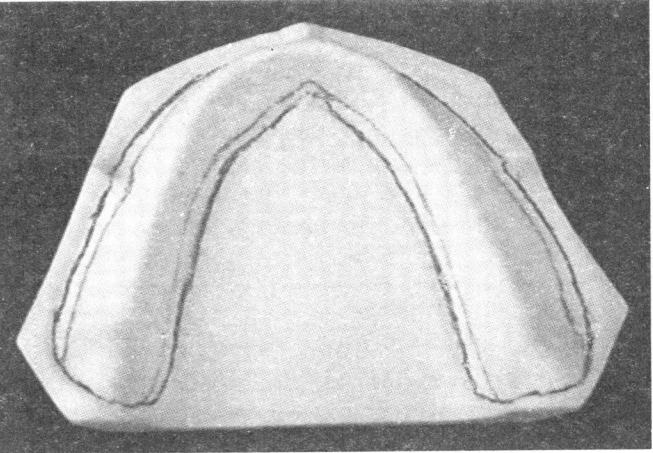

Fig. 2.4.26: Mandibular cast—Tray outline, top view

- Cure the impression tray under an inverted plaster bowl to reduce the porosity.
- Mix more resin in a paper cup and when it is in the dough stage, form handles and adapt them to the impression tray.
- Remove the set impression tray from cast and trim it with bur. Evaluate the completed tray and do necessary corrections.
- Store the impression tray on the cast until needed.

b. *Finger adapted dough method*
- As described for sprinkle on method, make outline of impression tray on the cast, block the undercuts, adapt relief wax and apply separating medium over the cast and relief wax.
- Proportion the acrylic impression tray material according to manufacturers recommendations and mix in a paper cup or other suitable container.
- Once it reaches dough stage, roll the resin to the desired thickness with a roller or use a special from to make the impression tray uniformly thick.
- Hand adapt the material to the cast carefully to avoid overthinning the resin on the convex portions of the cast.
- Remove excess tray material from borders. Make handles from excess material and adapt them to the tray.
- Cure the impression tray on the bench or under an inverted plaster bowl.
- Remove the set impression tray from cast, trim the borders, evaluate the completed tray to do necessary corrections and store the tray on the cast until needed (Figs 2.4.27 to 2.4.44).

2. Vaccum-adapted method
- After making the outline of impression tray on the cast, block the undercuts and place the relief on the cast with a material, such as a wet sheet of non asbestos casting ring lining material, that will not melt during heating of the thermoplastic resin sheet.
- Center the cast on the vacuum adapted plate and place a resin sheet of appropriate thickness in the heating frame, rotate the heating unit into position and continue heating until the specified sag in the material occurs.
- Lower the frame and resin sheet onto the cast and start vacuum adaptation. Once adaptation is completed, allow it to cool and remove the cast from the vacuum adapting unit. Remove the tray from cast and trim the borders.
- Add handles made of autopolymerizing acrylic resin or use preformed metal handles and store the tray on the cast until needed.

3. Shellac method.
- Once the tray outline is made on the cast, block out the undercuts on the cast with a plaster and pumice mix or with wet non asbestos casting ring lining material.
- Adapt a layer of wet non asbestos casting ring lining material to the cast for relief. Center a sheet of double thickness shellac base plate material over the cast and wilt it onto the cast with flame.
- Fold the excess shellac material at the borders back on to itself to make them of proper thickness. Continue adaptation until the shellac material makes intimate contact with the cast and relief material.
- Make a handle from shellac base plate material and adapt it to the impression tray. Remove the tray from cast once its cooled and trim the borders. Store the impression tray on the cast until needed (Figs 2.4.45 to 2.4.53).

c. *Tray handle*
- According to some authors only one handle in the anterior portion of the tray is placed irrespective of whether it is maxillary impression tray or mandibular impression tray.
- But some authors suggested one handle in the anterior portion for maxillary impression tray and three handles for mandibular impression trays; one in anterior region and two in the molar region.
- Handles on the impression tray should approximate the position of the teeth on the finished denture and should not interfere with lip movements of patients.
- Dimensions of tray handle should be approximately:
  Thickness  – 3 to 4 mm
  Length     – 8 mm
  Height     – 8 mm
- Place horizontal grooves across the facial and lingual surfaces of the handles to improve the grip (Fig. 2.4.54).

## EVALUATION AND CORRECTION

A. The maxillary special tray
- The buccal and lingual flanges should be 2 mm short of the tissue reflections.
- Gently move the cheek anteroposteriorly to observe clearance for buccal frenum attachments and extend lip directly forward to observe clearance for labial frenum attachment.
- The tray must contain both hamular notches and extend approximately 2 mm posterior to the

## SPECIAL TRAYS FABRICATED FOR MUCOCOMPRESSIVE OR DEFINITIVE PRESSURE TECHNIQUE (WITHOUT SPACER)

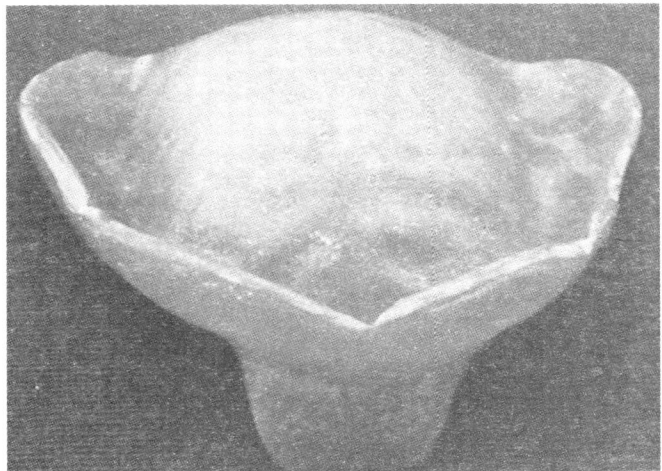

**Fig. 2.4.27:** Maxillary special tray fabricated for definitive pressure technique (tissue surface)

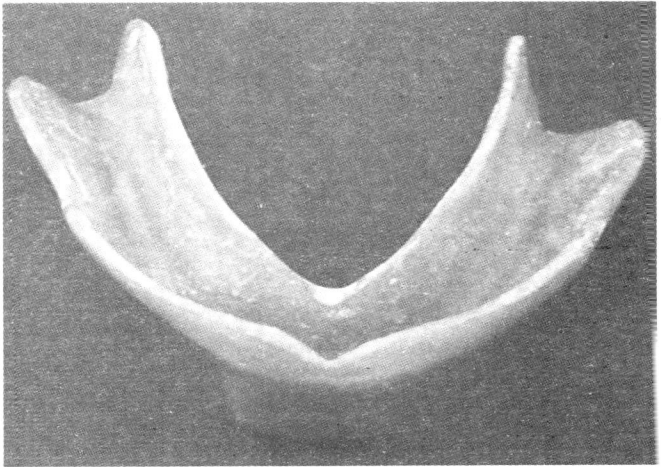

**Fig. 2.4.28:** Mandibular special tray fabricated for definitive pressure technique (tissue surface)

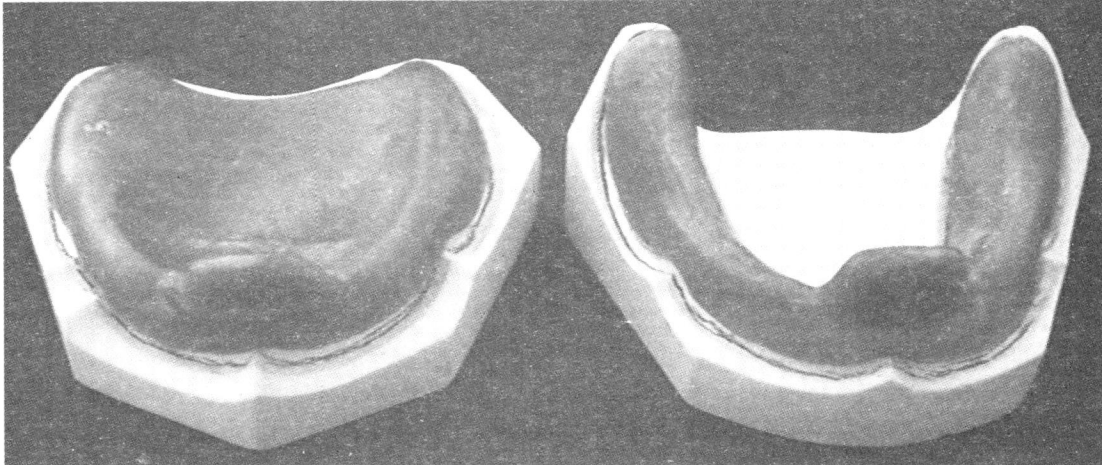

**Fig. 2.4.29:** Special trays adapted on maxillary and mandibular casts, front view

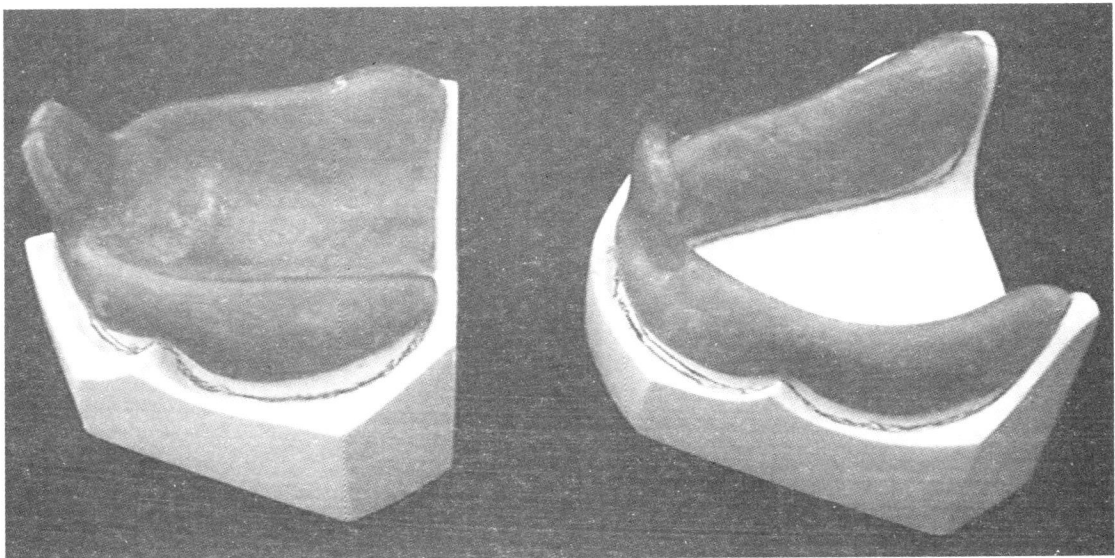

**Fig. 2.4.30:** Special trays adapted on maxillary and mandibular casts, side view

## SPECIAL TRAYS FABRICATED FOR MUCOSTATIC OR PRESSURE LESS TECHNIQUE

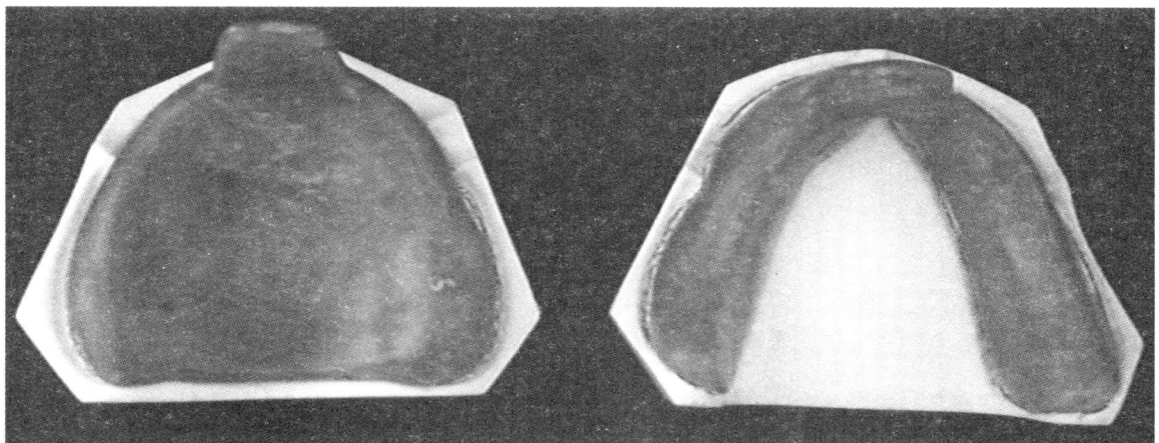

Fig. 2.4.31: Special trays adapted on maxillary and mandibular casts, top view

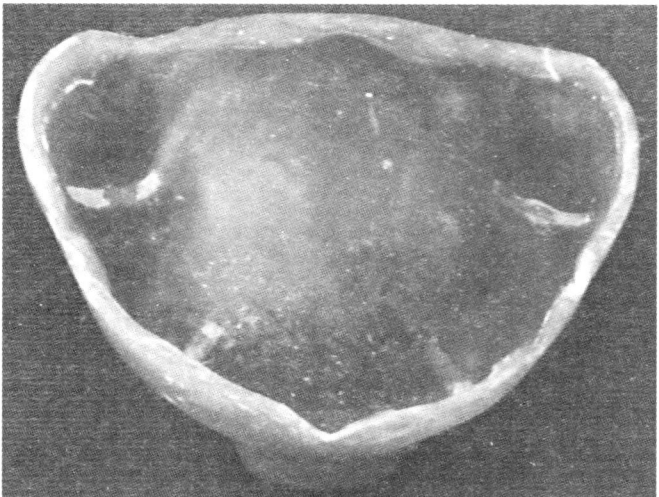

Fig. 2.4.32: Maxillary special tray fabricated for mucostatic and pressure less technique (tissue surface)

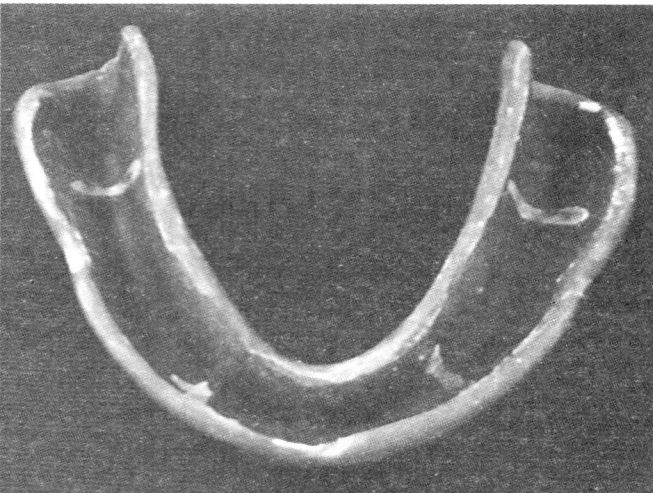

Fig. 2.4.33: Mandibular special tray fabricated for mucostatic and pressure less technique (tissue surface)

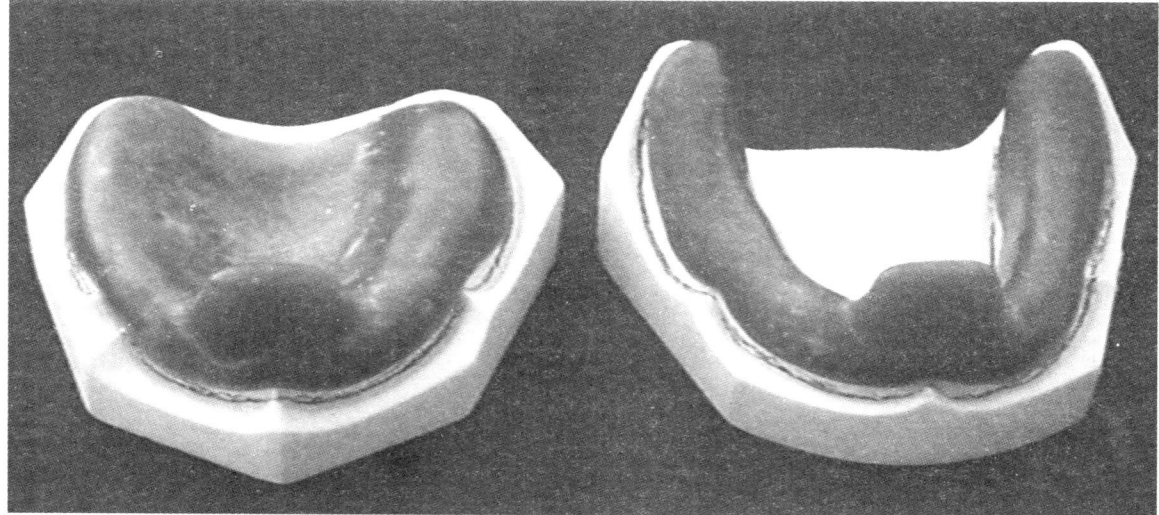

Fig. 2.4.34: Mandibular special tissue front view

## SPECIAL TRAYS FABRICATED FOR SELECTIVE PRESSURE TECHNIQUE

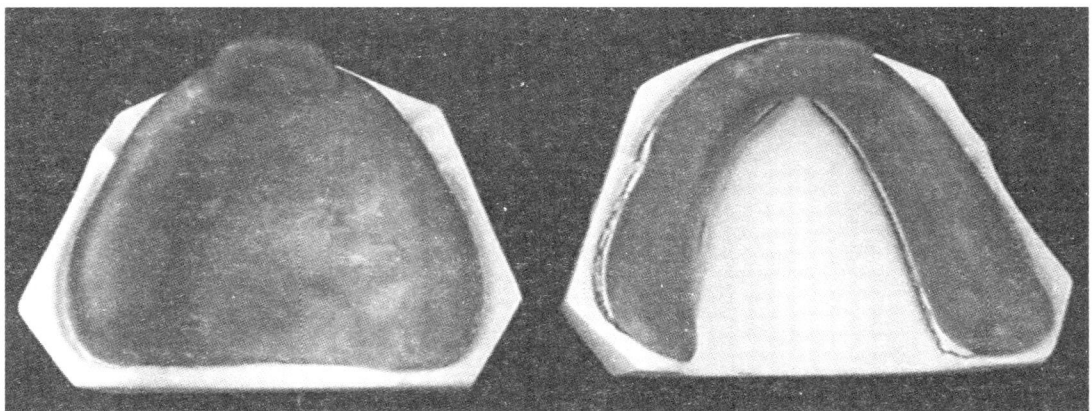

Fig. 2.4.35: Mandibular special tray top view

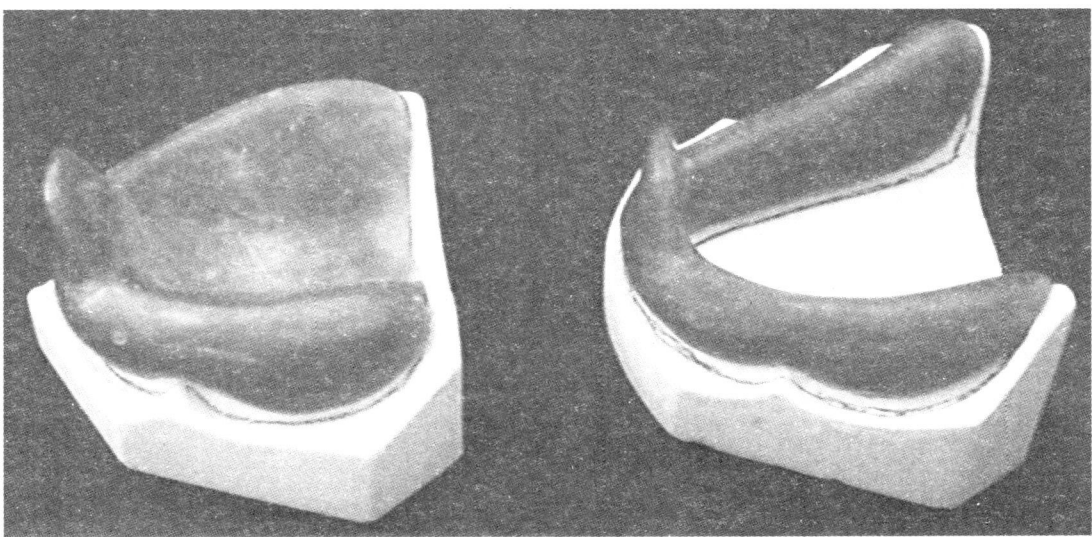

Fig. 2.4.36: Mandibular special tray side view

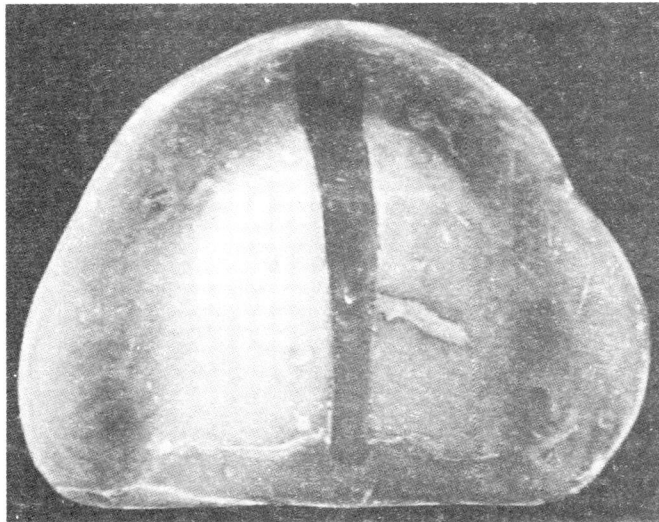

Fig. 2.4.37: Maxillary special tray fabricated for selective pressure technique (tissue surface)

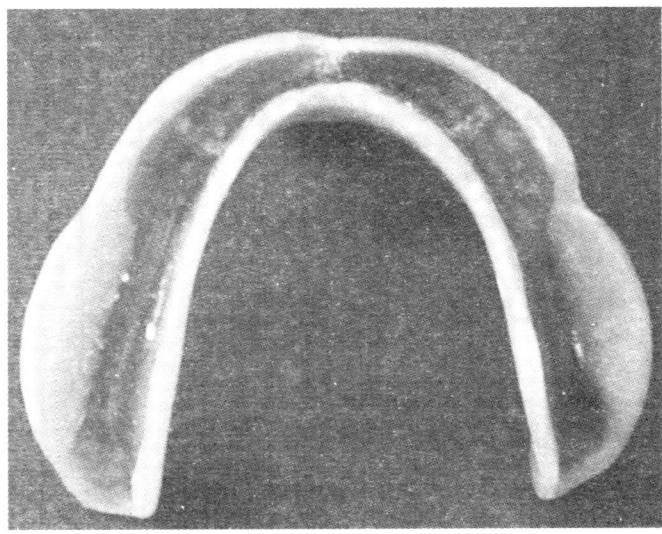

Fig. 2.4.38: Mandibular special tray fabricated for selective pressure technique (tissue surface)

## SPECIAL TRAYS FABRICATED FOR ANTERIOR FLABBY RIDGE SITUATIONS

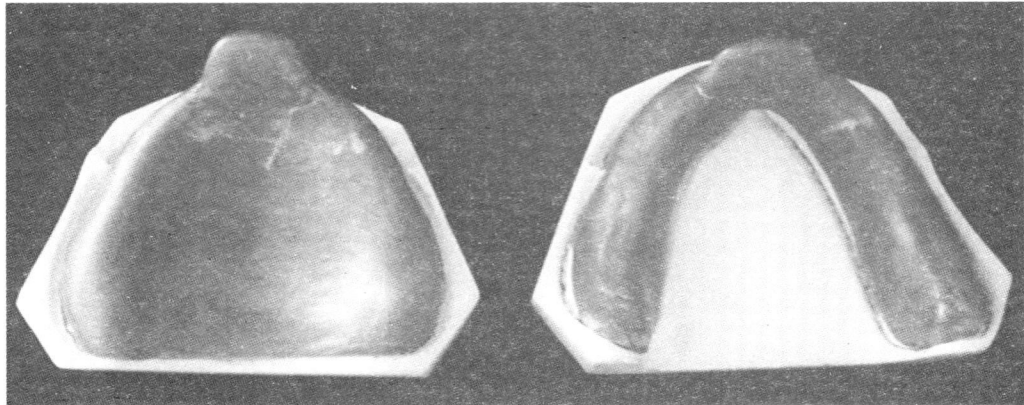

Fig. 2.4.39

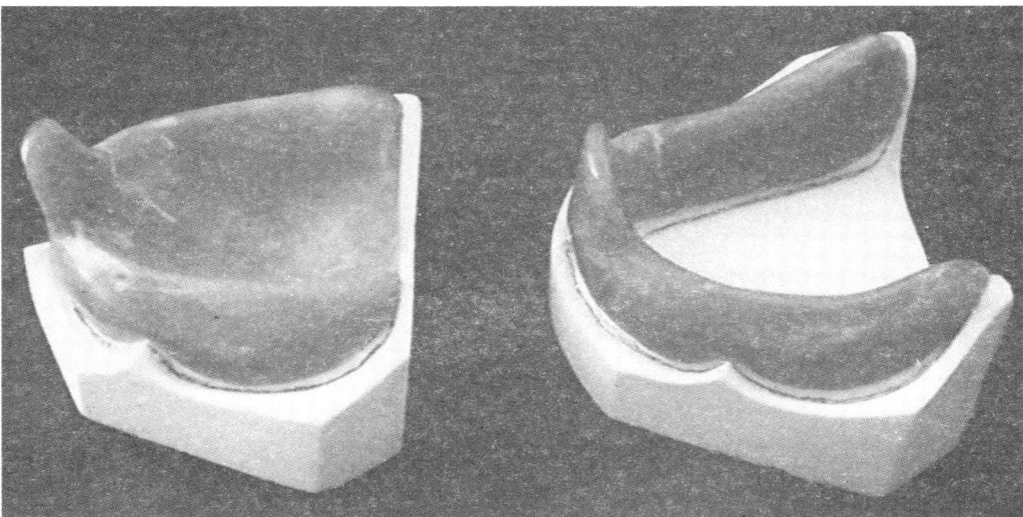

Fig. 2.4.40

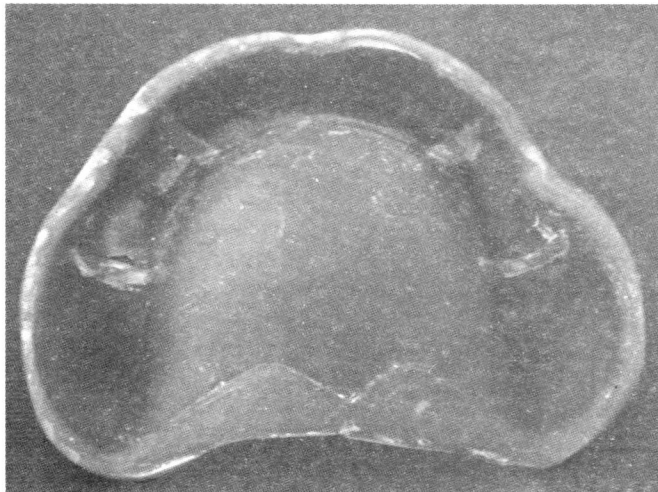

**Fig. 2.4.41:** Maxillary special tray fabricated for anterior flabby ridge situations (tissue surface)

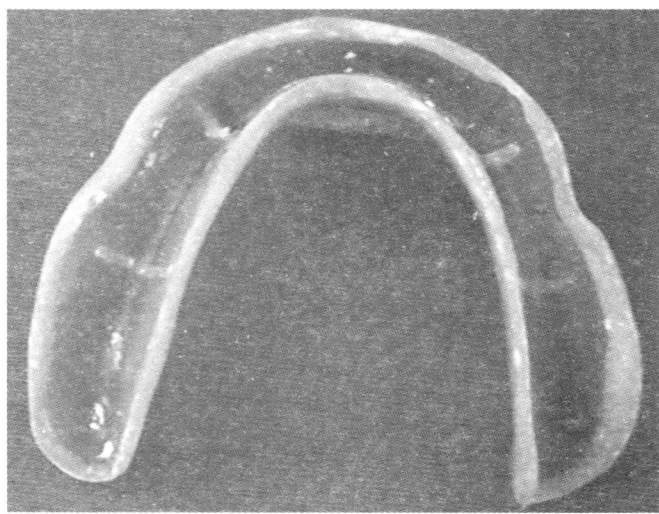

**Fig. 2.4.42:** Mandibular special tray fabricated for anterior flabby ridge situations (tissue surface)

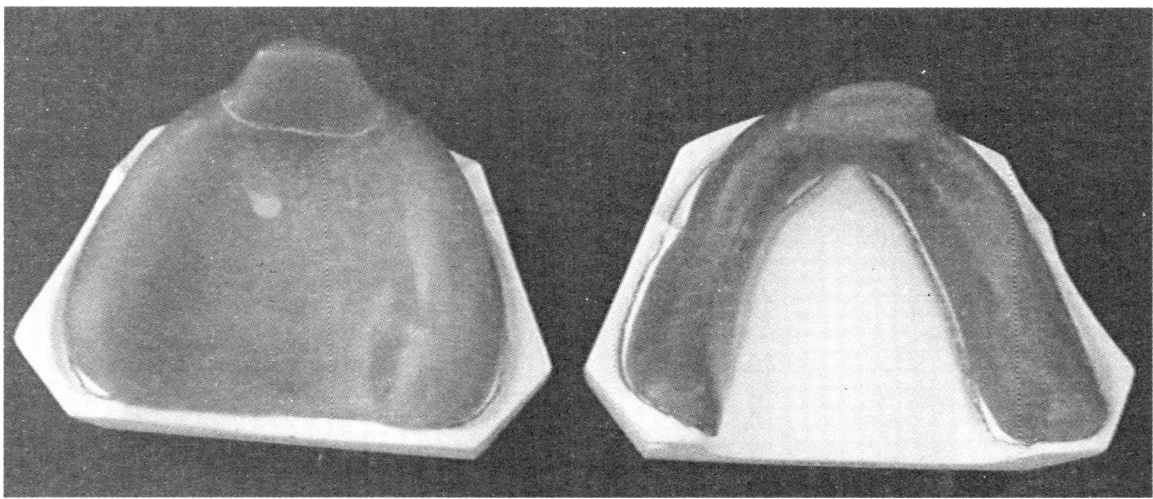

Fig. 2.4.43: Top view

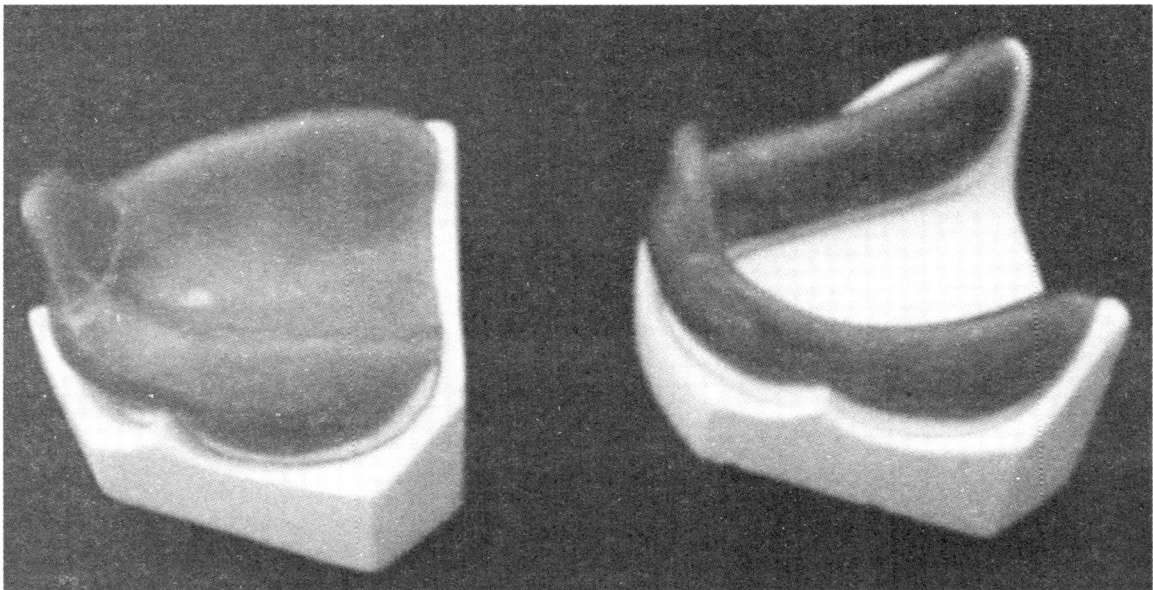

Fig. 2.4.44: Side view

vibrating line. The vibrating line is observed in mouth as patient says series of short "ahs". Posterior border of tray is marked with disposable indelible marker, palatal tissues dried quickly, tray is placed in mouth and patient is asked to say "ah". Now tray is removed and marking on tray are compared with hamular notches and vibrating line. If it is under extended, the length is corrected by addition of modelling compound.

- Place tray in mouth and ask patient to open their mouth wide. If this action causes displacement, the tray is over extended in the hamular notch area.
- Ask the patient to open jaw wide and do lateral movements in protrusion, if this movements cause displacement of tray, then thickness of tray is more in alveolar tubercle area and is being contacted by anterior border of ramus of mandible.

B. The mandibular special tray
- Adjust the buccal flange to a line parallel to the ridge crest and 2 mm short of the external oblique ridge. Check this by palpating external oblique ridge and edge of tray intraorally using the ball of index finger. One should feel the external oblique ridge and the tray border simultaneously. Adjust buccal frenum areas until there is no interference in its normal function.
- Adjust the labial flange of tray until there is no muscle or tissue interference and until tray is about 2 mm short of tissue reflections when the

## 86 Pre-Clinical Prosthodontics

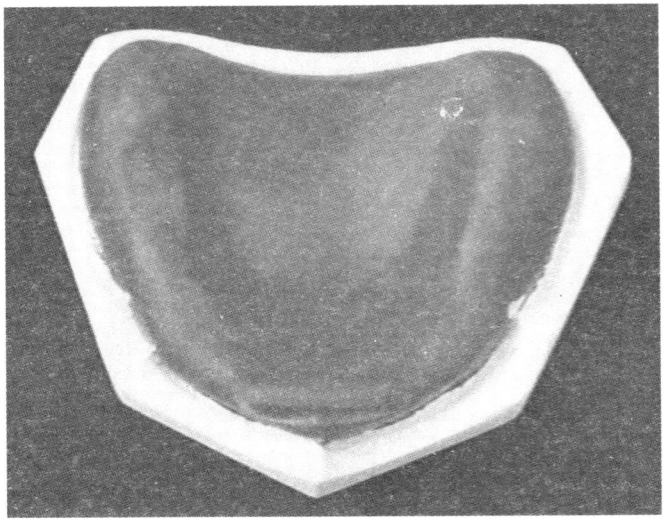

**Fig. 2.4.45:** Maxillary special tray in shellac

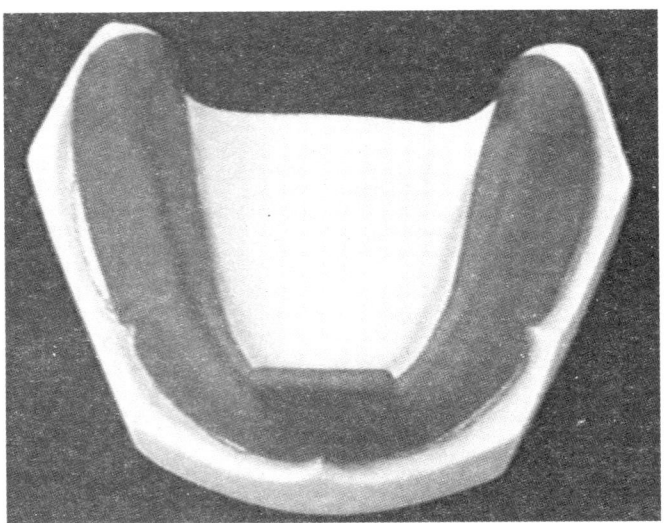

**Fig. 2.4.46:** Mandibular special tray in shellac

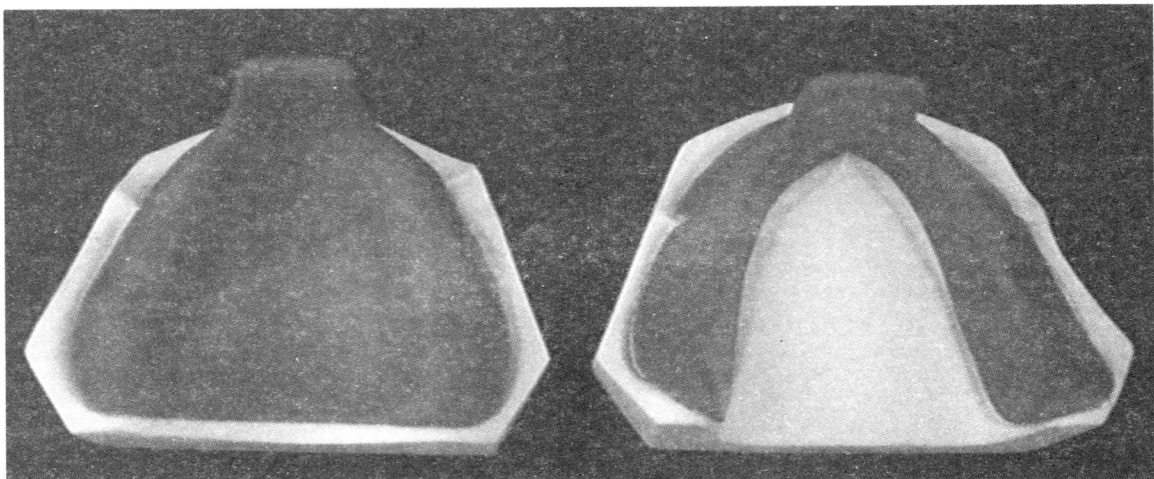

**Fig. 2.4.47:** Special trays with shellac top view

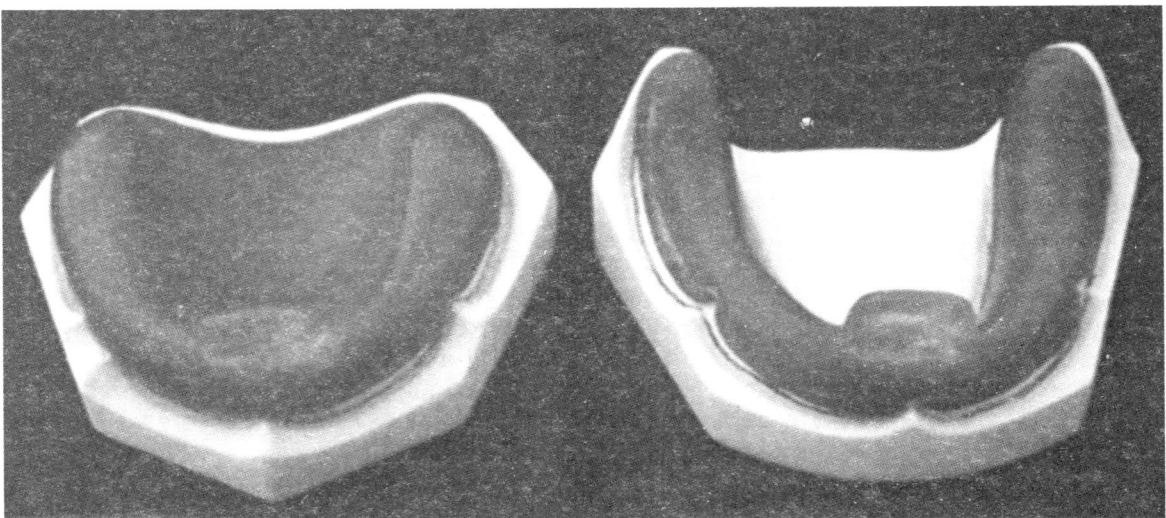

**Fig. 2.4.48**

# Impression Making

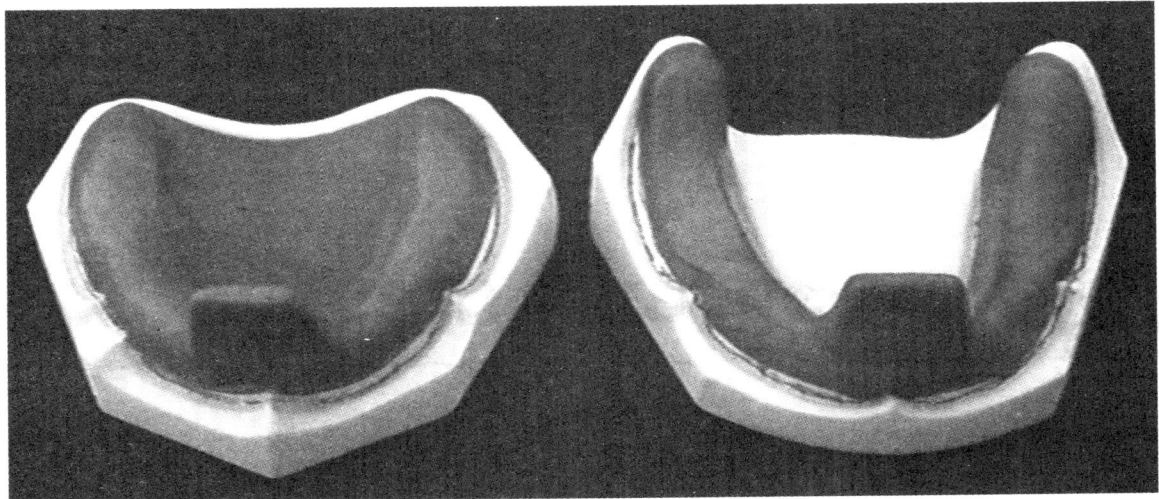
Fig. 2.4.49

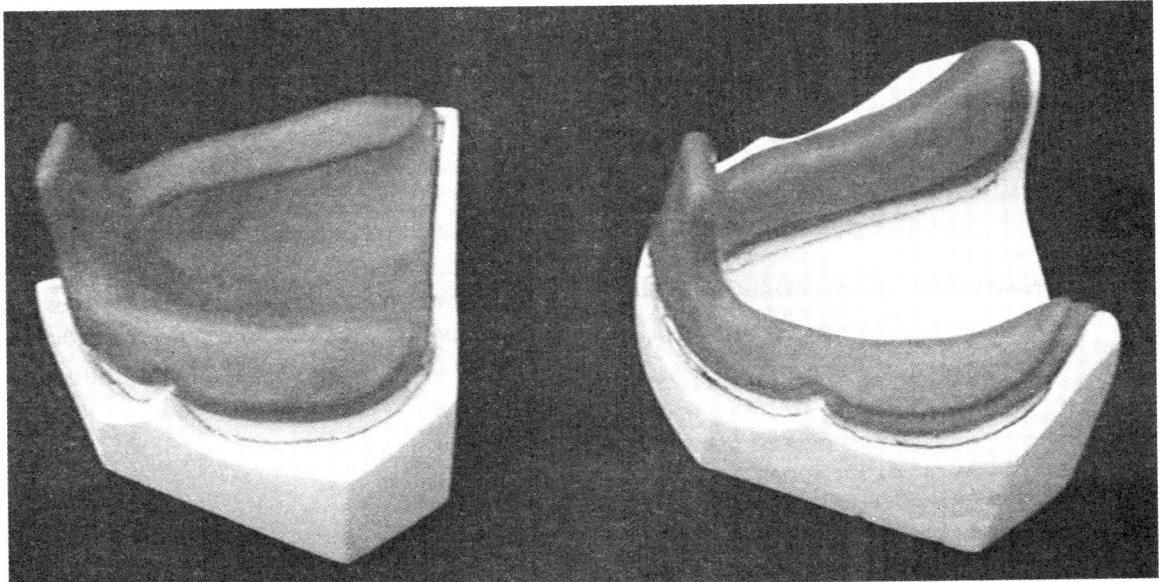
Fig. 2.4.50

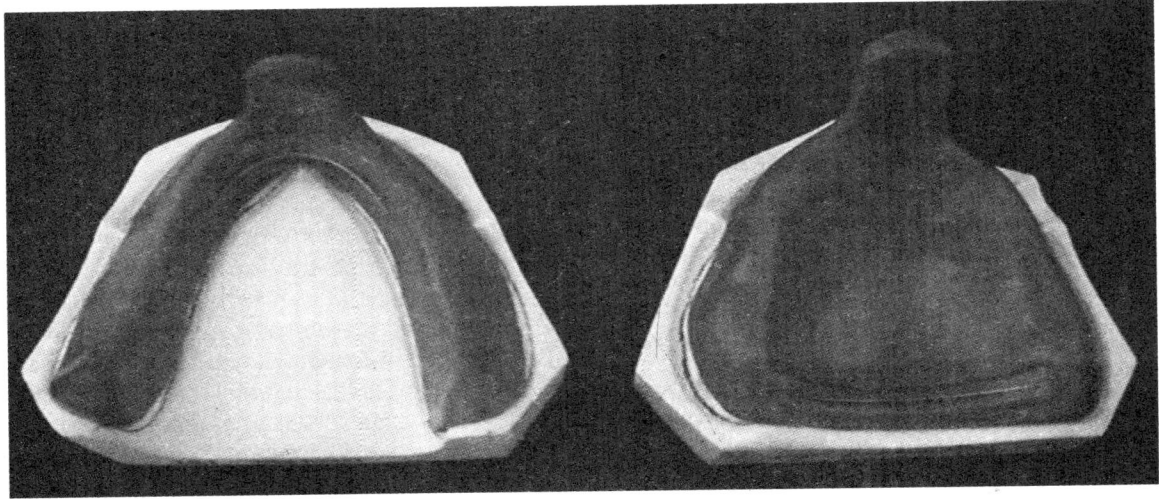
Fig. 2.4.51: Posterior view

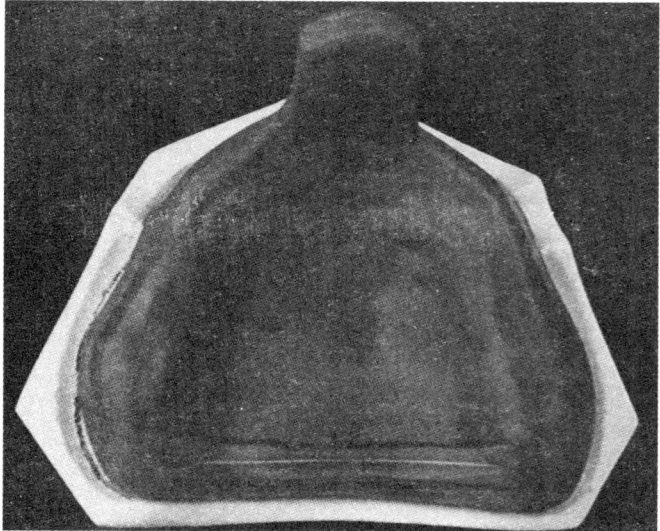

Fig. 2.4.52: Maxillary shellac special tray—reinforced type

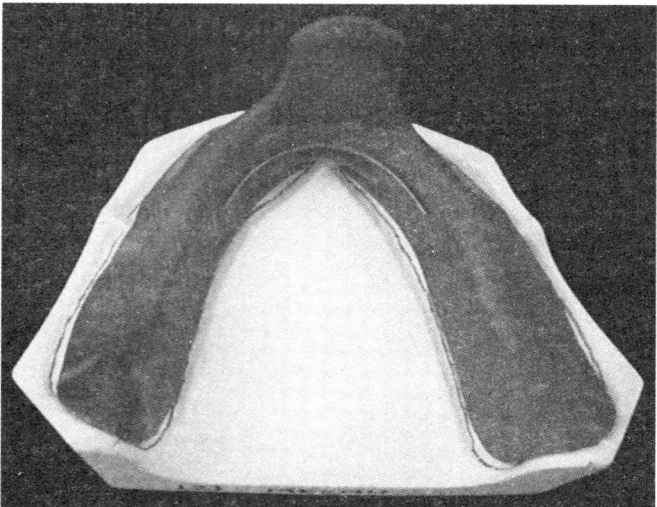

Fig. 2.4.53: Mandibular shellac special tray-reinforced type

lip is gently reflected horizontally. Adjust labial frenum area until there is no interference in its normal function.

- Place tray in mouth and ask patient to separate jaws widely. As the patient attempts to close, exert slight pressure downward on tray and note masseter groove area. Reduce the tray to allow a space of 2 or 3 mm short of buccinator muscle action.

- Ask patient to place their tongue in right buccal vestibule. Dislodgement of tray will indicate over extension of lingual flange on left side in the posterior one third region.
- Over extension of anterior two thirds of lingual flange is checked by asking patients to place their tongue well back on the palate.
- To check tray at lingual frenal attachment, ask patient to open their mouth wide and place the tip of tongue on margin of the upper lip.

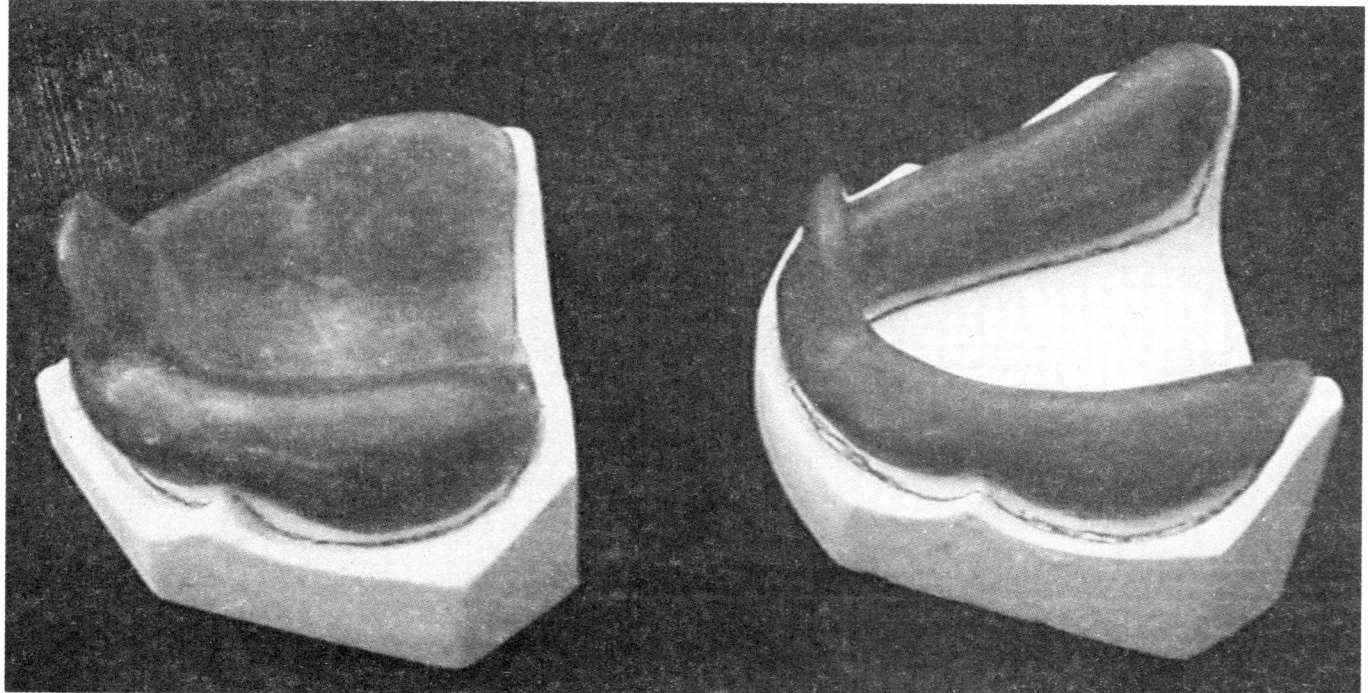

Fig. 2.4.54: Side view

# IMPRESSION BORDER MOLDING

### DEFINITION

- "The shaping of the border areas of an impression tray by functional or manual manipulation of the tissue adjacent to the borders to duplicate the contour and size of the vestibule"—GPT.
- "Determining the extension of a prosthesis by using tissue function or manual manipulation of the tissues to shape the border areas of an impression material"—GPT.

### RATIONALE/OBJECTIVES

- The two main objectives of border molding are:
  1. To shape the border of the impression in order to allow the muscles to function in harmony with the denture.
  2. To improve the border seal of the denture.

### REQUIREMENT OF MATERIALS USED FOR BORDER MOLDING

1. Should have sufficient body to remain in position on the borders during loading of the tray.
2. Should allow some preshaping of the form of the borders without adhering to the fingers.
3. Should have a setting time of 3 to 5 minutes.
4. Should retain adequate flow while seating in the mouth.
5. Should allow finger placement of material into deficient parts after seating the tray.
6. Should not cause excessive displacement of the tissues of the vestibule.
7. Should be readily trimmed and shaped so that excess material can be carved and the border shaped before the final impression is made.

### TYPES

1. Border molding with stick compound.
2. Border molding with autopolymerizing acrylic resin.
3. Border molding with polyether impression paste.
4. Border molding with impression waxes.
5. Border molding with periopak.
6. Border molding with tissue conditioners.

### EQUIPMENT AND MATERIALS (Fig. 2.4.55)

1. Modeling compound sticks.
2. Bunsen burner.
3. Alcohol torch.
4. Special tray.
5. Water bath at about 120°F or 48.9°C.
6. Border molding with stick compound.
7. 2 × 2 sponges.

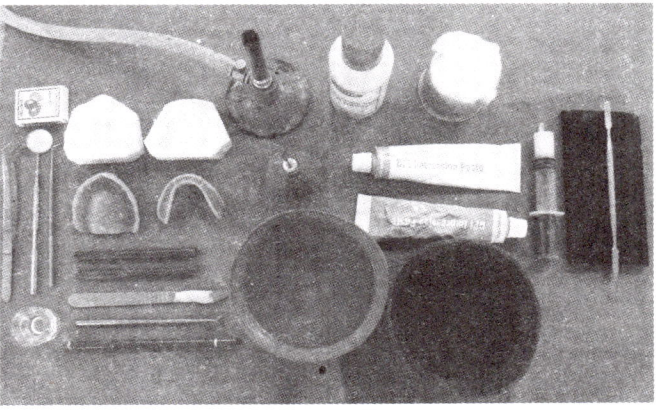

Fig. 2.4.55

8. Wet cotton.
9. Bard Parker blade.
10. Sharp curved scissors.
11. Petrolatum.
12. Mouth wash.

### METHODS

1. Based on manipulation
   a. Manual or digital manipulation
   b. Functional manipulation
   c. Combination of manual and functional manipulation.
2. Based on technique
   a. Open mouth technique.
   b. Closed mouth technique.
   c. Single step or simultaneous border molding.
   d. Incremental or segment wise border molding.

#### Manual or Digital Manipulation

- The contour of the denture borders is obtained by the dentist with digital (finger) manipulation of lips and cheeks of patient within functional limits.
- It is easy to perform and does not require much of patient co-operation.
- It is influenced by the direction of movement and force applied.

#### Functional Manipulation

- The contour of the denture borders is obtained by the functional movements provided by the patients.
- Hence the functional movements mold the borders in harmony with the natural functional movements that take place in daily life.
- Some of the functional movements helping in border molding are:
  i. Opening and closing movements of jaw— molds distobuccal flanges.
  ii. Side to side movements of jaw—molds disto buccal flanges.

iii. Smiling and whistling—molds labial and buccal borders.
iv. Sucking motion—molds buccal frenum and buccal borders.
v. Licking the lips—molds lingual borders.
vi. Occluding on occlusal rims to exert biting pressure.

**Combination of Manual and Functional Manipulation**
- This is the common procedure followed during border molding.
- Digital or manual manipulation of lips and cheeks of patients is done by dentist and patient provides the functional movements required for border molding.

**Open Mouth Technique**
- In this technique the tissues are recorded in their undisplaced position.
- It is most commonly used. The patients mouth is partly opened and tray is held in position.
- Dentist has better control of the procedure and can also see whether muscle trimming is done properly.

**Closed Mouth Technique**
- In this technique the tissues are recorded in their functional and displaced position.
- The patient applies pressure by closing against occlusion rims or teeth that are attached to the impression trays and executes muscle actions such as swallowing, grinning or pursing the lips while the impression material flows.
- Materials used are:
  - impression compound
  - waxes
  - soft liners in conjunction with old dentures
  - The disadvantages of this technique are:
    i. Once the pressure is released, tissues rebound to their original relaxed position and result in unseating of dentures.
    ii. Because of the pressure applied, the tissues are deprived of normal blood supply and results in resorption of residual ridges.

## PROCEDURE
- Border molding can be achieved either with incremental technique using stick compound or one step technique using rubber material such as polyether impression material.
- Incremental technique using stick compound also known as low fusing compound is the most common technique used for border molding. It is available in various colours like green, gray and white, among which green stick compound is most popular.
- Green stick compound is softened over flame by rolling repeatedly to prevent overheating and burning.
- The softened stick compound is flowed along the border of the required segment of the tray.
- The tray is tempered in warm water, placed carefully in patients mouth and necessary movements performed by dentist and patient as explained below.

**Maxillary Border Molding**
- Sequence of border molding
  i. According to Carl O Boucher
     - Labial vestibule
     - Buccal vestibule—Right side
     - Buccal vestibule—Left side
     - Posterior palatal area
  ii. According to Sheldon Winkler:
     Border molding is established in one third segments
     - Right posterior one third
     - Left posterior one third
     - Anterior one-third
     - Posterior palatal area
  iii. According to heart well
     - Distobuccal flange area of both sides including hamular notch and posterior palatal seal area.
     - Mesiobuccal flange right side.
     - Mesiobuccal flange left side.
     - Labial flange right side.
     - Labial flange left side.
- **Movements**
  1. Labial frenum and labial flange
     - Upper lip is elevated and extended:
       - outwards
       - downwards
       - inwards
  2. Buccal frenum
     - Cheek is elevated and pulled
       - outwards
       - downwards
       - inwards
       - backwards
       - forwards
  3. Buccal flange
     - Cheek is extended
       - outwards
       - downwards
       - inwards
  4. Distobuccal angle of buccal flange
     - Patient is asked to open wide and move the mandible from side to side with protrusive movements.
  5. Posterior palatal seal area
     - A strip of softened green stick compound is placed on tray over vibrating line through

hamular notches and tray is seated in mouth. Under pressure and patient is asked to say series of "Ahhh ------".

Mandibular border molding
- Sequence of border molding
  1. According to Carl O Boucher:
     – Labial flange
     – Right buccal flange
     – Left buccal flange
     – Anterior lingual border
     – Posterior lingual border on right side including retromolar pad
     – Posterior lingual border on left side including retromolar pad.
  2. According to Sheldon Winkler:
     i. Lingual border is completed in thirds
        – Right posterior third
        – Left posterior third
        – Anterior third
     ii. Buccal and labial borders completed in thirds
        – Right posterior third
        – Left posterior third
        – Anterior third
     iii. Retromolar pad
  3. According to Heartwall:
     – Distobuccal flange and buccal shelf area bilaterally.
     – Right distolingual flange and retromylohyoid space.
     – Left distolingual flange and retromylohyoid space.
     – Anterior lingual sulcus.
     – Remainder of buccal flange and labial flange of right side.
     – Remainder of buccal flange and labial flange of left side.
- Movements
1. Labial frenum and labial flange
   – Lifting the lower lip
     – outwards
     – downwards
     – inwards
2. Buccal frenum
   – Cheek is lifted
     – outwards
     – upwards
     – inwards
     – backwards
     – forwards
3. Buccal flange
   – Cheek is moved
     – outwards
     – upwards
     – inwards

– The effect of Masseter muscle on the border of impression is recorded by asking the patient to exert a closing force while dentist exerts a downward pressure on the tray.
4. Anterior lingual flange
   – Length of anterior lingual flange is determined by asking patient to protrude his tongue.
   – Thickness of anterior lingual flange is determined by asking patient to push the tongue against anterior part of palate.
5. Lingual flange of both sides in molar region
   – Length and slope of lingual flange in this area is determined by asking patient to protrude the tongue which activates mylohyoid muscle and raises floor of mouth.
   – Asking patient to make "K" sounds also activates mylohyoid muscle.
   – Tip of tongue alternatively touching right and left cheek.
6. Distolingual flange to distobuccal flange
   – Superior constrictor muscle which supports retromylohyoid curtain is activated by asking patient to protrude the tongue.
   – Patient is asked to close the mouth as dentist applies downward force on the tray. This records any effect that the contraction of medial pteryoid muscle has on retromolar curtain.
   – Patient is asked to open wide. If tray is too long, a notch will be formed at the postero medial border of retromolar pad due to the encroachment of tray on the pterygomandibular raphae and tray must be adjusted accordingly.

## SECONDARY IMPRESSIONS

### SYNONYMS
- Final impressions.
- Master impressions.
- Wash impressions.
- Secondary impressions.

### DEFINITION
- The impression that represents the completion of the registration of the surface or object—GPT.

### RATIONALE/OBJECTIVES
- To record as accurately as possible the shape of the mucosa overlying the alveolar ridges and hard

palate together with the functional depth and width of sulci.
- To produce a denture base that will be stable, retentive, comfortable and esthetic and that will pressure the remaining tissues.

## EQUIPMENT AND MATERIALS

1. Border molded impression trays.
2. Final impression material.
   - Zinc oxide eugenol paste.
   - Alginate
   - Silicone impression material.
   - Polysulfide impression material.
   - Polyether impression material.
   
   Normal zinc oxide eugenol is used as final impression material. But, if the patient has very dry mouth an elastomeric impression material should be used as ZOE paste is less likely to adhere to tissues. Elastomeric materials may also be used when there are severe undercuts.
3. Glass slab
4. Spatula
5. Petrolatum
6. Straight hand piece and burs
7. Lecron carver
8. T burnisher
9. Mouth mirror
10. Indelible pencil

## PREPARATION

Border molded impression tray is prepared to secure the final impression.
1. The relief and spacer wax is removed from inside the tray along with any border molding material that has flowed over it.
2. Any excess material on the outside of the tray is removed.
3. Thickness of labial flange should be adjusted to approximately 2.5 to 3 mm thickness from one buccal frenum to other.
4. Approximately 0.5 mm thickness of border molded material is removed from the inner, outer and top surface of border.
5. The border molded material over posterior area of maxillary tray is not adjusted to serve three functions,
   i. Enchances posterior palatal seal by slightly displacing soft tissues.
   ii. Serves as a guide for proper positioning of tray for making final impression.
   iii. Prevents excess impression material from running down the patients throat.
6. Holes are placed in impression trays to prevent air entrapment and to provide escape ways for final impression material.
   i. Maxillary tray
      - Over the center of palatal rugae area.
      - Over residual ridge sites where soft tissues are mobile and displaceable. This avoids recording tissues in displaced position.
   ii. Mandibular tray
      - In the center of alveolar groove, approximately 10 mm apart.
      - Over retromolar pads. This relieves pressure over crest of alveolar ridge and retromolar pads.
7. Tray adhesive is applied to inner surface of tray if materials like elastomers or alginate are used as final impression materials.
8. A light coating of petroleum jelly is applied to skin around the lips and mouth to prevent the zinc oxide eugenol paste from adhering to the skin.

## MAKING IMPRESSION

- The final impression material of choice is mixed according to manufacturers instructions. If material of choice is ZOE paste, disperse base and catalyst paste in a equal lengths over glass slab and make a smooth uniform mix, spread the mix over large area in a thin layer in order to reduce trapped air bubbles.
- Load the tray with impression material and spread out evenly to all parts of the tray, including the borders.
- Placement of tray
  a. **Maxilla**
     - The tray is centered as it is carried to position on upper ridge by observing position of labial frenum relative to labial notch in the tray. Once frenum is positioned within the notch, the index fingers of each hand are shifted to the first molar region and with alternating pressure tray is carried upward, without displacement of front end of tray downward, until posterior palatal seal of the tray fits properly in the hamular notches and across the palate. The tray is held in position with a finger placed in the palate immediately anterior to posterior palatal seal.
  b. **Mandible**
     - The tray is rotated into the mouth in a horizontal plane with the anterior handle, until it is over the residual ridge. Now, the patient is asked to raise the tongue slightly and the tray is moved downwards towards its final position. The index fingers of each hand are positioned over posterior handles of tray with alternating gentle pressure, the tray is seated until the buccal flanges come into contact with the mucosa covering the buccal shelf. Instruct the

patient to bring the tongue forward and touch the upper lip, while the impression material sets.
- Border molding movements are repeated until the impression material sets.
- When the final impression material has set, the tray is removed from the mouth and inspected for acceptability. For easy removal, the lip or cheek of patient is lifted on one side so that air goes beneath the dentures and breaks the seal.

## IMPRESSION EVALUATION

- The completed impression is examined and immediately placed in cold water for one to two minutes. Unless there are large undercuts, it is best to reinsert and evaluate the quality of the impression. It should exhibit excellent retention and stability, even more than the completed border molded tray, unless the ridge is very flat or thin.
- Small voids present in the impression can be ignored, as they can be best removed from the master cast.
- If there are large voids, due to insufficient material used then the impression should be repeated.
- Thin over extensions often seen over posterior borders due to free flow of impression material can be easily trimmed with sharp scissors.
- A thick buccal border on one side and a thin buccal border on opposite side indicates that the tray was out of position on the side of thick border and impression should be repeated.
- A thin labial border with tray exposed on inside surface of labial flange indicates placement of tray too posteriorly over anterior ridge and impression should be repeated.
- A thick lingual border on one side and a thin lingual border on opposite side indicates that the lower tray was out of position on the side of thin border and impression should be repeated.
- A thick labial border in the upper arch with tray exposed over the anterior slope of palate indicates placement of tray too far forward in relation to residual ridge and impression should be repeated.
- A thin anterior lingual border with tray exposed on inside surface of lingual flange indicates placement of lower tray too far forward in relation to residual ridge and impression should be repeated.
- Excess thickness of impression material over the fitting surface of the tray and material unsupported by borders of tray indicates that the tray was not seated down sufficiently on residual ridge and impression should be repeated.
- The tray exposed over the fitting surface and borders showing through the final impression material indicates that the tray has been seated on the residual ridge with too much pressure and impression should be repeated.
- The correct thickness of material over the fitting surface of the tray, but with the border showing through the final impression material, indicates that the tray is over extended in that area.

# BEADING AND BOXING OF FINAL IMPRESSION

## DEFINITION

- The enclosure of an impression to produce the desired size and form of the base of the cast and to preserve desired details.

## RATIONALE/OBJECTIVES

1. To preserve the functional width and depth of the sulcus in the final cast by beading the final impression.
2. To obtain a uniform, smooth and desired form and thickness of the base of cast by boxing the final impression.

## EQUIPMENT AND MATERIALS

1. Completed final impressions.
2. Beading materials
   - Beading wax (usually blue in colour) (or) orthodontic wax (or) utility wax (or)
   - Mix of dental plaster and pumice (or)
   - Caulking compound
3. Boxing materials
   - Boxing wax (usually white in colour) (or)
   Metal strips (or)
   Sheet of heavy lead foil
4. Base plate wax
5. Wax knife
6. Wax spatula
7. Bunsen burner
8. Plaster bowl
9. Plaster spatula
10. Plaster knife
11. Water
12. Bard Parker blade
13. Separating medium
14. A sheet of wax paper (or) glass slab.

## METHODS

1. Wax beading and boxing method.
2. Plaster of Paris and pumice beading and wax boxing method.
3. Caulking compound beading and paddle boxing method.

## FABRICATION

### (1) Wax beading and boxing method

- This method is especially suitable for impressions made in zinc oxide eugenol impression paste as it readily adheres to the beading wax.
  1. Place the impression on the bench with impression surface up. Align the ridge portion of impression approximately parallel to the bench top by using soft wax or modeling clay. Adjust the height until a boxing wax strip extends approximately 13 mm above the highest point on the impression.
  2. Place a base plate wax cut in desired form in the tongue space of mandibular impression and seal it approximately 3 to 4 mm below the border of the impression with hot wax spatula.
  3. Adapt beading wax around the periphery of the impression. This wax should be approximately 4 mm wide, 3 to 4 mm below the border of the impression and 6 mm past the posterior borders. Seal the beading wax to the impression with hot spatula.
  4. Place the beaded impression on the bench top, warm the boxing wax over bunser burner until flexible and fold it around the beaded impression. Seal the end of boxing strip to the underlying layer of beading wax. Seal the beading wax to the boxing strip on both the impression side and the underside to make it water tight.
  5. Fill the impression with cool water to check for leaks. Leakages can be filled by adding additional wax.
  6. Now fabricate the master cast by pouring mixed dental stone into the boxed impression. Once dental stone sets, peel of the wax and place the impression in warm water to recover the master cast (Figs 2.4.56 to 2.4.63).

### (2) Plaster of Paris and pumice beading and wax boxing method

- This method is especially suitable for impressions made in rubber base or silicone impression materials because unlike ZOE impression paste these materials do not adhere to the beading wax.
  1. The handles of the trays are cut off with a fissure bur or carborundum disc. Equal amounts of

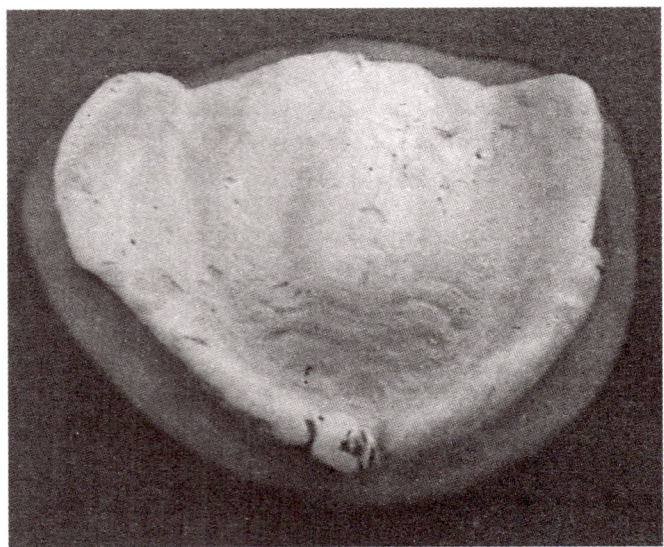

Fig. 2.4.56: Wax beading done for maxillary final impression

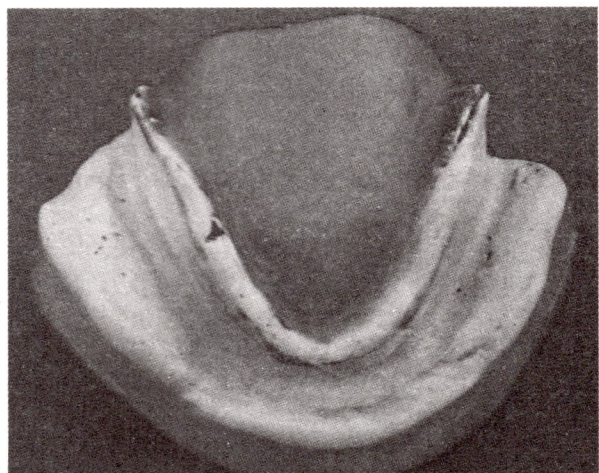

Fig. 2.4.57: Wax bending done for mandibular final impression

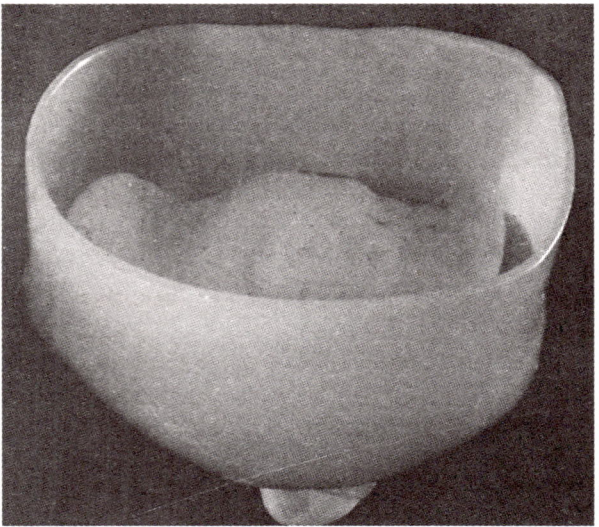

Fig. 2.4.58: Wax bending and boxing completed for maxillary final impression

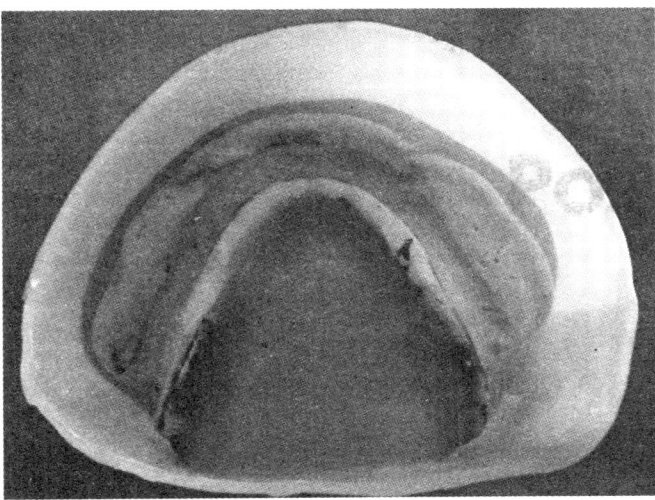

Fig. 2.4.59: Wax bending and boxing completed for maxillary final impression

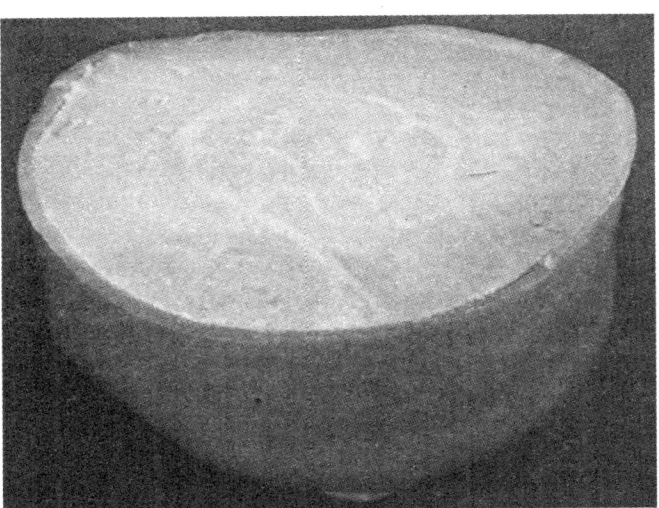

Fig. 2.4.60: Dental stone poured into the maxillary beaded and boxed final impression

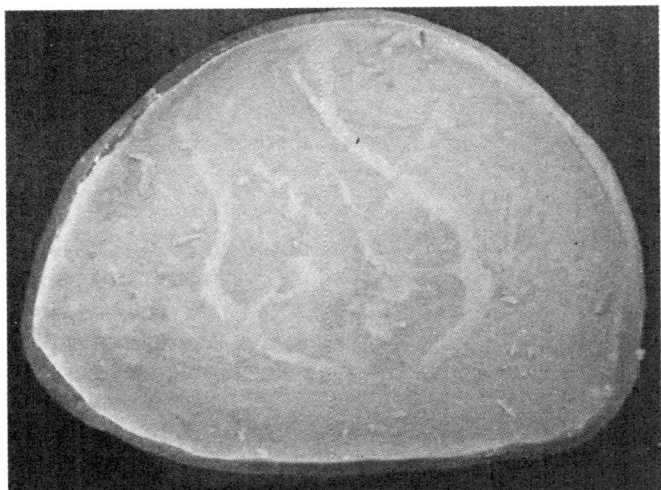

Fig. 2.4.61: Dental stone poured into the mandibular beaded and boxed final impression

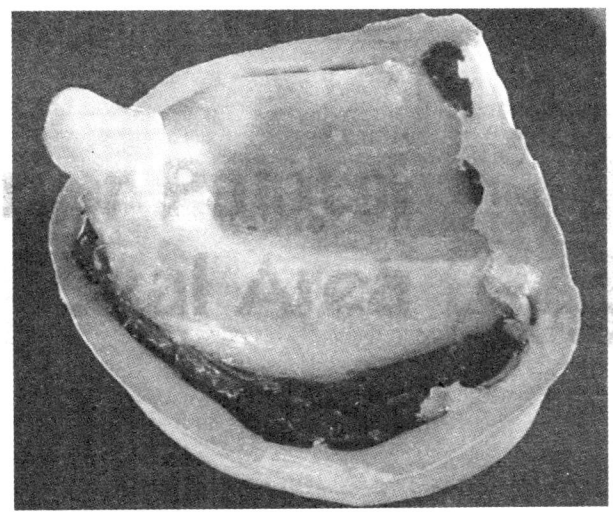

Fig. 2.4.62: Maxillary final impression along with master cast, after removal of bending and boxing wax

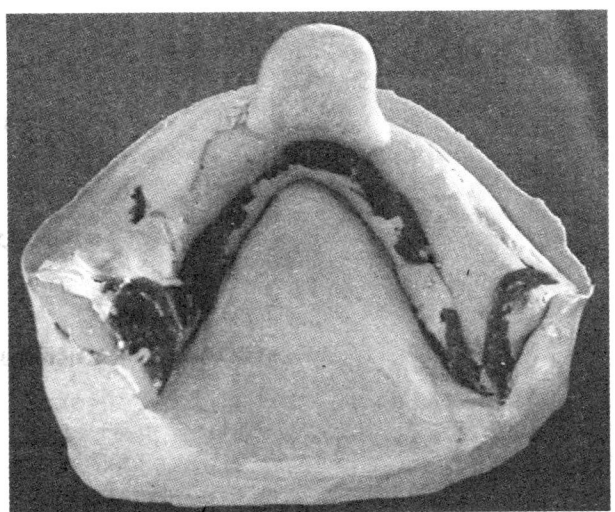

Fig. 2.4.63: Mandibular final impression along with master cast, after removal of beading and boxing wax

plaster of paris and pumice are combined and thoroughly mixed while dry to get a uniform mix. The pumice weakens the set plaster and facilitates easy separation of cast after pouring.

2. Water is added to plaster pumice mix to make a stiff mix. It should be spatulated thoroughly to reduce setting time. Place the stiff mix on a glass slab. Now place the impression over the stiff mix with impression surface facing upwards. Align the ridge portion of impression parallel to bench top. Use a spatula to draw the plaster mix around the impression until it is 3 to 4 mm below the border.

3. After the plaster–pumice is set, the land areas are trimmed so that they are about 4 mm wide and about 6 mm past the posterior borders.

4. Adapt the boxing wax to the beaded impression so that the wax extends at least 13 mm above the highest point on the impression. Seal the boxing wax to the plaster with a hot spatula. Paint the plaster surfaces with a separating medium.
5. Fill the impression with cool water to check for leaks. Leakages can be filled by adding additional wax.
6. Now fabricate master cast by pouring mixed dental stone into the boxed impression. After setting, cut away the plaster and pumice beading and place the impression in warm water to recover the master cast.

*(3) Caulking compound beading and paddle boxing method*

- This method of beading and boxing was described by Blank in 1961.
  1. Adapt a strip of caulking compound rope 3 to 4 mm below the borders of the impression. Seal the caulking compound to impression with a warm spatula.
  2. Fold a metal boxing strip around the beaded impression and secure it with a rubber band. Boxing strip should be approximately 13 mm above the highest point on the impression. With the help of warm spatula seal it to the caulking compound.
  3. Take a table tennis paddle and attach metal strips around the borders. Melt scrap wax into this metal enclosure to serve as a wax base for boxing the impression.
  4. Place the boxed impression over the paddle and seal the boxed impression to wax on the paddle.
  5. Now fabricate master cast by pouring mixed dental stone into the boxed impression. After setting, remove boxing strip and caulking compound and place the impression in warm water to recover the master cast.

*(4) Measurements*

- Beading wax
  - 4 mm wide
  - 3 to 4 mm below border of impression
  - 6 mm past the posterior borders
- Boxing wax
  - A height of 13 mm above the highest point on the impression.

# Record Bases 5
CHAPTER

To fabricate close fitting auto-polymerizing acrylic resin baseplates and wax occlusion rims that will be used later for obtaining the occlusal plane, vertical dimension, centric relation, and the face-bow transfer. When this is accomplished the task of recording jaw relations, the transfer of the models to the articulator, and the try-in of the trial denture are easier with marked improvement of the occlusion and vertical dimension of the final denture.

## RECORD BASES

### SYNONYMS
- Base plates
- Trial denture bases
- Transfer bases
- Temporary denture bases

### DEFINITION
- A material or device representing the base of a denture. It is used for making maxillomandibular relation records and arranging teeth—GPT.

### RATIONALE / OBJECTIVES
1. To retain the recording medium or device used for recording maxillomandibular relations.
2. To aid in transfer of accurate jaw relationships to an articulator.
3. To enable the setting of artificial teeth for the trial denture.

### REQUIREMENTS
- According to Elder (1955) record bases should have following requirements.
    1. The record base should adapt to the basal seat area as the finished denture base.
    2. The record base should have the same border form as the finished denture base.
    3. The record base should be sufficiently rigid to resist biting forces.
    4. The record base should be dimensionally stable.
    5. The record base as constructed should permit its use as a base for setting up teeth.
    6. It should be possible to construct record bases quickly, easily and inexpensively.
    7. Record bases should have no undesirable colour.

- Tucker (1966) added that the base plate should not abrade the cast during removal and replacement. He also stated that base plate should bond to the material used for blocking undercuts on the cast, so that it become part of the base plate.

## TYPES

1. **Temporary record bases**
   - Shellac base plates.
   - Cold cure acrylic resin.
   - Vacuum formed vinyl and polystyrene.
   - Base plate wax.
2. **Permanent record bases**
   - Heat cure acrylic resin.
   - Gold.
   - Chromium–cobalt alloy.
   - Chromium–nickel alloy.

### NOTE
- Temporary record bases are eventually discarded and replaced by denture base material, once their role in establishing jaw relation, teeth arrangement and try in is complete. Permanent record bases are not discarded and become part of the actual base of the finished complete denture.

## TEMPORARY RECORD BASES

### Shellac base plates

- Shellac which is derived from the resinous exudate of a scale insect, forms the basic constituent of shellac base plate. Fillers such as powdered talc or mica are added to increase the strength of shellac base plate.
- It is the commonly used material for fabrication of record bases. They are available in shapes of maxillary and mandibular arches.

*Advantages*

1. They will adapt to intimate contact with the master cast.
2. Record bases can be fabricated in minimal amount of time using shellac base plates.
3. Shellac base plates are inexpensive and can be easily adapted to master cast using readily available laboratory equipment.
4. If any mistakes occur during fabrication of record bases with shellac base plates can be corrected easily by reheating and readapting to the master cast.
5. Uniform thickness can be maintained all over the record base.

*Disadvantages*

1. Shellac base plates have less strength and require reinforcement with other materials to improve strength.
2. Shellac base plates are brittle materials and easily susceptible to breakage.
3. There are chances of loosing their initial adaptation to the master cast.
4. Shellac tends to warp when subjected to repeated changes in temperature, like during fabrication of occlusal rims and setting of artificial teeth over record bases.

### Cold Cure Acrylic Resin

- They consist of powder and liquid components.

*Powder*

- Unpolymerized methyl methacrylate monomer.
- Hydroquinone (inhibitor).
- Glycol dimethacrylate (cross linking agent).
- Dimethyl - para - toluidine (activator).
- It is one of the most commonly used material for fabrication of record bases.

*Advantages*

1. They have better strength and does not require any reinforcement.
2. They have better stability to heat and does not warp during fabrication of occlusal rims and setting of artificial teeth over record bases.
3. They are dimensionally stable and help in accurate recording of jaw relations.
4. They remain accurate close fit to the master cast.
5. Their handling characteristics are suitable for constructing record bases that are both serviceable and economical.

*Disadvantages*

1. When compared to shellac, it requires more time in fabrication of record bases.
2. It is difficult to control required thickness during fabrication of record bases.
3. Residual monomer present in record bases can cause irritation to oral tissues.

### Vacuum Formed vinyl or polystyrene

- A sheet of required thickness thermoplastic resin and a thermal vacuum machine is used to fabricate record bases.

*Advantages*

1. Simple technique and easy to fabricate record bases.

2. Minimal amount required in fabrication of record bases.
3. Uniform thickness can be maintained all over the record bases.
4. Adequate rigidity required for record bases can be obtained.
5. It can be adapted accurately to the master cast.

*Disadvantages*
1. Expensive due to more cost of the required equipment.
2. It is difficult to achieve intimate adaptation to cast in deep recesses and border reflections.
3. It is difficult to form smooth rounded borders from only one layer of resin sheet.

### Base Plate Wax

– Extra hard base plate wax can be used in fabrication of record bases. They are not the common materials used for fabrication of record bases.

*Advantages*
1. Fabrication of record bases using base plate wax is easy and rapid.
2. It is inexpensive and easily available.
3. It is pink in colour providing esthetic quality.
4. It is easy to gain more space to set teeth when inter ridge space is less.

*Disadvantages*
1. It lacks rigidity.
2. It lacks dimensional stability.

## PERMANENT RECORD BASES

### Heat Cure Acrylic Resin

- The composition of heat cure acrylic resin is almost similar to cold cure acrylic resin except for the activator used. In case of cold cure acrylic resin, tertiary amine such as dimethyl - para - toludine is used as activator and in case of heat cure acrylic resin, external heat supplied acts as activator.

*Advantages*
1. They can form rigid, accurate and dimensionally stable record bases.
2. It is possible to control thickness of the record bases during waxing up.
3. The record bases will subsequently become part of the denture.
4. Retention and stability can be tested in the mouth prior to processing of final dentures and if required, steps can be taken to improve retention and stability at jaw relation stage itself.
5. It requires only minimal finishing and polishing.

*Disadvantages*
1. It is more time consuming and expensive to wax, flask, process and finish the record base.
2. The master cast usually gets damaged during processing, so a duplicate cast (mounting cast) has to be constructed.
3. During second curing process for attachment of teeth to record base may cause dimensional changes in the record base.

### Cast Alloys

- Permanent record bases can be fabricated by using casting gold alloys or base metal alloys such as chromium-cobalt, chromium-nickel alloys.

*Advantages*
1. They form rigid, accurate and dimensionally stable record bases.
2. They add more weight to mandibular dentures and help in retention and stability.
3. They are good thermal conductors and help in improved oral feelings and sensitivity to heat and cold.
4. They subsequently become part of the final denture.
5. They can be adviced for patients who frequently break their dentures.
6. They are capable of withstanding the stresses and strains exerted during trimming.

*Disadvantages*
1. It takes more time for fabrication of record bases as casting procedures are involved.
2. It is more expensive because of costly materials and procedures involved.

## EQUIPMENT AND MATERIALS

### A. For Fabrication of Record Bases with Shellac Base Plates

1. Maxillary and mandibular shellac base plates
2. Master cast
3. Bunsen burner
4. Chip blow
5. Alcohol torch
6. Match box
7. Rubber bowl
8. Cold water
9. Wet cotton
10. Powdered talc
11. Pumice plaster mix (to block undercuts on cast)
12. Wax spatula

13. Pair of straight and curved scissors
14. Non clogging rubber abrasive wheels.

### B. For fabricating of Record Bases with Cold Cure Acrylic

1. Cold cure acrylic powder and liquid
2. Powder dispenser and liquid dropper
3. Master cast
4. Separating medium
5. Paint brush
6. Dapen dish
7. Base plate wax (to block undercuts on cast)
8. Wax spatula
9. Lecron carver
10. Bard Parker blade
11. Hot water
12. Plaster bowl
13. Pressure pot
14. Acrylic trimming burs
15. Base plate mold
16. Wooden roller
17. Silicone lubricant
18. Sheet of cellphane
19. Petroleum jelly
20. Cement spatula
21. Base plate wax
22. Large round bur
23. Boxing wax
24. Dental stone
25. Rubber bands
26. Rubber bowl
27. Straight spatula
28. Water.

### FABRICATION

- Shellac base plates and cold cure acrylic resins are the most common materials used for fabrication of record bases. Hence fabrication of record bases with these two materials is discussed in detail.

### A. Fabrication of Record Bases with Shellac Base Plates

- Soak the cast in clear slurry water or rub powdered talc on the cast inorder to avoid sticking of base plate to the cast when heated.
- Fill the undercuts on cast with a mix of one part flour of pumice to one part plaster.
- Soften the shellac base plate over bunsen burner flame and place it over the cast or place the shellac base plate on the cast and a brush flame from a bunsen burner is moved slowly over the surface of the shellac until it appears shiny and material slumps onto the cast.
- Firm pressure is applied with wet fingers or wet cotton to adapt the shellac base plate to the palatal portion of maxillary cast or to the lingual surface of mandibular cast.
- The material is now reheated and adapted over the crest of the ridge and into the reflections.
- While the material is still warm and soft, it is removed from the cast and trimmed with scissors, leaving approximately 5 mm beyond the edge of the cast.
- Now the shellac is again repositioned on cast, reheated and readapted. The trimmed edges are heated using alcohol torch, elevated from the cast, folded back on to the shellac base plate itself and burnished with a No. 7 wax spatula to form a smooth, rounded bur.
- Cool the shellac base plate and remove it from the cast. If necessary, trim the borders with non clogging rubber abrasive wheels, store the shellac base plates on the cast to minimise warpage before use (Figs 2.5.1 to 2.5.9).

### Reinforcement of record bases made with shellac base plates

- Shellac base plates should be reinforced to improve both the strength and rigidity.
- A steel wire of 12 to 14 group is embedded across the posterior palatal seal area in maxillary base plate and it is embedded lingually to the crest of the ridge from one premolar to other premolar area in mandibular base plate.

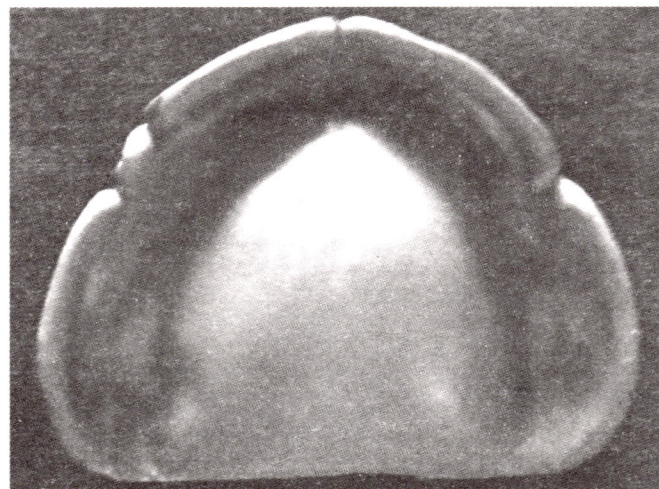

**Fig. 2.5.1:** Maxillary record base in shellac—tissue surface

## Record Bases 101

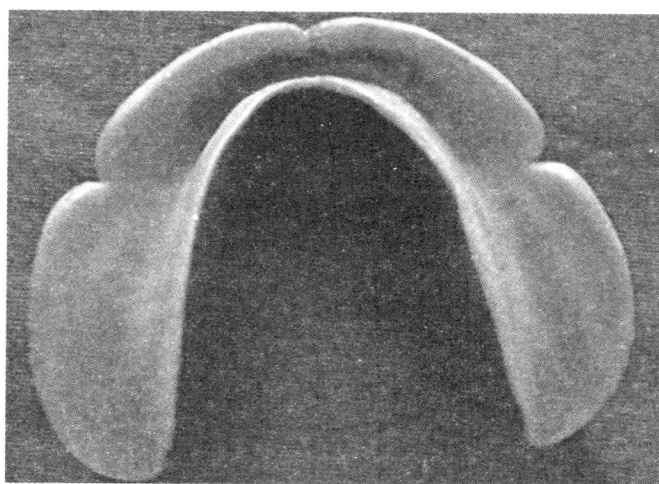

Fig. 2.5.2: Mandibular record base in shellac—tissue surface

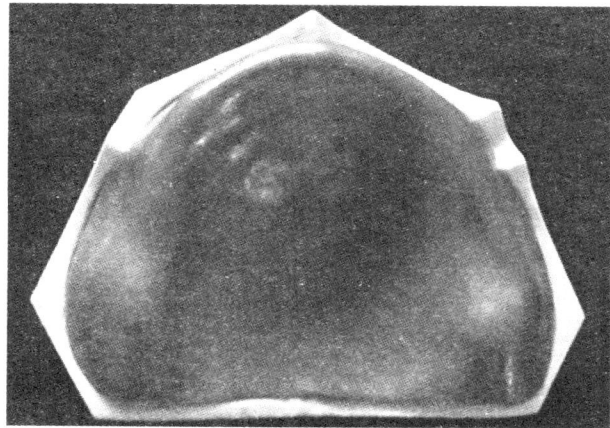

Fig. 2.5.5: Maxillary shellac record base fitted to master cast—top view

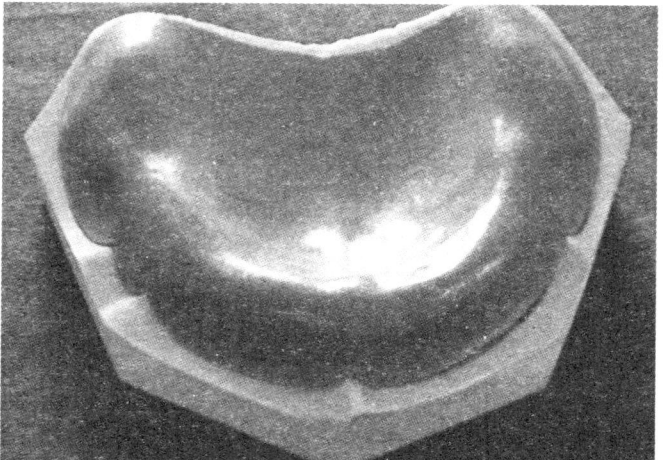

Fig. 2.5.3: Maxillary shellac record base fitted to master cast—front view

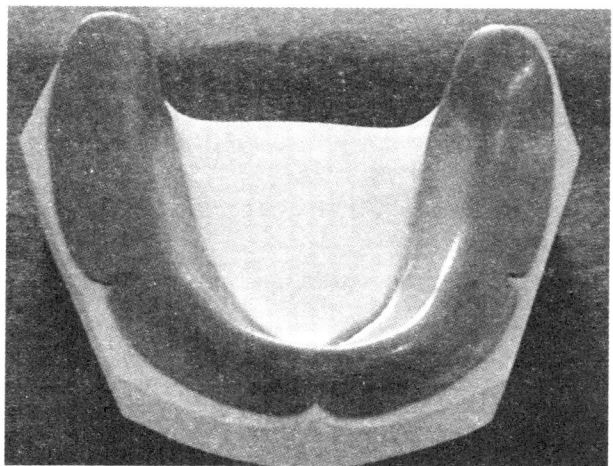

Fig. 2.5.6: Mandibular shellac record base fitted to master cast—front view

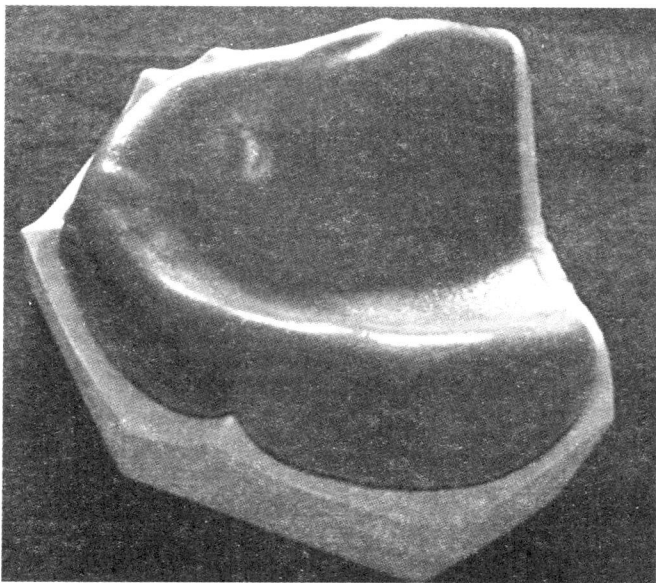

Fig. 2.5.4: Maxillary shellac record base fitted to master cast—side view

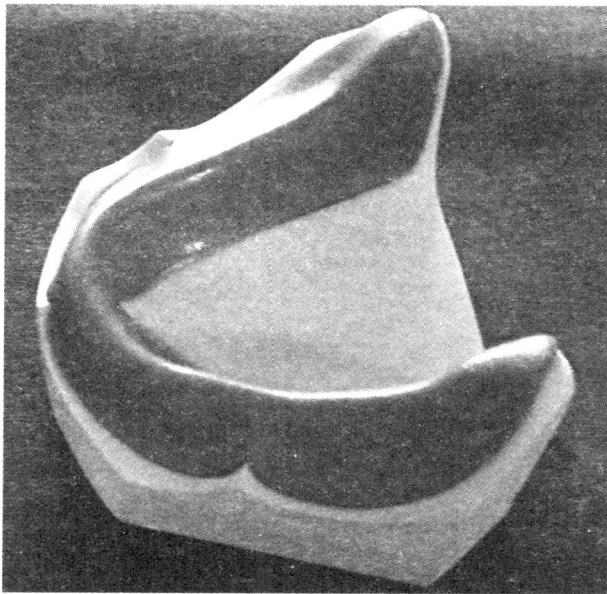

Fig. 2.5.7: Mandibular shellac record base fitted to master cast—side view

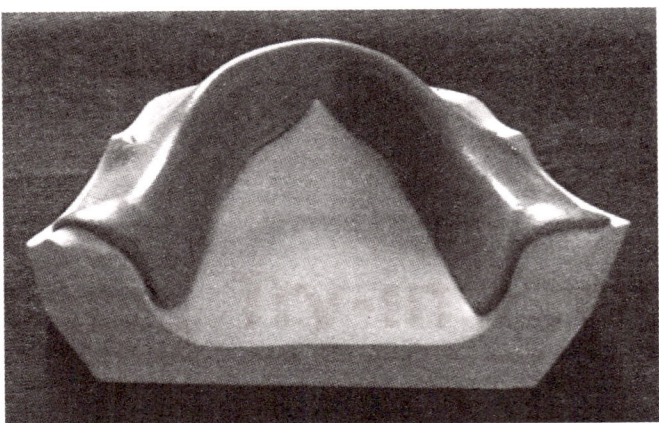

**Fig. 2.5.8:** Mandibular shellac record base fitted to master cast—posterior view

Stabilization of record bases made with shellac base plates
- Shellac base plates have a tendency to warp and to avoid this many materials and methods are used to stabilize them.
- Materials used to stabilize shellac base plates are
  - Lead foil.
  - Zinc oxide eugenol impression paste.
  - Elastomeric impression materials.
  - Autopolymerizing resins.

### B. Fabrication of Record Bases with Cold Cure Acrylic Resins

Methods
1. Sprinkle on method
2. Finger adapted dough method (non flasking method)
3. Flasking method
4. Stone-mold method
5. Wax-confined method

### 1. Sprinkle on Method
- It is the excellent method for producing well adapted record bases using cold cure acrylic resin polymerization shrinkage will be less with this procedure.
- Block out the undercuts on the master cast with base plate wax and apply separating medium (tinfoil substitute) to the cast. Undercuts are not severe, they can be blocked by applying soft curing resin with paint brush (or) sprinkle on method.
- Paint brush method is nothing but blocking the minor undercuts on cast by dipping the paint brush into liquid and then into powder and brushing this combination over the undercuts of the cast.
- Once undercuts are blocked and separating medium applied, a thin layer of powder (polymer) is sprinkled over small surface of cast and sufficiently wetted with liquid (monomer) to produce a slight flow. Alternate applications of powder and liquid are made until a thickness of 2 to 3 mm has been developed.
- Now allow the record base to cure under an inverted plaster bowl or in a pressure pot under warm water for 20 minutes at 20 Psi pressure. Record bases cured under pressure results in less porosity, but do not seem to fit as well as those curved at normal atmospheric pressure.
- The completed record base is then removed, trimmed and polished. Store the finished record base in water until ready for use.

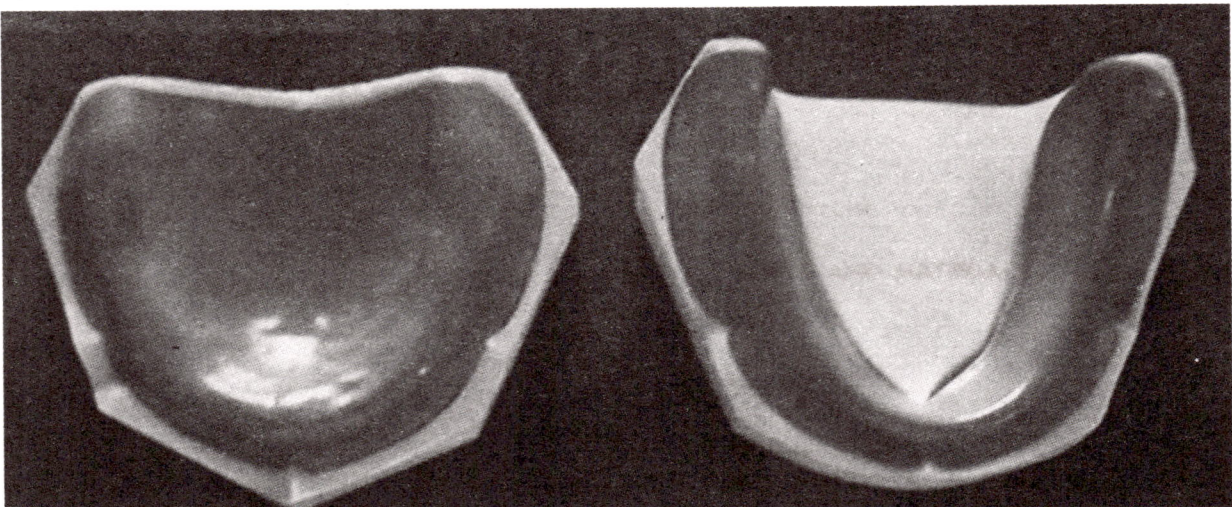

**Fig. 2.5.9**

## 2. Finger Adapted Dough Method (non flasking method)

- Block out undercuts on cast with wax or soft curing resin and apply separating medium (tin foil substitute) to the cast.
- Proportion and mix the cold cure resin powder and liquid according to the manufacturers recommendations when it reaches the dough stage, it is rolled into a cigar shape, placed on a roller board and rolled to the desired thickness of 2 to 3 mm.
- A thin film of petrolatum should be applied to roller board, roller and fingers to prevent resin from adhering. Wetting the fingers with water also prevents resin from adhering to fingers.
- Now the rolled resin sheet is placed over the cast, adapted to the hard palate area of maxillary cast or lingual surface of mandibular cast first and then onto the crest of the ridge and into the reflection area.
- Place the record base on cast under a plaster bowl or in a pessure pot for polymerization.
- After polymerization has been completed, remove the record base and do the trimming, finishing and polishing.
  **Trimming** – with arbor bands mounted on lathe
  **Finishing** – with acrylic burs and sand papers
  **Polishing** – with wet pumice and rag wheels
- Final dimensions of record base should be

  i. Maxillary record base
     - 1 mm thickness over crest and facial slopes of the ridge (for easy placement of teeth).
     - 2 mm thickness in hard palate area (for rigidity).
  ii. Mandibular record base
     - 1 mm thickness over crest and facial slopes of the ridge.
     - 2 mm thickness in the lingual flange area.

### Disadvantages of this technique

1. Repeated contact with resin during adaptation may lead to contamination of resin and also results in contact dermatitis.
2. It is quite difficult to achieve uniform thickness of record base by hand adaptation.
3. Continued finger adaptation throughout polymerization process results in distortion of resin.
4. Soft curing resin used to fill undercuts can be displaced by finger adaptation (Figs 2.5.10 to 2.5.16).

## 3. Flasking Method

- Duplicate the cast for fabrication of record bases with dental stone.
- Prepare wax pattern of desired dimensions of maxillary and mandibular record bases over the duplicated maxillary and mandibular casts.
- Invert the duplicated casts along with record bases in a flask with dental plaster and tighten the flask with clamps.
- Once plaster sets loosen the clamp of flask and keep the flask in hot water for 5 minutes for dewaxing. Separate the two halves of flask and eliminate all the wax with hot water.
- Once the two halves of flask are dried, apply separating medium to the cast and investment.
- Cold cure resin is mixed according to manufactured recommendations in a porcelain or glass jar and then covered with lid.
- Once the resin reaches dough stage, it is placed in to the mold created by elimination of wax pattern in the flask. Now close the flask and tighten the flask with clamps and allow it to polymerize for 20 to 30 minutes.
- The record base is removed from the flask, trimmed and polished as mentioned in finger adaptation method.

### Advantages
- Record bases obtained by flasking method are accurate and stable.

### Disadvantages
- Requires more time for fabrication of denture bases and hence expensive.
- Master cast may break during this procedure and therefore we should duplicate master cast and use one for fabrication of record bases and other for mounting to articulator after recording of jaw relations.

## 4. Stone-Mold Method

- Prepare wax patterns of desired dimensions of maxillary and mandibular record bases over the master casts with base plate wax.
- Make index indentations on the land area of the cast at four widely separated points with a large round bur. Apply separating medium to the master cast.
- Now box the casts along with wax patterns using boxing wax. The boxing wax should extend atleast 15 mm above the cast.
- Mix the dental stone according to manufacturers recommendations and vibrate it in to the boxed cast and wax pattern to form a stone mold. Once dental stone sets, separate stone mold from the master cast and remove the wax pattern from the cast.

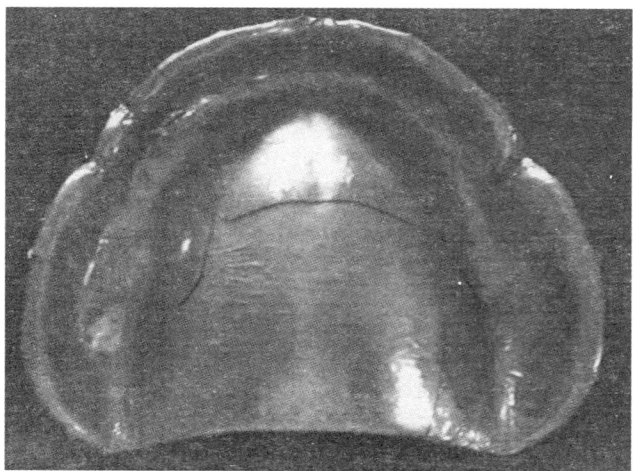

**Fig. 2.5.10:** Maxillary shellac record base—reinforced with lead foil—tissue surface view

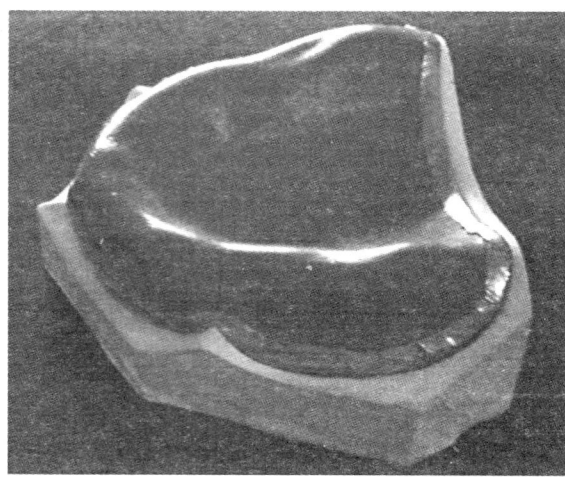

**Fig. 2.5.13:** Maxillary shellac record base—reinforced with lead foil—side view

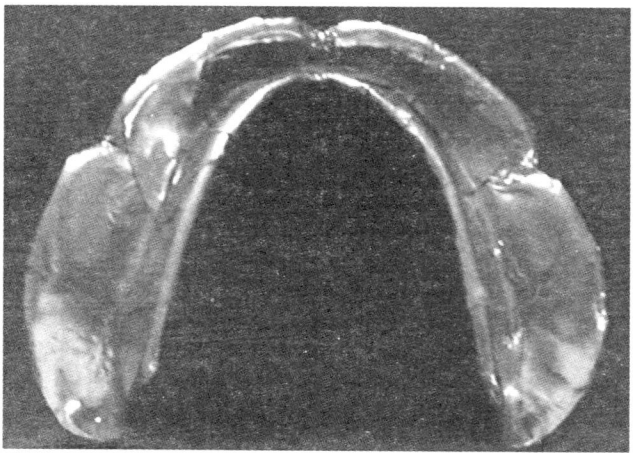

**Fig. 2.5.11:** Mandibular shellac record base—reinforced with lead foil—tissue surface view

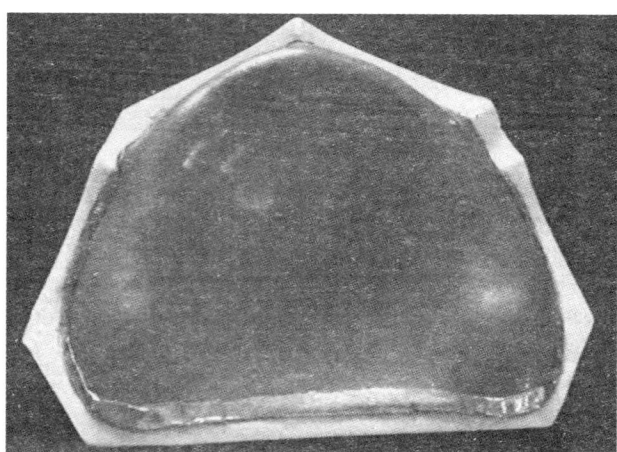

**Fig. 2.5.14:** Maxillary shellac record base—reinforced with lead foil—top view

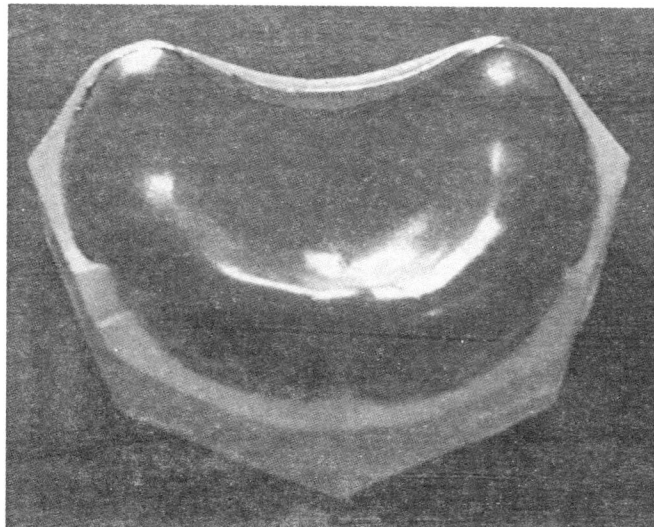

**Fig. 2.5.12:** Maxillary shellac record base—reinforced with lead foil—front view

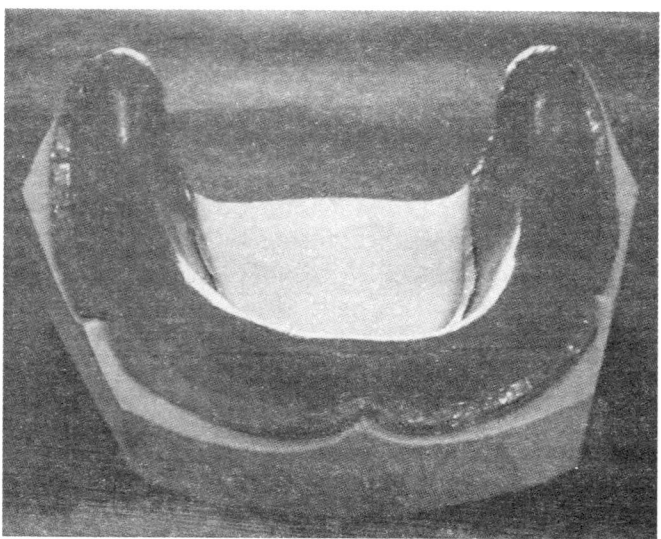

**Fig. 2.5.15:** Mandibular shellac record base—reinforced with lead foil—front view

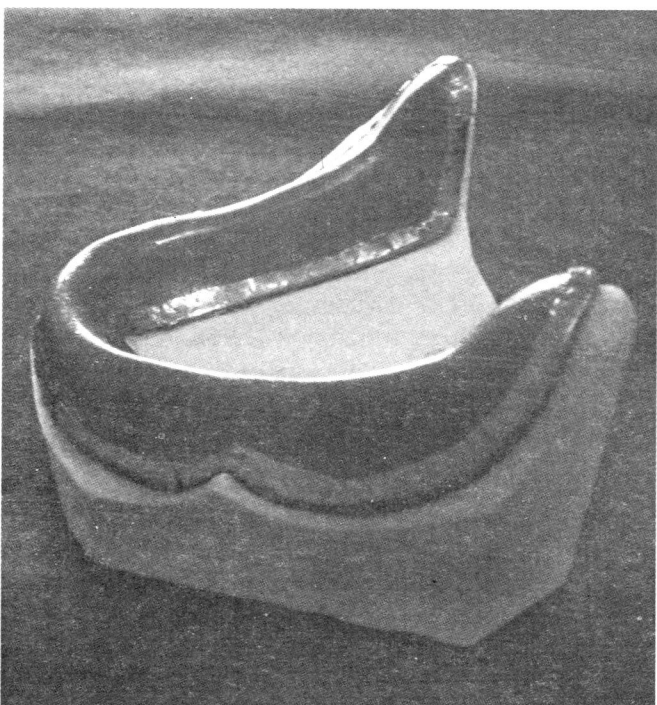

**Fig. 2.5.16:** Mandibular shellac record base—reinforced with lead foil

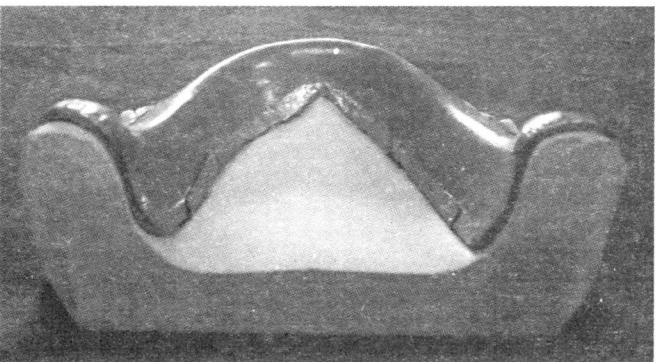

**Fig. 2.5.17:** Mandibular shellac record base reinforced with lead foil—posterior view

- Apply separating medium to both casts and stone molds and block out undercuts if any with wax or soft curing resin. Mix cold cure resin according to manufacturers recommendations and once it reaches dough stage, place it in the stone mold and reassemble the cast and stone mold and maintain tight closure with heavy rubber bands. Allow it to cure in a pressure pot.
- Once curing is over, separate the stone mold from master cast and remove the record base. Trimming, finishing and polishing done as mentioned in finger adaptation method.

Advantages
- Accurate and stable record bases can be fabricated.

- Less trimming and finishing is necessary.

Disadvantages
- The stone index may break under pressure when closing the mold.
- Requires more time to fabricate record bases.

5. **Wax Confined Method**
   - Lavere and Freda have described this method of making record bases from wax and autopolymerizing resin.
   - Block out undercuts on master cast and apply 3 coats of separating medium over the master cast. Allow last coat to set for 10 minutes.
   - Adapt one layer of base plate wax over the master cast to make a wax form or tray. Trim the wax 2 mm short of the borders of the cast.
   - Take two parts polymer to one part monomer of cold cure acrylic resin and mix to obtain a thin and uniform resin.
   - Add small amount of resin mix in the borders of the cast and on the palatal surface of maxillary cast. Pour the remaining resin mix on to the tissue surface of the adapted base plate wax and spread it evenly over the entire tissue surface.
   - Now invert the base plate wax (tray) with resin mix over the master cast and compress evenly till the resin attains a thickness of approximately 2 mm. Contour the excess resin over borders to obtain smooth and round borders.
   - Allow the acrylic resin to cure under pressure pot for 20 minutes. Once cured, remove the record base from cast, trim it and polish it as described previously.

Advantages
- Record bases of uniform thickness all over can be obtained.
- Outer wax surface makes the record base neat and pleasing in appearance.

**C. Fabrication of Record Bases using Vacuum Method**
- Block out the undercuts on master cast with wax or any other material which does not melt during heating.
- Take a sheet of base plate resin and insert in flame located below the electric heater coil and switch on the heater, continue heating until resin sheet begins to sag approximately one-half inch.
- Now lower the softened resin sheet on to the master cast with the help of supporting frame and turn on the vacuum. Resin sheet will be closely adapted to the cast.

- Switch off the heater and allow the record base to cool for one minute. Remove the record base from cast, trim it and do the finishing.

### D. Fabrication of Record Bases using Base Plate Wax
- Apply talcum powder to the cast or wet the cast, to prevent the wax from sticking to the cast. Soften the base plate wax over bunsen burner flame and adapt it to the master cast. Remove the excess wax with a sharp instrument and make the borders round and smooth.

### E. Fabrication of Record Bases using Heat Cure Resin
- Do not block the undercuts. Soften the base plate wax and adapt it to the master cast to obtain a wax pattern of record bases.
- Now invert the wax pattern in a flask with dental plaster. Once the plaster sets, do dewaxing by placing the flask in hot water. After removing the wax, allow the mold to become dry and then apply separating medium to the mold.
- Mix the heat cure resin according to manufacturers recommendations and once it attains dough stage, pack it into the mold and process it using short or long curing cycle. After completion of processing, remove the record base from cast, trim it and do the finishing.
- Now block the under cuts on the tissue side of processed record base with a plastic material and pour the dental stone into the tissue side of record bases to obtain maintaing casts for the transfer of jaw records to the articulator.

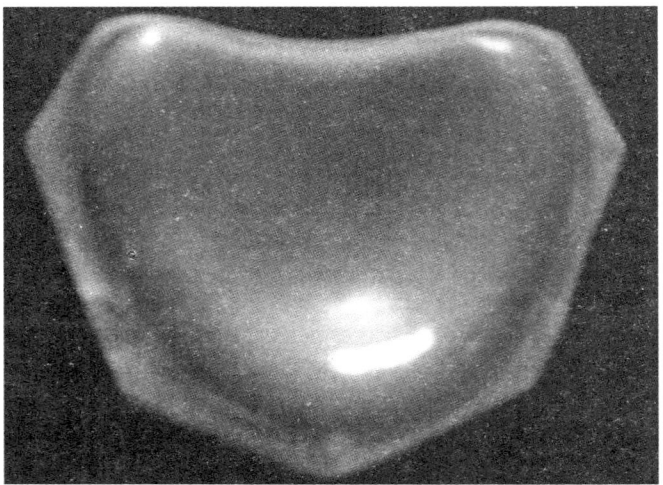

**Fig. 2.5.18:** Maxillary cold cure acrylic record base—front view

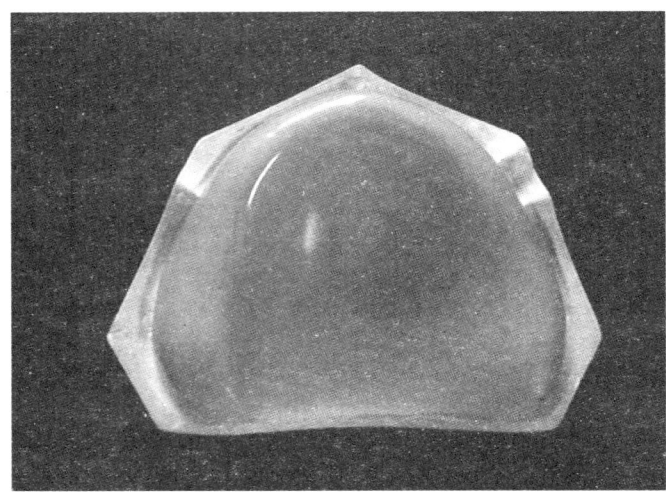

**Fig. 2.5.20:** Maxillary cold cure acrylic record base—top view

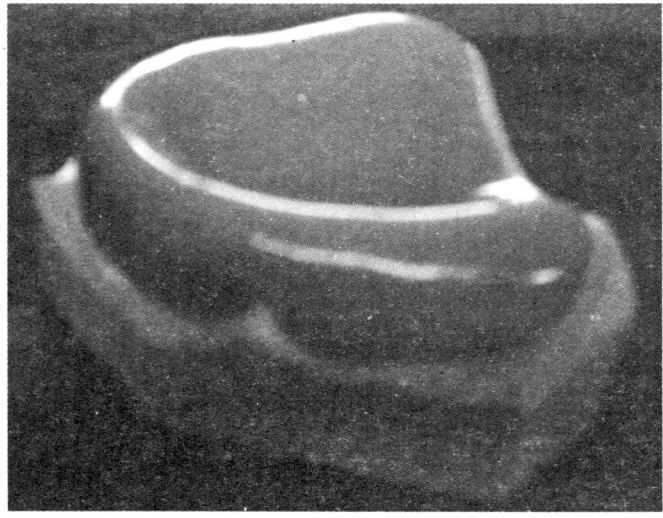

**Fig. 2.5.19:** Maxillary cold cure acrylic record base—side view

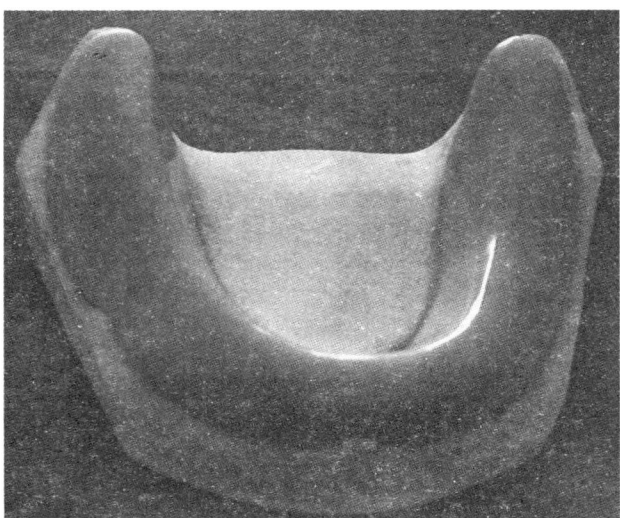

**Fig. 2.5.21:** Mandibular cold cure acrylic record base—front view

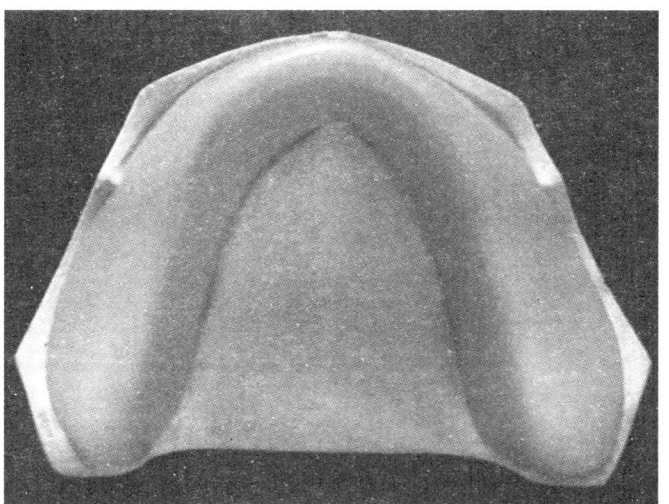

Fig. 2.5.22: Mandibular cold cure acrylic record base—posterior view

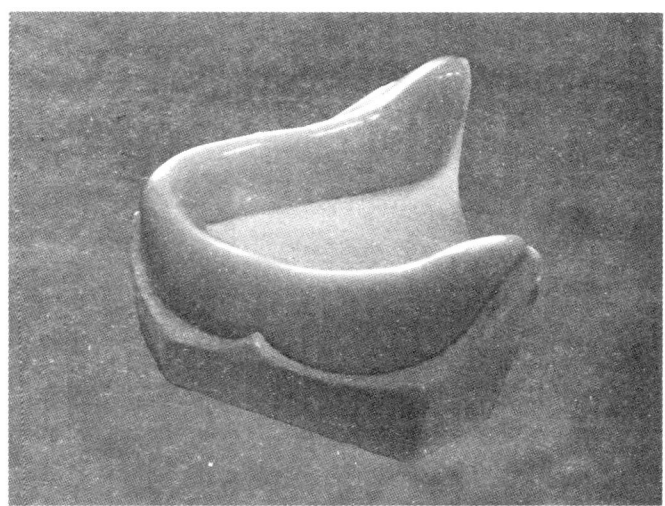

Fig. 2.5.23: Mandibular cold cure acrylic record base—side view

### F. Fabrication of Record Bases using Cast Alloys
- Refractory casts are prepared from the final cast wax pattern is fabricated over the refractory cast, which is sprued and invested in a suitable investment. Once the investment is set, the wax is burned out and molten alloy is cast into the mold cavity with the help of casting machine. On cooling, the casting (record base) is removed from the investment, finished and polished.

# CHAPTER 6
# Occlusion Rims

To construct a wax rim to be a substitute for the teeth. The occlusion rims are used for the occlusal plane, vertical dimension, centric relation, face-bow, and the placement of the teeth. The mid-line, high smile line, and canine to canine distance are recorded on the wax occlusion rims.

## OCCLUSION/RECORD/BITE RIMS/BITE BLOCKS

### SYNONYMS
- Occlusal rims
- Record rims
- Bite rims
- Bite blocks

### DEFINITION
- Occluding surfaces fabricated on interim or final denture bases for the purpose of making maxillomandibular relationship records and arranging teeth—GPT.

### RATIONALE/OBJECTIVES
1. To establish the level of occlusal plane.
2. To establish the neutral zone or arch form which is related to the activity of the lips, cheeks and tongue and includes preliminary circumoral and facial support.
3. To establish the preliminary maxillomandibular relation records, which include the vertical and horizontal jaw relationships and an estimate of the interocclusal distance.

### SHAPE
- The shape of occlusal rims generally follows the shape of the edentulous arch. So, the shape of occlusal rims can be in the form of.
  A. Square ('U' shaped)
  B. Tapering ('V' shaped)
  C. Ovoid

### POSITION
- The occlusal rims should be designed to confirm to the arch form that the patient had before the natural teeth and alveolar bone were lost. Hence

the best guide for determining the position of occlusal rims is to consider the pattern of bone resorption where the teeth are lost and the use of anatomical landmarks that are relatively stable in position.

a. **Mandibular arch**
   - Pattern of bone loss or resorption.
     Anterior region: More bone loss occurs on labial side (inwards and downwards).
     Premolar region: Bone loss occurs equally on buccal and lingual sides (centrally and downwards).
     Molar region: More bone loss occurs on lingual side (outwards and downwards).
   
   Position of occlusal rims
   - Hence the occlusal rims should be placed labial to the ridge in anterior region, over the ridge in premolar region and slightly lingual to the ridge in the molar region.

b. **Maxillary arch**
   - Pattern of bone loss or resorption.
     Anterior region: Bone loss occurs on labial side (inwards and upwards).
     Posterior region: Bone loss occurs on buccal side (inwards and upwards).

Position of occlusal rims
- The occlusal rims should be placed labial to the ridge in anterior region and buccally to the ridge in posterior region.

## DIMENSIONS

a. **Mandibular Arch**
   i. Occlusal rim height
      Anteriorly
      - 16 to 17 mm from the reflection of cast (deepest part of labial sulcus).
      - 6 to 8 mm from the crest of ridge.
      Posteriorly
      - Parallel to base of the cast (and residual ridge) on a plane intersecting the retromolar pad at 2/3 of the retromolar pad's height.
      - 3 to 6 mm from the crest of ridge.
      - Occlusal rim should end 8 mm short of posterior border of record base.
   ii. Occlusal rim width
      Anteriorly        –   3–5 mm
      Premolar region   –   5–7 mm
      Molar region      –   8–10 mm

b. **Maxillary Arch**
   i. Occlusal rim height
      Anteriorly
      - 20–22 mm from the reflection of cast (deepest part of labial sulcus).
      - 10–12 mm from the crest of ridge.

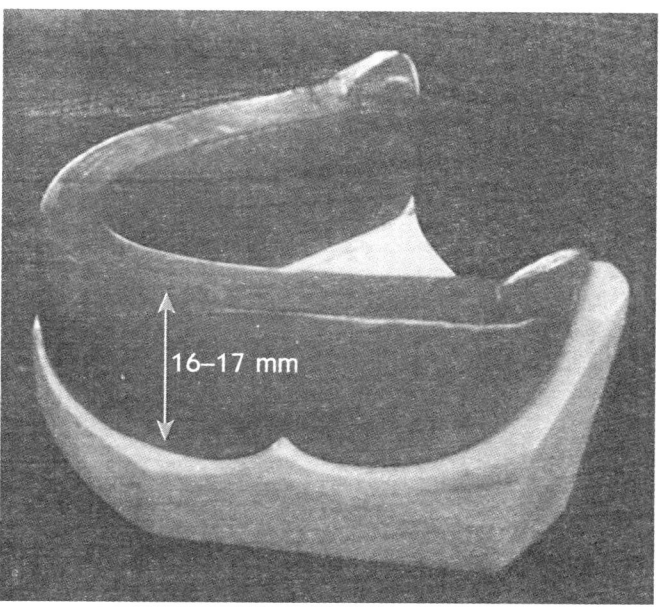

Fig. 2.6.1

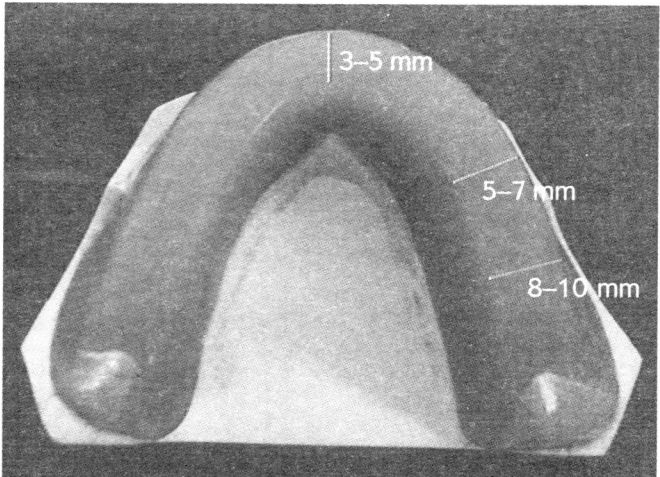

Fig. 2.6.2

   Posteriorly
   - 16–18 mm from the reflection of cast (from the depth of buccal sulcus in the molar region).
   - 5–7 mm from the crest of ridge.
   - 10 mm anterior to the hamular notch.
   ii. Occlusal rim width (Figs 2.6.1 and 2.62)
      Incisal region    –   3–5 mm
      Premolar region   –   5–7 mm
      Molar region      –   8–10 mm
   iii. Inclination
      - Labial surface of occlusal rim should be approximately 8 to 10 mm anterior to center of incisive papilla.
      - Posteriorly, the occlusal rim should be inclined 2 to 5 degree towards the lingual direction.

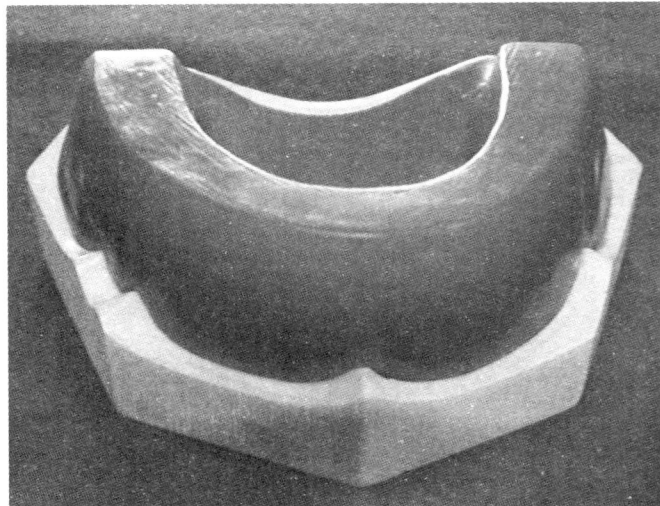

Fig. 2.6.3

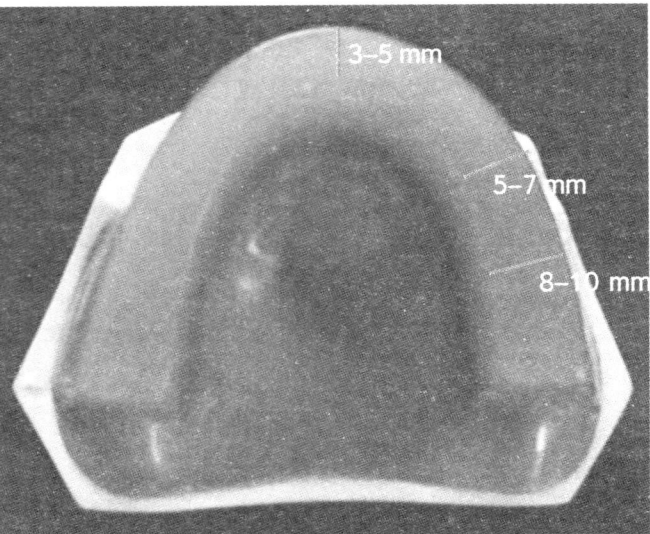

Fig. 2.6.4: Maxillary occlusal rim showing the widths of incisal, premolar and molar regions

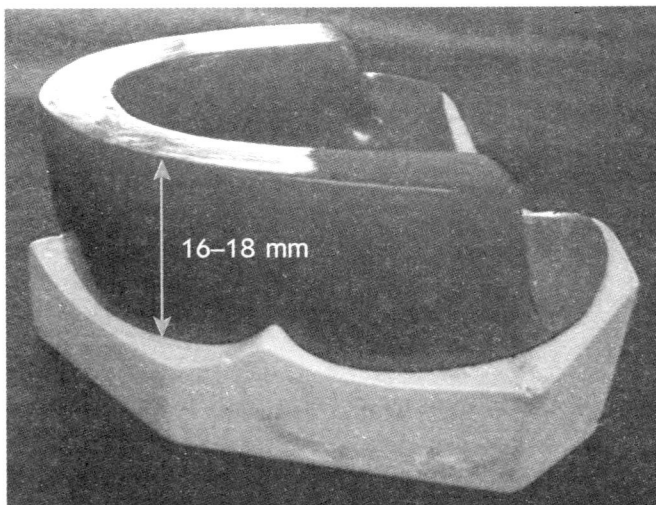

Fig. 2.6.5: Maxillary occlusal rim showing height anteriorly and posteriorly

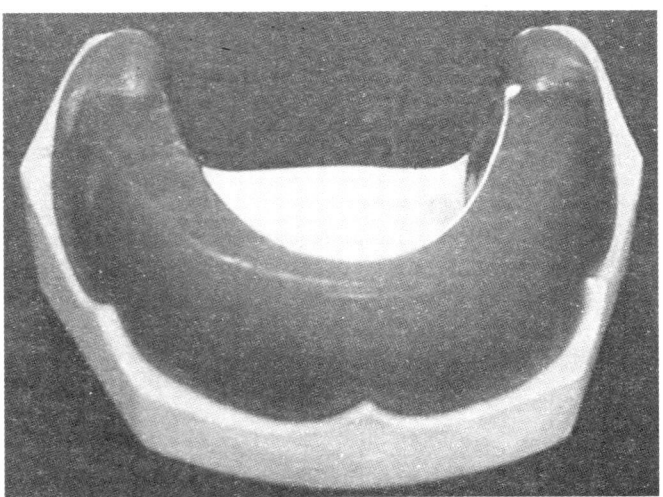

Fig. 2.6.6

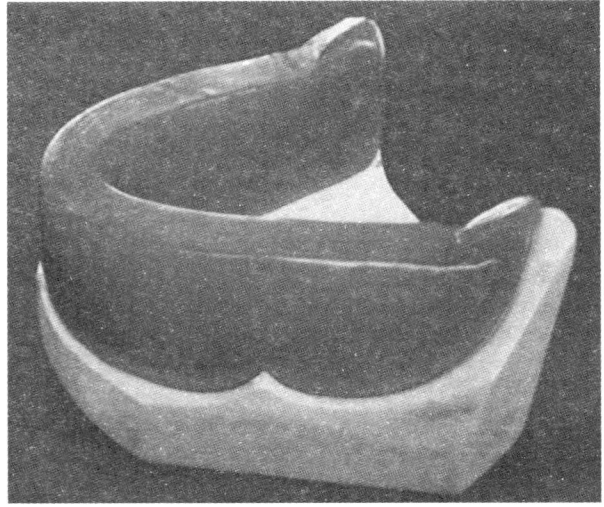

Fig. 2.6.7

## EQUIPMENT AND MATERIALS

- Maxillary and mandibular record bases on master casts.
- Base plate wax (or) modelling compound.
- Bunsen burner and matches.
- Wax knife.
- Wax spatula.
- Hot plate.
- Hanau torch (blow torch).
- Chip blow.

## FABRICATION

### MAXILLARY OCCLUSION RIM

Materials needed:

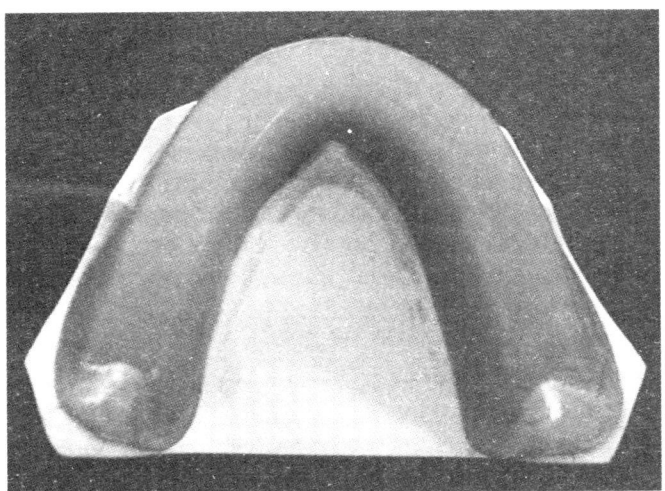

Fig. 2.6.8

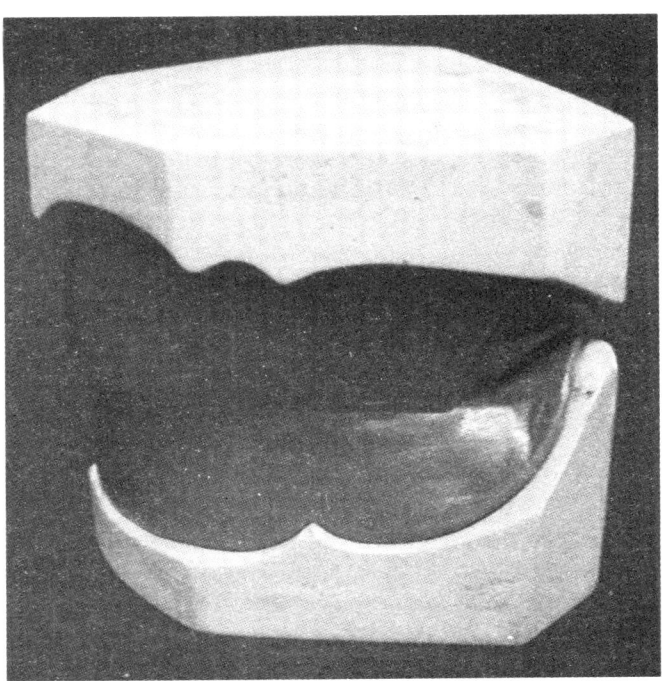

Fig. 2.6.9

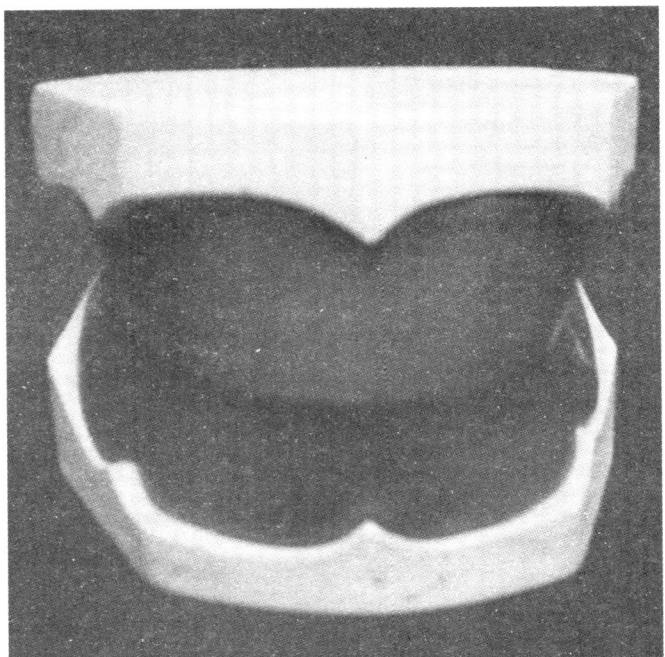

Fig. 2.6.10

1. Pink baseplate wax
2. Hot plate
3. Spatula
4. Knife
5. Alcohol torch
6. Stone casts of previous dentures

1. Apply a thin layer of sticky wax to the baseplate on the crest of the ridge.
2. Use only clean pink baseplate wax. Do not use the harder set-up wax. Warm by flaming 1 to 2 sheets of baseplate wax carefully. Roll tightly lengthwise, flatten on table, fold 1 inch of each end over (to shorten length) and adapt to the baseplate as follows.

4. Flame the underside of the wax rim and position it on the baseplate. Seal it to place with a hot spatula.
5. Warm a sheet of baseplate wax over a Bunsen flame and fold it into a rectangle; 4 to 5 mm. thick and long enough to extend around the wax. Adapt the softened wax on the labial and buccal areas to properly build out the contour. Mold the canine areas to give a slight eminence. Smooth and finish shaping the contours with the occlusal plane former. The posterior width is about 6 mm. and the anterior portion 3–4 mm.

   *Note:* Most occlusion rims are far too wide and crowds the tongue space. Study the stone casts of the previous dentures (especially if they were satisfactory) and simulate the arch form and occlusal widths.
6. The anterior length of the rim should be about 22 mm. from the highest area of the labial flange to the occlusal edge.
7. Construct the maxillary occlusion rim so it will be over the probable position of the teeth. The anterior portion is always labial to the crest of the ridge. In addition, the anterior portion must have a slight labial inclination. The posterior areas have a lingual inclination. All the lingual walls are 90° to the occlusal plane. The distal end of the rim runs at an angle toward the posterior border, starting at about the distal of the 2nd molars.

## MANDIBULAR OCCLUSION RIM

The procedures for making the mandibular rim are very similar to the maxillary rim except that less time is spent contouring since the lower rim will be contoured to match the upper rim as a patient procedure. Make the height of the rim about 20 mm. from the labial border to the incisal edge, all at straight angles except the posterior edge which angles down, and in front of the pear-shaped pad.

# Posterior Palatal Seal Area

**CHAPTER 7**

A complete maxillary denture requires a posterior seal that will maintain the denture during movements of the soft palate. The maxillary denture is primarily retained by negative atmospheric pressure. This requires an intact peripheral seal. After processing, the volumetric shrinkage is as high as 7%. This causes the resin to lose contact from the critical posterior area with a resulting loss of seal. A correct posterior palatal seal will maintain firm contact and thus the peripheral seal.

### DEFINITION

Posterior palatal seal area is defined as the *soft tissues along the junction of the hard and soft palates on which pressure within the physiologic limits of the tissues can be applied by a denture to aid in the retention of the denture*—GPT.

### SYNONYM

Post dam

### LOCATION

Along the posterior border of the maxillary denture.

### SIGNIFICANCE/IMPORTANCE

1. Serves primarily in denture retention by making contact with anterior portion of soft palate and by preventing passage of air between the tissues and denture base.
2. Maintains contact with the moving soft palate and reduces the patient's awareness and thus reduces gag reflex.
3. Prevents food accumulation between posterior borders of dentures and the soft palate.
4. Compensates for polymerization shrinkage of denture base resin.
5. Reduces tongue irritation as posterior border merges better with palate.

### COMPONENTS

The posterior palatal seal is divided into two separate but confluent areas based upon anatomic boundaries.
1. Pterygomaxillary Seal
   - It is defined as that band of loose connective tissue lying between the pterygoid hamulus of the sphenoid bone and the distal portion of the maxillary tuberosity.
   - It extends through the pterygomaxillary notch (hamulus) continues 3–4 mm anterolaterally to

end in the mucogingival junction on the posterior part of the maxillary ridge.
- Hamular process, located 2 to 4 mm posteriorly and medial to the distal limit of the maxillary residual ridge, should not be covered by denture as patient would experience pain if the hard denture base were to cover them.

2. Post Palatal Seal
- It determines the posterior limit of maxillary dentures and extends medially from one maxillary tuberosity to the other.

## BOUNDARIES

The posterior palatal seal area has the following boundaries:
Anteriorly: anterior vibrating line
Posteriorly: posterior vibrating line
Laterally: Pterygomaxillary notch (hamular notch)

## VIBRATING LINE

- It is defined as *the imaginary line across the posterior part of the palate marking the division between the movable and immovable tissue of the soft palate which can be identified when the movable tissues are moving*—GPT.
- The two components of vibrating line are *anterior vibrating line and posterior vibrating line*.

### 1. Anterior Vibrating Line

Definition: It is defined as *an imaginary line located at the junction of the attached tissues overlying the hard palate and the movable tissues of the immediately adjacent soft palate.*

#### Methods of Identification

1. Valsalva maneuver: Ask the patient to perform valsalva maneuver, which requires that both nostrils be held firmly while the patient blows gently through the nose. This will position the soft palate inferiorly at its junction with the hard palate.

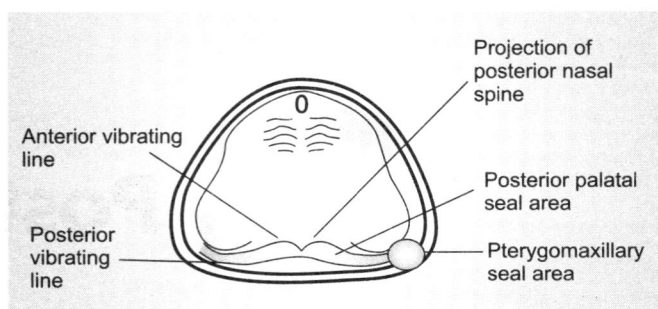

Fig. 2.7.1: Posterior palatal seal area

2. The anterior vibrating line can also be approximated by visualizing the area while instructing the patients to say "ah" with short vigorous bursts.

Shape: Anterior vibrating line is not a straight line but assumes the shape of "cupids bow due" to the projection of posterior nasal spine.

Note: Anterior vibrating line is always located in soft palate and should not be confused with the anatomic junction of the hard and soft palate.

### 2. Posterior Vibrating Line

Definition: It is defined as *an imaginary line at the junction of the aponeurosis of the tensor veli palatine muscle and the muscular portion of the soft palate.*

Methods of Identification
- The posterior vibrating line is visualized by instructing the patient to say "ah" in short bursts in a normal, unexaggerated fashion.
- It represents the demarcation between that part of the soft palate that has limited or shallow movement during function (quivers) and the remainder of the soft palate that is markedly displaced during functional movements.

Shape: Posterior vibrating line is usually straight
Note: Posterior vibrating line marks the most distal extension of the denture base.

# Jaw Relations/ Maxillomandibular Relationships

## CHAPTER 8

This is the most important step in the fabrication of a CD and success of your prosthesis depends on how accurately you recorded these relation. If the jaw relations are incorrect, the denture will move to occlude with each other and thus be dislodge from the ridges during occlusion

### DEFINITION
- Any spatial relationship of the maxillae to the mandible; any one of the infinite relationships of the mandible to the maxillae—GPT.

### MAXILLOMANDIBULAR RELATIONSHIP RECORD
- A registration of any positional relationship of the mandible relative to the maxillae. These records may be made at any vertical, horizontal or lateral orientation—GPT.

### RATIONALE/OBJECTIVES
1. To contour the occlusion rims and establish the plane of occlusion.
2. To record centric relation.
3. To determine vertical relation of rest position and occlusion.
4. To establish face-bow transfer record.
5. To develop the posterior palatal seal.
6. To select the artificial teeth.

### CLASSIFICATION
Boucher classified jaw relations into three groups
1. Orientation jaw relations.
2. Vertical jaw relations
   A. Vertical dimension of rest position (VDR).
   B. Vertical dimension of occlusion (VDO).
   C. Freeway space (VDR - VDO).
3. Horizontal jaw relations
   A. Centric relation
   B. Eccentric relations
      i. Protrusive relations
      ii. Lateral relations
         Left
         Right.

# ORIENTATION JAW RELATIONS

## DEFINITION

- The orientation jaw relations are those that orient the mandible to the cranium in such a way that, when the mandible is kept in its most posterior position the mandible can rotate in the sagittal plane around an imaginary transverse axis passing through or near the condyles.

- As the patients opens and closes the jaws, the posterior border of its movement, at least in the earliest phases, is the area of a circle in the sagittal plane around an imaginary transverse axis passing through or near the condyles. The same is true of the articulator. Similarly, other movements of the jaws occur in arcs. For an accurate reproduction of these movements, the axes of these arcs should be coincident between patient and instrument, particularly where the vertical dimension has to be changed. The axis of the arcs can be located when the mandible is in its most posterior position with the help of kinematic face bow or hinge bow or it can be approximated with the help of arbitrary type of face bow and same orientation relation can be transferred to the articulator.

## FACE BOW

- The hinge-like action in the lower compartment of the temporomandibular joint was described in the earliest editions of Gray's anatomy. Snow recognised the importance of hinge axis in mandibular movements and developed a face-bow to be used to transfer the position of the axis to the articulator.

- When the mandible opens and closes, rotation occurs around a transverse axis, which is more commonly called the hinge axis. This axis is called the terminal hinge axis when the mandible undergoes pure rotation while in centric relation, the maximum range of terminal hinge rotation averages about 12° and creates a range of 18 to 25 mm of interincisal opening.

- The face bow helps to relate the jaws to the hinge axis of mandible and transfer the relation to articulator, simulating some of the jaw movements of the patient. This inturn helps in developing occlusion with greater accuracy.

## DEFINITION

- Face bow is a caliper-like instrument used to record the spatial relationship of the maxillary arch to some anatomic reference point or points and then transfer this relationship to an articulator; it orients the dental cast in the same relationship to the opening axis of the articulator—GPT.

## OBJECTIVES

- To record the relationship of the jaws to the opening axis of the jaws and to orient the casts in this same relationship to the opening axis of the articulator.
- To support the maxillary cast while it is being mounted on the articulator.

## INDICATIONS

1. During complete denture fabrication while balanced occlusion is desired.
2. During fixed partial denture fabrication to obtain accurate crowns and bridges.
3. When cusp form of teeth are used for complete denture fabrication.
4. When interocclusal check records are used.
5. During full mouth rehabilitation when accurate occlusal restorations are to be made.
6. When vertical dimension at occlusion is to be changed during teeth setting.
7. In gnathological studies and treatment.
8. For making occlusal corrections after denture processing.

## TYPES

1. Arbitrary face bows
   a. Fascia type
      Ex  Hanau fascia type face bow
          Denar fascia face bow
   b. Ear piece type
      Ex  Hanau ear piece type face bow
          Hanau spring bow
          Hanau twirl bow
          Whip mix quick mount face bow
          Denar slidematic face bow
2. Kinematic face bow or hinge bow
   Ex  Hanau kinematic face bow
       Denar kinematic face bow

## ARBITRARY FACE BOWS

- Arbitrary face bows are used to locate the hinge axis or opening axis of jaw approximately or arbitrary and transfer the record to the articulator.
- While doing the face bow records, three points are considered in the skull. Two points are located

posterior to the maxilla called posterior reference points and one point is located anteriorly called the anterior reference point. The spatial plane formed by joining the anterior and posterior reference points is called the plane of orientation.
- Posterior reference points represent the terminal hinge axis position or opening axis of jaws and can be determined approximately by using arbitrary face bow or can be determined absolutely by using kinematic face bow.
- Anterior reference point determines the level at which occlusal plane to be placed in the articulator.
- Arbitrary face bow is the one generally used in the construction of complete dentures.
- Arbitrary face bow is attached to maxillary occlusal rim while taking face bow records.

## HANAU FASCIA TYPE FACE BOW

- Posterior reference points—marked bilaterally 13 mm anterior to external auditory meatus on the canthotragal line (runs from outer canthus of eye to the top of the tragus of ear). This is done using Richey Condylar Marker. By this method, posterior reference points are located within 2 mm of the true center of the opening axis of the jaws.
- Anterior reference point—orbitale (50 mm superiorly from incisal edge of maxillary central incisor 18 mm inferiorly to inner canthus of eye).

## HANAU EAR PIECE TYPE FACE BOW

Posterior reference points—External auditory meatus.
By this method posterior reference points are located within 5 mm of the true center of the opening axis of jaws.
Anterior reference point—orbitale.
- It is most commonly used type of face bow during construction of complete dentures. Its design allows easy manipulation clinically.

## HANAU TWIRL BOW

Posterior reference points—External auditory meatus.
Anterior reference point—orbitale.

### Special features
1. Both ear pieces can be closed simultaneously and equidistantly.
2. Face bow is not needed to mount the maxillary cast in the articulator. A mounting guide (transfer jig) allows the mounting of maxillary cast to articulator.

## WHIP-MIX QUICK MOUNT FACE BOW

Posterior reference points—External auditory meatus.
Anterior reference point—Nasion.

### Special features
1. Nasion relator of face bow positioned against bridge of nose determines anterior reference point.
2. Intercondylar scale present infront of the face bow indicates the intercondylar distance as small, medium and large (S, M and L).

## DENAR SLIDEMATIC FACE BOW

Posterior reference points—External auditory meatus.
Anterior reference point:
- 43 mm superior to lower border of upper lip in relaxed state for edentulous patients.
- 43 mm superior to incisal edge of right maxillary central incisor for dentulous patients.
- The anterior reference point is marked using a denar reference plane locator. It is marked on right side of patient.

### Special features
1. It has an electronic device, which gives a reading that can be seen in the anterior region. This reading denotes the one - half of the patients intercondylar distance.
2. Face bow is not required to mount the maxillary cast in the articulator. Transfer zig allows the mounting of maxillary cast to the articulator.

## KINEMATIC FACE BOWS

- The kinematic face bows are used to locate the true terminal hinge axis and transfer this record to the articulator.
- The kinematic face bow is attached to mandibular occlusal rim while taking face bow records.
- It is generally used for fabrication of fixed partial dentures and during full mouth rehabilitation.
- It is generally not used for construction of complete dentures due to complex and time consuming procedures involved.
  E.g. Hanau kinematic face bow.
       Denar kinematic face bow.

## PARTS OF FACE BOW

1. U-shaped frame or assembly.
2. Condyle rods / Ear pieces.
3. Bite fork
4. Locking device
5. Orbital pointer
6. Nasion relator assembly
7. Intercondylar scale
8. Electronic device
9. Transfer zig

## U-SHAPED FRAME OR ASSEMBLY

- It is the main part of face bow to which all other parts are attached with the help of clamps.
- It should be large enough that extend from the region of one TMJ around the front of the face (5 to 7.5 cm in front of it) to the other TMJ and wide enough to avoid contact with sides of face.

## CONDYLE RODS AND EAR PIECES

- They are attached on either side of the free end of U-shaped frame.
- They are positioned on the patient at the approximate or absolute location of the hinge axis or opening axis of jaws.
- Fascia type of arbitrary face bows and kinematic face bows have condylar rods. Ear piece type of arbitrary face bows have ear pieces.

## BITE FORK

- It is the part of the face bow that attaches to the occlusal rims.
- It is horse shoe shaped with stem attached to it.
- Bite fork of arbitrary face bow is attached to maxillary occlusal rim and bite fork of kinematic face bow is attached to mandibular occlusal rim.

## LOCKING DEVICE

- Locking device helps in attaching bite fork to the face bow.
- It also serves to support the face bow, the maxillary occlusion rim and the maxillary cast while the casts are being attached to the articulator.
- It consists of vertical transfer rod and horizontal transverse rod. Vertical transfer rod is attached to U shaped frame and horizontal transverse rod connects the vertical transfer rod with the stem of the bite fork.

## ORBITAL POINTER

- It is present in Hanau arbitrary face bows.
- It marks the anterior reference point, which is orbitale in case of Hanau arbitrary face bows.

## NASION RELATOR ASSEMBLY

- It is a part of whip-mix quick mount arbitrary face bow.
- It marks the anterior reference point, which is Nasion in case of whip-mix quick mount arbitrary face bow.

## INTERCONDYLAR SCALE

- It is a part of whip-mix quick mount arbitrary face bow.
- It is present infront of face bow and indicates the intercondylar distance as small, medium and large (S, M, L).

## ELECTRONIC DEVICE

- It is a part of Denar slidematic face bow.
- It gives the reading that can be seen in anterior region. This reading denotes the one-half of the patients intercondylar distance.

## TRANSFER JIG

- It is a part of Hanau twirl-bow and Denar slidematic face bow.
- Transfer jig allows the mounting of the maxillary cast to the articulator without attaching the face bow (Fig. 2.8.1).

## ADVANTAGES OF FACE BOW

1. Avoids errors in occlusion of finished prosthesis.
2. Allows minor changes in the occlusal vertical dimension in articulator without having to make new maxillomandibular relations.
3. Most helpful in supporting the maxillary cast while it is being mounted on the articulator.
4. Allows more accurate programming of the articulator.

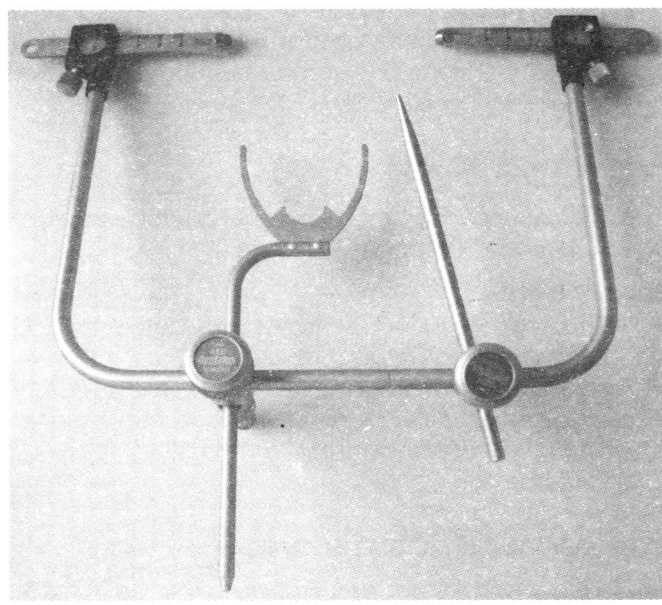

**Fig. 2.8.1:** Parts of face bow

# VERTICAL JAW RELATIONS

## DEFINITION

- It is defined as the distance between two selected points, one on a fixed (maxilla) and one on a movable member (mandible)—GPT.
- The vertical jaw relations are expressed in the amount of separation between the maxillae and mandible under specified conditions. It depends on the TMJ and the tone of muscles of mastication. Vertical jaw relations should be recorded accurately for the proper comfort, health and function of the oral and surrounding associated structures. Increased or decreased vertical dimension results in complications as mentioned below and ultimately lead to failure of prosthesis.

## EFFECTS OF INCREASED VERTICAL DIMENSION

1. Discomfort to the patient.
2. Trauma to denture bearing area and underlying mucosa.
3. Increased lower facial height (elongated face).
4. Stretching of facial muscles which results in strained appearance.
5. Pain and clicking in the TMJ.
6. Clicking of teeth which results in rapid wear of acrylic teeth.
7. Increased resorption of alveolar bone.
8. Difficulty in swallowing and speech.
9. Increased volume of oral cavity.

## EFFECTS OF DECREASED VERTICAL DIMENSION

1. Decreased lower facial height.
2. Cheek biting.
3. Angular cheilitis due to folding of corners of the mouth.
4. Loss of lip fullness, thinning of vermillion borders of lip and deepend wrinkles on face result in aged appearance.
5. Elevation of soft palate due to elevation of tongue or mandible results in obstruction of opening of the eustachian tube.
6. Decreased masticatory efficiency (chewing).
7. Pain and clicking in TMJ accompanied with headaches and neuralgias.
8. Decreased volume of oral cavity.

## TYPES

A. Vertical dimension of rest position (VDR).
B. Vertical dimension of occlusion (VDO).
C. Free way space (VDR - VDO).

## VERTICAL DIMENSION OF REST POSITION (REST VERTICAL DIMENSION)

Definition: The distance between two selected points measured when the mandible is in physiologic rest position—GPT.

### Physiologic rest position

- It is defined as the postural position of the mandible when an individual is resting comfortably in an upright position and the associated muscles are in a state of minimal contractural activity.
- The mandible is considered to be in its physiologic rest position when all the muscles that close the jaws and all the muscles that open the jaws are in a state of minimal tonic contraction sufficient only to maintain posture.
- The vertical dimension of rest position is a measurable distance, a repeatable reference within an acceptable range and a useful reference when establishing the vertical dimension of occlusion. When used as a reference point in recording the vertical dimension of occlusion, rest position should be determined first and then reduced or closed to the vertical dimension of occlusion.

### Factors affecting physiologic rest position

1. The position of the mandible is influenced by gravity. Hence, while recording vertical jaw relations patient should be asked to sit upright or stand with the head erect, looking straight ahead.
2. Rest position is a relaxed position of the mandible. The measurements vary when a patient is tense, under strain, nervous, tired or irritable. Dentist also should be relaxed while making jaw relations. If dentist is tense, nervous, tired or under strain, it influences patients reactions and even patient becomes tense and nervous. Hence the procedures are advisably postponed until both the patient and dentist are in relaxed frame of mind to obtain accurate recordings.
3. It is difficult to determine the rest position in patients suffering from neuromuscular disturbances. Dentist should have patience and devote considerable time while recording jaw relations for such patients.
4. Rest position is a position in space, which cannot be maintained for definite periods of time. Hence, dentist should make measurements without delay once the rest position is assumed.
5. Failure to establish rest position as a reference point may result in increased or decreased interocclusal distance, which cause damage to supporting structures or TMJ.

## VERTICAL DIMENSION OF OCCLUSION

### Definition
- The distance measured between two selected points when the occluding members are in contact—GPT.
- The vertical dimension of occlusion is established by the natural teeth when they are present and in occlusion. In edentulous patients vertical dimension of occlusion is established by the vertical height of the two dentures when the teeth are in contact. Hence the vertical dimension of occlusion must be established for edentulous patients so that denture teeth will come into contact at approximate height. This is achieved during jaw relations with the help of occlusal rims, by various methods and procedures.

## FREEWAY SPACE (INTEROCCLUSAL DISTANCE)

### Definition
- It is defined as the distance between the occluding surfaces of the maxillary and mandibular teeth when the mandible is in physiologic rest position.
- It is the difference between the vertical dimension of rest position and vertical dimension of occlusion. Free way space = vertical dimension of rest–vertical dimension of occlusion.
- Space between teeth is essential when mandible is at rest. If there is no space present between teeth during rest position, leads to discomfort, pain and hyperemia until the resorption of bone establishes the necessary interocclusal distance. Interocclusal space (free way space) permits the supporting hard and soft tissues to rest and aid in maintaining normal physiology of oral cavity.
- Freeway space ranges between 1 to 8 mm in natural dentition. In complete denture fabrication for edentulous patients, free way space of 2 to 4 mm at premoalr region is usually advocated.

## HORIZONTAL JAW RELATIONS

- Horizontal jaw relations are the relations of mandible to maxilla in a horizontal plane or in antero posterior direction.
- Philip pfaff was the first to describe the technique of "taking a bite" also known as "mush" or " biscuit" or "squash bite" in 18th century.

### A. CENTRIC JAW RELATION

### Definition
- It is defined as the maxillomandibular relationship in which the condyles articulate with the thinnest avascular portion of their respective discs with the complex in anterior-superior position against the slopes of the articular eminences. This position is independent of tooth contact. This position is clinically discernible when the mandible is directed superior and anteriorly. It is restricted to a purely rotatory movement about the transverse horizontal axis—GPT.
- In general, centric relation is the most posterior relation of the mandible to the maxillae at the established vertical dimension and at the antero-superior relation of condyle to the glenoid fossa.
- Centric relation is a guided, retruded posterior border position rather than a habitual position presented by patient. Hence patient should be trained to retrude mandible during making centric jaw relation records.
- Centric relation is a bone to bone relation. Hence it is a constant, repeatable and recordable position and taken as a reference point for establishing centric occlusion.

### Significance of centric relation
- Normally mandibular movements are guided by proprioceptive impulses obtained from peridontal ligament, surrounding natural teeth. But in edentulous patients, periodontal ligament is absent due to absence of teeth. So, in edentulous patients mandibular movements are guided by proprioceptive impulses obtained from tempero mandibular joint. The centric relation position acts as proprioceptive center to guide the mandibular movements.
- Centric relation position acts as a centric from which all centric and eccentric movements can be made.
- It is the most unstrained position, hence functional movements like chewing and swallowing are performed in this position.
- If centric relation and centric occlusion of artificial teeth do not coincide results in instability of dentures and causes pain and discomfort to the patient.
- An accurate centric relation record properly orients the mandibular cast to the opening axis of articulatory and the mandible.
- Using centric relation records, condylar guidance in an articultor can be adjusted to produce balanced occlusion.

### Methods of retruding the mandible
- The mandible should be in most retruded position while recording centric jaw relations. The following methods help in retruding the mandible to most posterior position.
    1. Ask the patient to relax the jaws, pull it back and close slowly on back teeth.
    2. Instruct the patient to bring upper jaw forward while occluding on the posterior teeth. This

automatically results in retruding the mandible as maxille is immobile.
3. Instruct the patient to move the lower jaw forward and backward repeatedly while holding his or her fingers lightly against the chin.
4. Patient is instructed to touch the posterior border of the upper record base with his or her tongue.
5. Instruct the patient to tap the occlusal rims repeatedly. This automatically results in retruding the mandible.
6. Relax the temporal and masseter muscles by palpating them.
7. Instruct the patient to open wide and relax, move the jaws to left and relax, move the jaws to right and relax and move the jaws forward and relax. This helps in coordination of movements and patient easily follows dentists instructions.
8. Tilt the patients head backwards while the exercises listed above are carried out.

## B. ECCENTRIC JAW RELATION

### Definition

- Any relationship of the mandible to maxilla other than the centric relation—GPT.
- Eccentric jaw relation denotes the relationship of mandible to maxilla when the mandible is at any position other than the centric relation position.
- Eccentric jaw relation records are used to programme the articulator to simulate the patients jaw movements. A programmed articulator is helpful in constructing a balanced denture occlusion.

    i. Protrusive jaw relations
       - As the mandible moves forward in protrusive movements, the condyles move downward and forward. These downward movements of posterior part of mandible results in downward movement of mandibular teeth and disocclusion of maxillary and mandibular posterior teeth creating a space between them. This phenomenon of disocclusion of posterior teeth when anterior teeth come in contact with each other during protrusive movements is called as the Christensen phenomenon. To provide the patient with smooth, continuous contact of the denture teeth throughout the functional range of jaw motion, the Christensen phenomenon should be included in development of occlusion.
       - Protrusive jaw relations can register the influence of condylar paths over the movements of mandible in protrusive movements and enables us to programme the articulator in the same path.

    ii. Lateral jaw relations
       - The relations of mandible to maxilla when mandible is moved to the left or right side of centric relation are called as lateral jaw relations.
       - As mandible moves laterally to one side, the condyle on the opposite side (balancing side) moves downward, forward and inward creating disocclusion and space between arches of opposite side. This is also called as Bennett movement.
       - Lateral jaw relations are used to programme the lateral condylar guidance of articulator which together with incisal guidance guides the lateral movements of the articulator.
       - Hanau was of opinion that individual lateral registrations were of little value and derived a formula to set the condylar posts.

       $$L = \frac{H}{8} + 12$$

       $L$— Lateral condylar inclination.
       $H$— horizontal condylar inclination (established by protrusive relation record).

### Instruments and Materials Required for Making Jaw Relations

1. Gloves, mouth mask and eye protection
2. Patients drape
3. Master casts with stable record bases and occlusal rims
4. Base plate wax
5. Hanau torch and matches
6. Wax spatula
7. Wax knife
8. Hot plate
9. Lecrons carver
10. Mouth mirror and periodontal probe
11. Face bow
12. Aluwax or impression plaster or ZOE paste
13. Dental floss
14. Pencil marker
15. Fox occlusal plane
16. Rubber bowls with hot and cold water
17. Metal scale
18. T burnisher
19. Cement spatula
20. Mixing pad
21. Gothic arch tracers
22. Articulator (Fig. 2.8.2).

### Sequence of Procedures Followed During Recording of Jaw Relations

1. Customizing the occlusion rims.
2. Recording orientation jaw relations and face bow transfer.

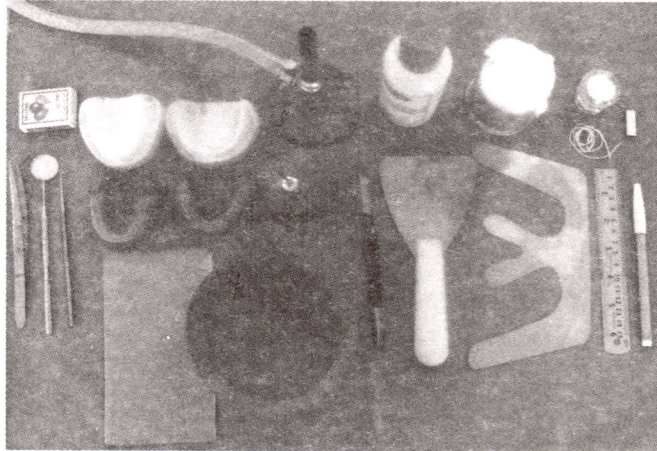

Fig. 2.8.2

3. Recording vertical dimension of rest.
4. Recording vertical dimension of occlusion and free way space.
5. Recording centric jaw relation.
6. Recording eccentric jaw relations.
7. Transfer of recorded jaw relations to the articulator for teeth arrangement.

**Customizing the Occlusion Rims**
1. Try in of the occlusion rims.
2. Establishing labial form of occlusion rims.
3. Establishing the buccal and lingual form of occlusion rims.
4. Establishing the overjet.
5. Establishing the level of occlusal rims.
6. Establishing the plane of occlusal rims.

1. Try in of the occlusion rims
   - Place the occlusal rims in patients mouth and cheek for retention, stability and interferences.
   - Occlusal rims with record bases should be stable to obtain accurate jaw relation records.
   - The stability and retention of unstable record bases can be improved by lining the tissue surface with a thin layer of zinc oxide eugenol paste or elastomeric impression material.
   - If there are interferences in the upper and lower record bases during closing or lateral movements should be correct. If not corrected results in pain and injury to the tissues. Occasionally these interferences are seen in the posterior portion between upper and lower record bases.

2. Establishing the labial form of occlusion rims
   - The occlusal rim should provide adequate lip support and labial fullness or inadequate or excessive labial support will seriously affect the facial appearence and aesthetics of the denture.
   - Inadequate support makes the upper lip look flabby and unsupported. There is deepening of nasolabial creases or folds which give aged appearance.
   - Excessive labial fullness results in stretched look. The philtrum appears shallow and nasolabial fold appears smooth.
   - Lip support is determined by amount of wax in the incisal edge of occlusal rim.

3. Establishing the buccal and lingual form of occlusion rims
   - The space between the buccal surface of the posterior teeth and inner surface of the cheeks is called the buccal corridor.
   - The occlusion rims should be placed within neutral zone and adequate buccal corridor should be present.
   - If buccal corridor is less, i.e. if occlusal rims are placed more buccally results in cheek biting and displacement of dentures by buccal musculature.
   - If buccal corridor is excessive, i.e. if occlusal rims are placed more lingually or palatally results in unaesthetic appearance due to dark spaces created.
   - In case of mandibular occlusal rims one should see that enough space is available for accomodation and free movements of tongue. If occlusal rims placed too lingually results in restriction of tongue movements and displacement of dentures. Hence the occlusal rims should be placed in the neutral zone, where the forces of buccal, lingual musculature are balanced.

4. Establishing the overjet
   - The incisal edge of maxillary occlusal rim should be placed 2–3 mm anterior to the incisal edge of the mandibular occlusal rim in cases of class I malocclusion. Overjet is increased in cases of class II malocclusion. In cases of class III malocclusion incisal edge of maxillary occlusal rim should be placed in flush with incisal edge of mandibular occlusal rim.

5. Establishing the level of occlusal rims
   - In most individuals, upper incisors are visible by 1 or 2 mm when lips are at rest and mouth is slightly open. This is known as incisal visibility. Hence, level of upper occlusal rims anteriorly should be 1 to 2 mm below the level of upper lip at rest. The posterior level of upper occlusal rim should be one-fourth inch below the level of opening of Stensen's duct.
   - The level of lower occlusal rim anteriorly should be at the level of lower lip and angle of mouth. Posteriorly, the level of lower occlusal rim should be at two-third the height of the retromolar pad.

6. Establishing the plane of occlusal rims
   - The plane of occlusal rim should be parallel to the plane of the maxilla. The plane of maxilla is determined anteriorly by interpupillary line and posteriorly by ala tragus line, which extends from ala of nose to the upper border of tragus of ear. Ala-tragus line is also known as campers line. Hence, the anterior portion of occlusal rim should be parallel to inter-pupillary line and posterior portion of occlusal rim should be parallel to ala-tragus line.
   - After adjusting the anterior part of upper occlusal rim parallel to the inter-pupillary line, the level of posterior part is adjusted parallel to ala-tragus line using fox occlusal plane. The ala-tragus line is marked on patients face using a thread dipped in dental plaster or pumice. The bite fork of fox plane is placed over the maxillary occlusal rim inside the mouth and the level of outer rim is compared with ala tragus line. Occlusal rim is adjusted by removing or adding wax until the level of outer rim of fox plane is parallel to ala tragus line (Figs 2.8.3 and 2.8.4).

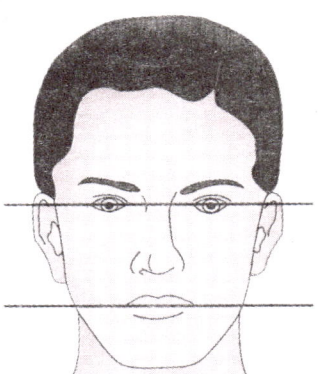

Fig. 2.8.3: The horizontal occlusal plane is parallel to the pupils of the eyes

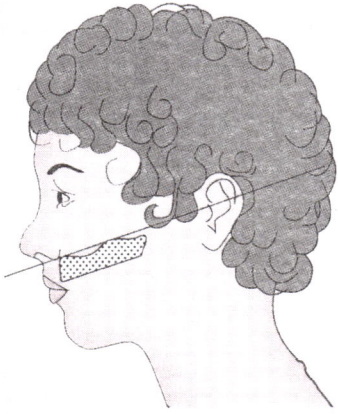

Fig. 2.8.4: The sagittal occlusal plane is parallel to the ala-tragus plane (Camper's Line)

# METHODS OF RECORDING JAW RELATIONS

## RECORDING ORIENTATION JAW RELATIONS AND FACE BOW TRANSFER (USING HANAU FASCIA AND EAR PIECE TYPE FACE BOW)

- When using Hanau fascia type of face bow, posterior reference points are marked 13 mm anterior to the tragus on the tragus-canthus line. The condylar rods are positioned over this mark and locking screws are tightened.
- When using Hanau ear piece type of face bow, there is no need to mark the posterior reference points and ear pieces of face bow are positioned directly in the external auditory meatus.
- The bite fork is heated and inserted into the maxillary rim parallel to the occlusal plane. The recording base is inserted into the mouth and extension rod of the bite fork is passed through the locking device of the face bow.
- The U-shaped flame is slipped over the stem of the bite fork. The stem of the bite fork should be parallel to the sagittal plane. The locking screws tightened to secure the bite fork to face bow assembly.
- The tip of orbital pointer is placed over the orbitale and locks are tightened to secure it to the face bow.
- The condylar lock nuts are then released in case of fascia type of face bow and the face bow and attached occlusal rims are transferred to the articulator.
- The condylar rods of face bow are inserted over the condylar ball extensions and centered before being locked in position by tightening the lock nuts.
- The face bow is adjusted by elevating screw to align the occlusal plane with the groove marked around the half way point of the incisal pin.
- The upper cast is attached to upper record base and secured to the upper arm of articulator with dental mounting plaster.
- Later, the lower occlusal rim is related to upper occlusal rim recording to centric relation records made and lower cast is attached to lower record base and secured to lower member of articulator with dental mounting plaster.
- Now the articulator is ready with occlusal rims for programming and teeth arrangement.

## METHODS OF RECORDING VERTICAL DIMENSION OF REST POSITION

1. Facial measurements after swallowing and relaxing
2. Tactile sense
3. Measurements of anatomic landmarks
4. Speech
5. Facial expression

### 1. Facial measurements after swallowing and relaxing
- Instruct the patient sit upright comfortably in a dental chair with eyes looking straight ahead at same level. Place the maxillary record base with occlusal rim in the patients mouth.
- Two reference points are selected with either an indelible marker or a triangle of adhesive tape, reference point is placed over tip of nose in upper jaw and at the point of chin in lower jaw.
- Now the patient is asked to wet the lips, swallow and relax the shoulders. By doing so, mandible attains the rest position, measure the distance between the reference points with a metallic scale. Repeat the procedure until consistent measurements are obtained. This measurement corresponds to vertical dimension of rest position.

### 2. Tactile sense
- Ask the patient to sit erect and mark the reference points as mentioned above. Now ask the patient to open the jaws wide until strain is felt in the muscles. Instruct the patient to close the jaws slowly and stop closing once jaws reach comfortable and relaxed position. The distance measured between reference points at this position denotes the vertical dimension of rest position.

### 3. Phonetics
- Ask the patient to repeat the name Emm and stop all jaw movements once the lips touch each other. Now the distance measured between reference points gives the vertical dimension of rest position.
- Engage the patient in conversation. Once patient stops talking followed by drop of mandible indicates that mandible attained rest position. Now measure the distance between the reference points.

### 4. Facial expression
The following facial expressions indicate mandible is in physiologic rest position.
- In normally related jaws the lips will be even anteroposteriorly and in slight contact. In protruded mandible lower lip will be anterior to upper lip and not in contact. In retruded mandible lower lip will be posterior to upper lip and not in contact.
- The skin around the eyes and over the chin will be relaxed.
- Relaxation around the nares aids in unobstructed breathing.

### 5. Anatomic landmarks
- The willis guide is used to measure the distance from the pupils of the eye to rima oris (corner of mouth) and distance from the anterior nasal spine to lower border of mandible. When these two measurements are equal, the jaws are considered to be in a state of physiologic rest position.

## METHODS OF RECORDING VERTICAL DIMENSION OF OCCLUSION

### 1. Mechanical methods
a. Pre extraction records
- **Profile radiographs:** The radiographs taken while teeth in occlusion are compared with radiographs taken while occlusal rims are in occlusion and occlusal rims are adjusted accordingly.
- **Casts of teeth in occlusion:** Impressions of both upper and lower arches made before extraction of teeth and casts fabricated. Maxillary cast is related in its correct anatomic position on an articulator with a face bow transfer and an occlusal record with jaws in centric relation is used to mount the mandibular cast. Once all the teeth have been extracted, impressions made and edentulous casts mounted on another articulator. The interarch measurements of both articulators are compared during recording of vertical dimensions.
- **Facial measurements:** Two tattoo points are placed, one on the upper part of face and one on lower part of face before teeth extraction and distance measured between these points. After extraction of teeth, the distance between these points is used in recording vertical dimensions. Usually one point is marked on tip of the nose and another point is marked on chin and distance between these two points is measured with the help of calipers.
- **Profile photographs:** Profile photographs of patient are taken and enlarged to life size. Measurements of anatomic landmarks on photographs are compared with measurements of same anatomic landmarks on face while recording the vertical dimension of occlusions.
- **Profile silhouettes:** Silhouettes literally means shape of something or some body seen against a light back ground. Lead wires are adapted

to the patients profile before extraction. The some outline is transferred to card board and cut out. After extraction the cut out of card board is placed against patients profile and vertical relations are recorded.
- Resin facemasks: Resin facemasks are made before extraction of teeth using a facial impression and cast.

b. Ridge relations
- Incisive papilla to mandibular incisors:
  - The distance between incisive papillae and incisal edges of maxillary central incisors is approximately 6 mm.
  - The distance between incisive papillae and incisal edge of mandibular anterior teeth is approximately 4 mm.
  - These measurements help in recording vertical jaw relations.
- Parallelism of the ridges
  - According to sears, parallelism of maxillary and mandibular ridges together with 5-degree opening in the posterior region gives a clue to the appropriate amount of jaw separation.
  - But, in most people loss of teeth occurs at different times and when a person becomes completely edentulous, it is often noted that residual ridges are no more parallel to each other because of resorption of residual ridges.

c. Measurement of the former dentures
  - The former dentures are measured between the ridge crests in the maxillary and mandibular dentures with the help of Boley gauge. These measurements are correlated with observations of patients face to determine the amount of change required in vertical dimension.

2. **Physiologic Methods**
a. Physiologic rest position tests
- Parting the lips after swallowing: Patient is asked to swallow and relax without making any further movements. The lips are separated by dentist to observe the amount of interocclusal space present between the occlusal rims. These should be 2–4 mm of interocclusal space at the premolar region.
- Niswongers method: Two points are marked one over the tip of nose and one over the chin. The patient is asked to swallow and relax. The distance between the two points is measured. This gives the vertical dimension of rest position. Now the occlusal rims are adjusted till the distance between two points become 2–4 mm less than the measurement obtained between these two points during rest position. This gives the vertical dimension of occlusion.

b. Phonetics
- Using the M sound: Ask the patient to say 'M' several times and stop all jaw movements once lips touch each other. Measure the distance between two reference points as mentioned above this gives vertical dimension of rest position. Adjust occlusal rims till measurement of 2–4 mm shorter than at rest position is obtained.
- Using ch, S and J sound: The production of ch, S and J sounds brings the anterior teeth close together. When correctly placed, the lower incisors move forward to a position nearly directly under and almost touching the upper incisors. If the distance is too large indicated decreased vertical dimension and if teeth touch and make clicking sounds indicates increased vertical dimension.
- Silverman's closest speaking space: It measures vertical dimension when the mandible and muscles involved are in physiologic function of speech. When sounds like ch, S and J are pronounced, the maxillary and mandibular anterior teeth come close to each other without contact. This minimal amount of space between maxillary and mandibular teeth in this position is called Silvermans closer speaking space.

c. Esthetics
- According to Willis, the distance between the outer canthus of eye and corner of mouth should be equal to the distance between lower border of septum of nose and the lower border of the chin (facial proportions).
- Tone of the facial skin should be same throughout. The nares and skin around the chin and eyes are relaxed. If corners of mouth are drooping it indicates decreased vertical dimension.
- Lip support and labial fullness should be adjusted to obtain natural appearance.

d. Swallowing threshold
- It is based on the theory that teeth come together with a very light contact at the begining of swallowing. Hence swallowing threshold is used to record vertical dimension of occlusion. The technique involves placement of wax cones on lower denture base in such a way that they contact upper occlusal rim when the jaws are open too wide. Salivation is stimulated by food such as candy and patient is instructed to swallow. The repeated action of swallowing the saliva gradually reduce the height of the wax cones

to allow the mandible to reach the level of vertical dimension of occlusion.

e. Tactile sense and patient perceived comfort
- The patients tactile sense can be used as a guide for determination of occlusal vertical dimension.
- In this method a central bearing plate is attached to upper occlusal rim and central bearing screw is attached to lower occlusal rim. The central bearing screw is progressively tightened. This tightening will bring both the occlusal rims towards each other. Tighten till patient feels discomfort in his jaws due to over tightening and note this point.
- The same procedure is repeated with central bearing plate in lower rim and central bearing screw in upper rim. The central bearing point is slowly reduced till patient indicates comfortable jaw relationship.

f. Boos bimeter (power point)
- Boos stated that maximum biting force occurs at vertical dimension of occlusion. Bimeter is the device used to measure the biting force. Bimeter is attached to mandibular record base and central bearing point (a metal plate) is attached to maxillary record base. Screw is turned to adjust vertical dimension of occlusion. The point of which highest biting force occurs is called power point and it indicates the vertical dimension of occlusion.

## METHODS OF RECORDING CENTRIC JAW RELATIONS

### 1. Physiologic Methods

a. Pressure method with nick and notch indexing.
- As explained earlier, centric relation is the most posterior relation of the mandible to the maxillae at the established vertical dimension. So, the next step to follow after establishing the vertical dimensions is to record the centric followed by eccentric jaw relations.
- This is the most common method used in recording centric jaw relations. The other methods like inter occlusal check records, graphic tracings and radiographic methods are used to verify whether the centric relations recorded by pressure less records give accurate centric jaw relations.

Procedure
- After establishing vertical jaw relations, remove about 3 mm of mandibular occlusal rim from first premolar area distally to the end of the wax rim both on the right and left sides.
- 2 or 3 notches are made on each side of maxillary occlusal rim from first premolar area distally to the end of the wax rims. Notch is a 'V' shaped valley running totally across the width of the occlusal rim. It prevents antero posterior movement.
- One nick is made anterior to the notch on both sides of maxillary occlusal rim. This prevents lateral movement. Nick is also a 'V' shaped valley but it does not extend throughout the width of the occlusal rim.
- Slightly lubricate the areas of nick and notches with petrolatum.
- Make the patient sit upright in dental chair and insert the prepared maxillary and mandibular occlusal rims.
- The patient is trained, instructed and guided to close the mouth in centric relation. The best way to assist the patient in retruding the mandible is to place the index fingers on the buccal flanges of the mandibular occlusion rim in both premolar regions with the thumbs under patients chin. The recording base is held firmly to the lower jaw and patient is asked to close his mouth slowly and gently on the back teeth under the guidance of the dentist. Another method is to place the occlusal rims in patients mouth and ask the patient to swallow and not to make any movements after that the mandible attains centric relation during swallowing cycle.
- Scribe the midline, canine line and high lip line on the occlusal rims in the recorded centric relation position with lecron carver. Midline on occlusal rims should coincide with midline of face except in cases of facial asymmetry. Canine line is scribed vertically on occlusal rims coinciding with the ala of the nose. Patient is asked to smile and the high lip line is scribed horizontally marking the level of exposure of occlusion rims during smiling.
- Remove the mandibular record base from patients mouth and place soft Aluwax from the first premolar region to distal end of occlusal rim on both sides, where you have removed 3 mm of wax previously. The Aluwax should be 1½ mm above the original height of the occlusal rim. Now place the mandibular record base in warm water so that Aluwax on both right and left sides is evenly and thoroughly softened.
- Place the mandibular record base in patients mouth and guide to attain the same retruded mandibular centric relation position as attained previously. See that the mid line, canine line scribed on upper and lower occlusal rims will coincide with each other. The closure should continue until the anterior

occlusal rims are within 1/2 mm of the original accepted vertical dimension.
- Remove the record bases from mouth and place them in cold water till wax hardens.
- With the help of centric relation record, now mount the lower cast to the articulator. Remember that upper cast is already mounted to articulator during orientation jaw relations and face bow transfer.
- Note that instead of Aluwax, we can also use impression plaster or bite registration paste such as zinc oxide eugenol paste.
- Instead of using nick and notch method to seal the upper and lower occlusal rims in centric relation, we can also seal the upper and lower occlusal rims once centric relation is attained by placing heated stapler pins through upper and lower occlusal rims posteriorly on both sides.

b. Pressure method
- In this method, once the vertical jaw relation records are made, mandibular occlusal rim is removed and height of mandibular occlusal rim is increased approximately by 1 to 2 mm.
- Now place the mandibular occlusal rim in warm water for uniform softening of wax. Now place the mandibular occlusal rim back in patient mouth, guide the patient to close his mouth in centric relation position till the previously measured vertical dimension is obtained.

c. Tactile or interocclusal check records
- It is a two step procedure in which during first step tentative centric jaw relations are recorded and trial dentures fabricated. In the second step, interocclusal check records are made with trial dentures and tentative centric jaw relations recorded earlier were verified and errors are corrected.

Indications
- Abnormally related upper and lower jaws.
- In cases of displaceable flabby tissues.
- In cases of large tongue.
- In cases of uncontrolled mandibular movements.
- In case of patients already using complete dentures.

Procedure
- As mentioned earlier, in the first step tentative centric jaw relations recorded. Mandibular occlusal rim is reduced to create extra space for interocclusal material.
- Upper and lower occlusal rims are mounted on articulator, teeth arrangement done and trial dentures are fabricated. These trial dentures are used in second step for making interocclusal check records.
- In the second step, upper and lower trial dentures are placed in patients mouth. Aluwax or any other bite registration material is loaded on to the occlusal surfaces of teeth lower trial denture. Now patient is asked to slowly retrude the mandible and close on the wax till tooth contact takes place. Once tooth contact takes place trial dentures are removed from patients mouth, wax is allowed to cool and both trail dentures are placed on their articulated casts and compared with tentative centric relation records.
- If both the condylar elements of articulator contact against the centric stops (centric position of condyle in glenoid fossa) indicates that tentative centric relation records are accurate and need not be changed.
- If any one of the condylar elements of articulator do not contact against the centric stops indicates that tentative centric relation records are inaccurate.

2. Functional Methods (Chew-in Methods)
- Functional methods utilize the functional movements of jaws to record the centric jaw relation. Patient is instructed to perform protrusive and lateral movements to identify the most retruded position of mandible.

a. Needle house method.
- This is the most commonly used functional method for recording centric jaw relations.
- This method requires fabrication of occlusal rims with impression compound. Two metal beads or styli on each side are embedded into premolar and molar areas of maxillary occlusal rim made of impression compound.
- Now both the occlusal rims are placed in patients mouth and instructed to do protrusive, retrusive, right lateral and left lateral movements of mandible. During this procedure, the metal styli attached to upper occlusal rim will create a diamond shaped markings on mandibular occlusal rim. The posterior most point of this diamond pattern represents the centric jaw relation.

b. Patterson method
- In this method, a trench is made in a wax mandibular occlusal rim and filled with a mixture of plaster and carborundum paste.
- The occlusal rims are placed in patients mouth and instructed to perform all mandibular movements. These movements produce compensating curves on plaster carborundum mix.

- Patient is asked to do mandibular movements till required vertical dimension is obtained and finally occlusal rims are sealed with staples in most retruded position.

c. Meyer's method
- This method uses soft wax to establish a generated path. A plaster index is made of the wax path and used to set the teeth.

3. **Graphic Methods (Excursive Methods)**
  a. **Arrow Point Tracing (Gothic arch Tracing).**
- It is a one dimensional graphic tracing made with the help of gothic arch traces. It is usually recorded in a horizontal plane. The mechanism involved is that a pen like pointer is attached to one occlusal rim and recording plate is attached to other occlusal rim. During mandibular movements the pointer draws characteristic patterns on the recording plate. The pointer is called as the central bearing point and the recording plate is known as the central bearing plate.
- Graphic methods are used to verify the centric jaw relations recorded by other methods and also to record the centric jaw records.
- In all graphic methods, tentative centric relation records are made in the begining and casts are mounted on an articulator. Now the tracing devices are attached to occlusal rims while they are on the articulator.
- Based on location of tracers, arrow point tracers are classified as intraoral and extraoral tracers.

  i. Intraoral tracing
  - In this type of tracer, central bearing plate is attached to maxillary rim and central bearing point or stylus is attached to mandibular rim. The central bearing plate is covered with a marking substance such as carbon, ink or wax. The stylus is adjusted by screw till it touches the central bearing plate.
  - Occlusal rims along with tracer assembly is placed in patients mouth and instructed to perform protrusive, right lateral and left lateral movements several times with light pressure. Central bearing device consisting of small fixed ball and a plate present between two occlusal rims helps in maintaining vertical relation while patient performs various mandibular movements. The stylus traces an arrow point on the central bearing plate corresponding to the movements. In intraoral tracing arrow points posteriorly. A short apex represents accurate centric relation records. Remove occlusal rims from patients mouth along with tracer assembly return to articulator and verify accuracy of previous tentatively recorded central jaw relations. If stylus coincides with the apex in the articulator indicates tentative records are accurate.
  - Disadvantages of intraoral tracers are, it is diffcult to see the tracing and hence guiding the patient is difficult. As intraoral tracing is small, it is difficult to locate the apex.
  - Advantage of intraoral tracers is they are strong enough to resist biting pressure.

  ii. Extraoral tracing
  - Extraoral tracer is always combined with intraoral tracer to equalize pressure. Here, the central bearing plate is attached to lower occlusion rim and centered bearing pin or stylus is attached to upper occlusal rim. The procedure is similar to that of intra oral tracing.
  - Advantages are tracing is visible and hence patient can be guided to do proper movements. The tracing point is larger, so apex is clearly seen.

  b. Pantograph
- It is defined as the "graphic record of mandibular movement in three planes as registered by the styli on the recording tables of a pantograph; tracings of mandibular movement recorded on plates in the horizontal and sagittal planes"—GPT.
- It is the most accurate method of recording centric jaw relations.
- It is generally not used for fabrication of complete dentures. It is used for full mouth rehabilitation of dentulous patients.

4. **Terminal Hinge Axis Method**
- In this method, a kinematic face bow is used to locate the terminal hinge axis. As the mandible rotates around hinge axis and occludes with the wax rims, it automatically sets in centric relation.

5. **Other Methods**
  a. Strips of celluloid placed between rims
- Strips of celluloid are placed between occlusal rims and pulled out. The patient is asked to close on strips of celluloid and restrain the celluloid from slipping away. In doing so, patients mandible automatically attains centric relation postion.

  b. Heating the surface of one of the rims
- Deep heating of posterior portion of mandibular occlusal rim and leaving the anterior portion cold in order to maintain vertical dimension of occlusion.

c. Deep heating or pooling method
   - Soft wax is placed on mandibular occlusal rims and patient is instructed to bite in centric relation.

d. Occlusal surfaces of lower posterior teeth covered with softened wax
   - Conical blocks of wax are placed on mandibular record base and patient is asked to swallow. This establishes both vertical and centric jaw relation.

e. Placement of soft cones of wax over lower denture bases

## METHODS OF RECORDING ECCENTRIC JAW RELATIONS

- Eccentric jaw relations are made to adjust the horizontal and lateral condylar inclinations in the articulator. This helps the articulator in reproducing eccentric movements of mandible and establish balanced occlusion.
- Methods used
  - Functional methods
  - Graphic methods (excursive methods)
  - Direct check records
- The procedures followed to record eccentric jaw relations are similar to those followed for recording centric jaw relations.

# CHAPTER 9
# Teeth Selection

Teeth selection is not simply a mechanical procedure, but require dexterity and knowledge of biology. Selection of teeth forms an important step before teeth arrangement as it creates a dentofacial harmony.

Selection and placement of artificial teeth is based on the knowledge of anatomy, histology, physiology, pathology and biomechanics. The nature of the mucosa and submucosa, the form and relationship of the residual ridge, the general systemic condition of the patient, the tone of mandibular musculature, esthetic factors and patient past experiences can all relate to the size, form and number of artificial posterior teeth that may be used on the denture bases.

The dentist is solely responsible for the selection of the teeth as he/she alone possesses the necessary information required in this regard.

## DEFINITION

- The selection of a tooth or teeth of a shape, size and colour to harmonise with the individual characteristics of a patient—GPT.

## OBJECTIVES OF TEETH SELECTION

1. The anterior teeth selected should create a esthetically pleasing appearance while simultaneously maintaining oral function.
2. The posterior teeth selected should aid in denture base stability and should be efficient for mastication rather than merely reproducing natural forms.
3. They should maintain correct vertical dimension and should allow the patient to speak normally.
4. They should not abuse the tissues over residual ridges.
5. Patient should be given enough information and assistance and should be guided toward a limited selection of anatomically possible tooth selections so that they can choose the teeth that make them happy.

## TYPES OF TEETH

1. *Based on size of teeth*
    a. Large teeth
    b. Small teeth
    c. Long teeth
    d. Short teeth
    e. Wide teeth
    f. Narrow teeth
    g. Medium or regular size teeth

2. *Based on shape of teeth*
    a. Square teeth
    b. Ovoid teeth
    c. Tapering teeth
    d. Square tapering teeth

3. *Based on colour of teeth*
    a. Dark shade teeth
    b. Light shade teeth

4. *Based on occlusal form of posterior teeth*
   a. Anatomic teeth (cusp teeth)
      i. With 33° cuspal angulation.
      ii. With 30° cuspal angulation (Pilkington-Turner teeth).
   b. Semianatomic teeth (low cusp teeth)
      i. With 20° cuspal angulation.
      ii. With 10° cuspal angulation (functional or anatoline teeth).
   c. Non anatomic teeth (cuspless teeth)
      i. with 0° cuspal angulation (mono plane teeth).
5. *Based on material used*
   a. Acrylic teeth
   b. Porcelain teeth
   c. Composite teeth
   d. Porcelain acrylic combination scheme
   e. Acrylic teeth with amalgam inserts
   f. Acrylic teeth with gold occlusal surface
6. Hollow-ground teeth (used over retained tooth root or implant abutment in cases of overdenture fabrication).

## GUIDELINES FOR ANTERIOR TEETH SELECTION

- Esthetics plays a very important role in selection of anterior teeth. Every one sees the anterior teeth and everyone has an opinion. Patient should be given enough information and should be guided toward selection of anatomically possible and esthetically pleasing teeth that make them happy.
- The various parameters considered during anterior teeth selection are as follows:
  1. Size of the teeth.
  2. Shape or form or mold of the teeth.
  3. Colour on shade of teeth.
  4. Tooth material.

### I. SELECTION OF TEETH SIZE

- The factors considered during selection of teeth size are:
  1. Mesiodistal width
  2. Incisogingival length
  3. Faciolingual thickness.
- The selection of teeth size can be done using pre-extraction records or based on post extraction records or by following various methods during examination of completely edentulous patient.

**A. Based on Pre Extraction Records**
1. **Diagnostic Casts**
   - The diagnostic casts with patients natural or restored teeth help in selection of tooth size and form. But, these casts cannot guide in selection of tooth colour. These are most reliable guides in selection of tooth size and form.

2. **Photographs of Patient**
   - The photographs of patients before loss of teeth helps in selection of tooth size, shape and also colour to some extent. It depends on the amount of teeth visible in photographs.
   - Facial photographs are also helpful in determining the placement of anterior teeth, arch form and lip support.

3. **Radiographs of Patient**
   - They help in selection of tooth size (especially incisogingival length) and tooth shape. But, most of the radiographs cannot exactly determine the size and shape of tooth due to inherent radiographic errors. So, radiographic errors like elongation of crown and shortening of crown should be compensated during taking measurements from radiographs.

4. **Previous Partial Dentures**
   - Most of the patients would have the history of wearing partial dentures at some period of time before becoming completely edentulous. So, if available the partial dentures are of more help in selection of tooth size, shape and colour.

**B. Based on Post Extraction Records**
1. **Extracted Teeth**
   - In case patients preserved their extracted teeth, they are the exact best guides in selection of size and shape of the teeth. The extracted teeth discolour and hence should not be used for selection of colour or shade of the teeth.

2. **Old Dentures of Patient**
   - If patient was already a denture wearer, his / her previous dentures can guide in selection of teeth upto some extent only. They cannot exactly guide in selection of teeth of proper dimensions if the teeth are worn out or attrited. They are especially useful in selection of teeth in cases of replacement of immediate dentures with new conventional dentures.

**C. Based on various methods used during examination of Completely Edentulous Patient**
- When the pre and post extraction records are not available or not useful in selection of anterior teeth, then the following methods can be used during examination of completely edentulous patient.

1. **Mesiodistal Width**
   A. **Based on Anthropometric Measurements**
   a. Using bizygomatic width—Face bow is used as calipers to measure the distance between zygoma.

i. width of maxillary central incisor

$$= \frac{\text{Bizygomatic width}}{16}$$

ii. total width of maxillary anteriors

$$= \frac{\text{Bizygomatic width}}{3.3}$$

iii. Width of maxillary lateral incisor is 2 mm less than central incisor
iv. Width of maxillary canine is 1 mm less than central incisor
v. Total width of mandibular anteriors

$$= \frac{4}{5} \times (\text{Total width of maxillary anteriors})$$

b. Using cranial circumference—cranial circumference is measured at the level of forehead using a measuring tape.
Total width of maxillary anteriors

$$= \frac{\text{Cranial circumference}}{10}$$

c. Using length of face (only in case of dentulous patients)—length of the face is the distance measured between hairline and the tip of chin. (width of maxillary central incisor)

$$= \frac{\text{Lenght of face}}{20}$$

### B. Based on Anatomic Landmarks
a. *Using size of maxillary arch*
   - Three points are marked, one on crest of incisive papilla and one each on both hamular notches. Three points joined to form a triangle. Each side of triangle is measured and combined to get a total value. The total value obtained equals the total width of all the maxillary anteriors and posterior teeth.
b. *Using corners of mouth as guide*
   - Make the marks on maxillary occlusal rims corresponding to corners of mouth during rest position. These marks denote the distal surface of canine hence the distance between these two points along the contour of occlusal rims gives the total width of maxillary anterior teeth.
c. *Using incisive papilla and canine eminence or buccal frenum as guide*
   - If canine eminences are clearly seen in edentulous ridges, then measure the distance from the distal of one canine eminence to the distal of other canine eminence with a flexible ruler. The ruler should follow the contour of the ridge and as it reaches the midline, it should be placed on the anterior border of the incisal papilla because the maxillary central incisors are situated labially to the papilla. The measurement obtained indicates the total width of maxillary anterior teeth.
   - If the canine eminences are not seen clearly, the attachments of buccal frenum can be used. A line placed slightly anterior to the frenum attachments will be distal to the canine eminence.
d. *Using ala of nose as guide*
   - One point is marked between center of the right and left eye brows and two points, one each on lateral most aspect of ala of nose are marked. When these three points are joined to extend on to maxillary occlusal rims marks the corners of mouth. Thus the distance measured between corners of mouth gives the total width of maxillary anterior teeth.

### 2. Selection of Incisogingival Length
a. *Using length of face as guide*
Length of face is the distance measured between hairline and the tip of chin.

$$\text{Length of maxillary central incisor} = \frac{\text{lenth of face}}{16}$$

b. *Using smile line as guide*
Patient is asked to smile with occlusal rims in place and a line is drawn on the rims at the point to which lip elevates. In general, the maxillary lip comes close to the gingival neck of the teeth when a patient smiles broadly. Hence, the teeth selected should have incisogingival length slightly above the smile line so that denture base won't be visible during smiling.
c. *Inter arch space as guide*
If the inter arch space is less then teeth with less incisogingival length should be selected and in cases of more inter arch space, teeth with more incisogingival length should be selected.

### 3. Selection of Faciolingual Thickness
Teeth with more faciolingual thickness are preferred when compared to teeth with less faciolingual thickness. This is because, thicker teeth can be rotated and spaced out to give a more realistic appearence.

## II. SELECTION OF TEETH SHAPE
- The factors considered during selection of shape of the teeth are:
  - Facial form of teeth.
  - Proximal form of teeth.
  - Incisal form of teeth.
  - Curvature of teeth.

### A. Based on Pre Extraction Records
1. Diagnostic casts
2. Photographs

3. Radiographs
4. Preserved partial dentures

**B. Based on Post Extraction Records**
1. Preserved extracted teeth.
2. Old complete dentures.

**C. Based on Examination of the Patient**

**1. Facial Form of Teeth**
- Williams and House and Loop classified the outline forms of face and selected anterior teeth which were in harmony with facial form. According to them, the shape of the teeth should be inverse of the shape of the face.
- The form of face is identified by connecting the following points on the lateral aspect of face: the forehead, the zygomatic arch and the angle of mandible.
- Accordingly, 3 basic forms of face and corresponding facial forms of teeth are (Fig. 2.9.1):
  a. Square form
  b. Ovoid form
  c. Tapering form

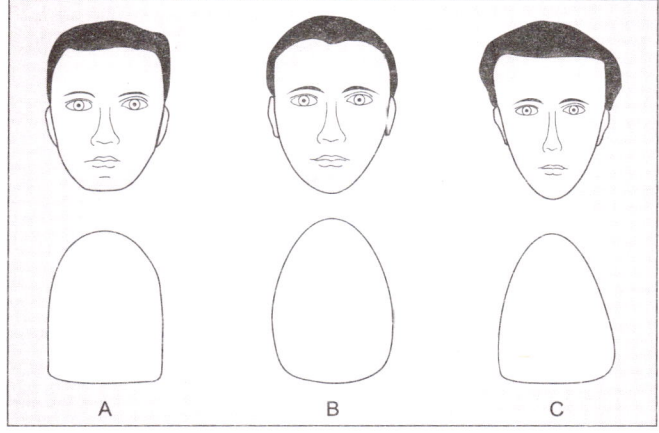

**Fig. 2.9.1:** Basic forms of face

- The shape of the maxillary central incisor should resemble the shape of the face if it were placed upside down.
- Selection of teeth based on theory of form of faces is known as the geometric theory.

**2. Proximal Form of Teeth**
- Based on the profile of patient, proximal form of teeth can be
  – straight
  – convex

**3. Incisal Form of Teeth**
- Based on the profile of patient, incisal form of teeth also can be
  – straight
  – convex.

**4. Curvature of Teeth**
- The tooth may curve in both mesiodistal direction and inciso gingival direction. The mesiodistal incisogingival curvature of tooth selected should complement the profile curvatures of the face.

### III. SELECTION OF COLOUR OF THE TEETH

- Light is electromagnetic radiation that can be detected by the human eye. The eye is sensitive to wavelengths from approximately 400 (violet) to 700 nm (dark red). A specific colour of object is recognised by human eye when that particular object reflects a specific colour and absorbs all the other colours of the incident light.

  E.g. A yellow object will absorb all the colours of the incident light but reflects the yellow colour which falls on retina of eye and recognised as yellow colour. Cone-shaped cells in the retina are responsible for colour vision.

### THREE DIMENSIONS OF COLOUR

- To accurately describe our perception of a beam of light reflected from a tooth and restoration surface, their basic dimensions of colour should be measured.

**1. Hue**
- Hue describes the dominant colour of an object such as red, green or yellow. It is basically the colour of an object. The hue of teeth is usually in the yellow range.

**2. Value (Brilliance)**
- Value is the lightness or darkness of a colour, which can be measured independently of the hue. For example, the yellow of a lemon is lighter than the red of a cherry. The value increases as an object becomes light or more nearly white. So, greater the value greater the lightness.

**3. Chroma (saturation)**
- Chroma represents the degree of saturation of a particular hue or colour of an object. For example, the yellow colour of a lemon is more intense than that of a banana which is dull yellow. So, lemon has more chroma than banana. Similarly, in natural teeth the canine and the incisor might have the same hue but a different chroma, canine is usually more saturated with colour hence it has more chroma.

## OTHER PROPERTIES OF COLOUR

### 1. Opacity
- Opacity is property of material that prevents the passage of light. When all the colours of the spectrum from a white light source such as sun light are reflected from an object with the same intensity as received, the object appears white. When all the colours of the spectrum are absorbed equally, the object appears black when an opaque object absorbs most of the colours of spectrum of light and reflects a particular colour, the object appears as the colour of reflected light.

### 2. Transluency
- Transluency is a property of substance that permits the passage of light but disperses the light, so objects cannot be seen through the material. Incisal edges and mesial and distal areas of teeth are some times translucent and when selecting artificial teeth for dentures this property should not be neglected, in order to get the natural appearance of teeth.

### 3. Transparency
- Transparency is the property of material that allows the passage of light in such a way that little distortion takes place and objects may clearly seen through them, e.g. glass.

### 4. Metamerism
- The objects that appear to be colour matched under one type of light may appear different under another light source. This phenomenon is called as the metamerism. Thus, if possible colour matching should be done under two or more different light sources, one of which should be day light and lab procedures should be carried out under the same lighting conditions.

### 5. Flourescence
- Apart from visible light, natural tooth also absorbs light at wavelengths too short to be visible to human eye (between 300 to 400 nm known as near ultraviolet radiation) and converts into light with longer wavelengths, in the process tooth actually becoming a light source. This property of converting the energy absorbed from light at lower wavelengths to light at longer wavelengths and becoming a light source is called flourescence. The emitted light, a blue - white colour, is primarily in the range of 400–450 mm. Flourescence makes a definite contribution to the brightness and vital appearance of human tooth.

## SELECTION OF COLOUR OF THE TEETH

### A. Based on Pre Extraction Records
- Photographs of patient.
- Preserved partial dentures.

### B. Based on Post Extraction Records
- Preserved extracted teeth (help in providing information about stains present but does not help in slection of colour).
- Old complete dentures.

### C. Based on Examination of the Patient

1. Age
   - In young patients requiring complete dentures, lighter shade teeth (high value) should be selected and for old patients darker shades of teeth should be selected as teeth becomes yellower and darker colour with advanced age.

2. Colour of the face
   - The tooth colour selected should be in harmony with colour of the face. For patients with fair complexion light colour teeth with high value should be selected and for patients with dark complexion dark colour teeth with low value should be selected.

3. Colour of the eye and hair
   - There is a relative proximity between colour of eye and hair to the complexion of face. Hence, in earlier days these factors were also considered during tooth selection. But, nowadays due to pollution and other factors like colouring the hair with various dyes and application of henna to hair will mislead us in selection of tooth colour and hence should not be considered.

## SHADE GUIDE

- A shade guide consists of various colour tabs resembling natural tooth with difference in hue, value and chroma, shade guide helps in selecting the correct shade of tooth for particular patient based on various factors. These are used in much the same way as paint chips are used to select the colours for house paint.

## STEPS IN SELECTION OF TEETH COLOUR

- Shade guide is used to select the colour of the teeth. A popular system for visual determination of colour is the Munsell colour system.
- According to Munsell colour system, the order of colour selection is as follows,
  a. 'Value' (lightness and darkness) is determined first by selection of tab that most nearly corresponds with complexion of particular patient. Value ranges from white (10) to black (0).
  b. Chroma (saturation) is determined next with tabs that are close to the measured value but are of increasing saturation of colour. Chroma ranges from achromatic or gray (0) to highly saturated colour (18).

c. 'Hue' is determined last by matching with colour tabs of the value and chroma already determined. Hue is measured on a scale from 2.5 to 10.

- Selection of colour of teeth is done in three steps,
    1. Shade tabs are placed at the side of the nose. This step establishes the basic value, chroma and hue of the teeth corresponding to the complexion of face.
    2. In the second step, shade tabs are placed under the lips with only incisal edge showing. This step simulates the tooth exposure when the mouth is relaxed.
    3. In the third step, shade tabs are placed under the lips with only cervical edge covered and remaining part of shade tab exposed. This step simulates the tooth exposure when patient smiles.
- Colour matching should be done under two or more different, light sources, one of which should be day light and the laboratory procedures should be performed under the same lighting conditions.
- If one looks at a particular colour for reasonably long time, receptor fatigue causes a complimentary colour to be seen when one looks at white back ground. Blue is the complimentary colour of yellow. Hence a blue back ground helps in better selection of tooth colour towards yellow.
- Patients with bright make up or lip stick may influence the teeth selection in wrong way and hence request the patients to remove make up and lip stick before teeth selection.

- **Squint Test**
    - This test helps in selection of tooth colour which will be in harmony with complexion of face. Hold the shade tabs to the patients skin near to his / her lips. Now dentist should slowly close the eyes, the shade that disppears first is the closest to the complexion of the patient. Hence, this shade should be selected.
    - For class I cases, same tooth shade is selected for both maxillary and mandibular anteriors. In class II cases, lighter shade is selected for mandibular anteriors to create illusion that teeth are more anterior than they really are in class III cases darker shade (lower value) is selected for mandibular anterior so that they wont be prominently seen as anteriorly placed.

## DENTOGENIC CONCEPT

- Frush and Fischer suggested guidelines for selection and arrangment of anterior teeth based upon the patients age, sex and personality. These guidelines help in enchancing the natural appearance of many patients teeth.

1. **Age**
    - Frush and Fischer stated that the dignity of the advancing age can be successfully portrayed in the denture by careful tooth colour selection and mold (shape) refinement.
    - With increasing age the interocclusal distance decreased and hence mandibular anterior teeth are more visible than maxillary anterior teeth. The amount of maxillary central incisors exposed when lips are gently parted is + 3 mm at 29 years of age and no exposure at 60 years of age. The opposite occurs for mandibular incisors, with approximately 0.5 mm showing at age 29 and 3 mm showing at age 60.
    - By varying the long axis of teeth, using diastema and grinding the incisal edges, the appearance of anterior teeth can be transformed from youthful to advanced in age.
    - In young age, the interdental papillae are pointed, closely adapted to teeth and stippled with age, they become shortened, blunted, edematous and smooth, with signs of gingival recession around necks of some of the teeth.
    - Natural teeth wear with age in most of the patients and this wear can be simulated by grinding the incisal edges of the denture teeth.
    - The colour of teeth also becomes darker with age and attains a yellow brown colour.

2. **Sex (Table 2.9.1)**

3. **Personality**
    - Frush and Fischer used a personality spectrum consisting of 3 ranges
        1. Delicate personality
        2. Vigorous personality
        3. Medium personality
    - *Delicate personality:* Delicate personality is fragile and frail. Round, light coloured femine looking teeth are selected for this personality.
    - *Vigorous personality:* This personality is hard and aggressive. Broad teeth with sharp angles and dark coloured teeth with masculine characters are selected for this personality.
    - *Medium personality:* This personality is moderate and somewhat robust. Majority people have medium personality. Teeth with medium characters are selected (blend of vigorous and delicate characters) for this personality.

## GUIDELINES FOR POSTERIOR TEETH SELECTION

- The various factors considered during selection of posterior teeth are:
    1. Size of the teeth.
    2. Shape of the teeth.

## Table 2.9.1

| Character | Male | Female |
|---|---|---|
| 1. Tooth form | 1. Square of cuboidal | 1. Spherical |
| 2. Labial surface | 2. Flat mesiodistally and incisogingivally | 2. Curved mesiodistally and incisogingivally |
| 3. Incisal angles | 3. Sharper mesioincisal and distoincisal angles | 3. Rounded mesioincisal and distoincisal angles |
| 4. Wideth | 4. Broader lateal incisors | 4. Narrower lateral incisors |
| 5. Arch form | 5. Broad and central incisors slightly turned in on mesial side | 5. Tapered or curved and central incisors turned in at distoincisal edge |
| 6. Cervical region | 6. More prominent | 6. Less prominent |
| 7. Incisal plane | 7. Incisal edge of lateral incisal is at some level as central incisor | 7. Incisal edge of lateal incisor raised compared to central incisor and canine |
| 8. Canines | 8. More prominent and turned out at incisal edge | 8. Less prominent and turned in at the incisal edge (inclined palatally). Hence only mesial third of canine are visible |
| 9. Colour | 9. Darker shade | 9. Ligher shade |

3. Colour of the teeth.
4. Tooth material.

## I. SELECTION OF TEETH SIZE

- Various factors considered during selection of teeth size are
  1. Mesiodistal width
  2. Buccolingual width
  3. Occlusogingival length.

### 1. Mesiodistal Width

- Posterior teeth for maxillary arch should be selected in such a way that all the posterior teeth occupy the space between the distal of canine to the maxillary tuberosity. If teeth are placed beyond the tuberosity results in cheek biting and tipping of the denture.
- Posterior teeth for mandibular arch should be selected in such a way that all the posterior teeth occupy the space between the distal of canine to the beginning of the retromolar pad, if teeth are placed over displaceable tissues like retromolar pad results in tipping of dentures during function.

### 2. Buccolingual Width

- A narrow occlusal table reduces the amount of forces acting on the denture during mastication, helping in decreasing the rate of residual ridge resorption.
- A narrow occlusal table allows the buccal and lingual flanges to slope towards the occlusal table, which helps the cheek and tongue to maintain the position of denture.
- A narrow occlusal table also provides proper path of escapement of food during mastication. For all the reasons explained above, the buccolingual width of artificial teeth should be selected slightly less than that of the corresponding natural teeth.

### 3. Occlusogingival Length

- The occlusogingival length of artificial teeth should be selected based on the amount of interarch space present to accomodate the teeth (i.e. vertical dimension at occlusion). The occlusal plane should be located at the half way between inter arch space.
- Hence, the artificial teeth with long occluso gingival length should be selected in cases of more interarch space and teeth with short occlusogingival length should be selected in cases of less interarch space.

## II. SELECTION OF SHAPE OF THE TEETH

- Shape of the posterior teeth should be selected based on various clinical situations and which is best for that particular situation.
- Based on occlusal form, posterior teeth are classified as:
  A. Anatomic teeth (cusp teeth)
    i. with 33° cuspal angulation.
    ii. with 30° cuspal angulation (Pilkington-Turner teeth).
  B. Semianatomic teeth (low cusp teeth)
    i. with 20° cuspal angulation.
    ii. with 10° cuspal angulation (functional or anatoline teeth)
  C. Non anatomic teeth (cuspless teeth)
    i. with 0° cuspal angulation (mono plane teeth)
  D. Special forms of teeth

### A. Anatomic Teeth (cusp teeth)

Indications

- Well formed ridges which offer good support and retention to dentures.

- When teeth to be arranged both in centric and eccentric relations to attain balanced occlusion using semiadjustable articulator.
- Patients with good neuromuscular control.

Advantages
- Better chewing efficiency.
- More natural appearence (better esthetics).
- Balanced occlusion can be provided with greater ease.
- Provides greater resistance to rotation of dentures.

Disadvantages
- Most time consuming and complex procedures involved in obtaining balanced occlusion.
- Restriction of posterior tooth positions to that allowed by cuspal anatomy.
- Harmonious balanced occlusion is lost when settling (stabilization of occlusion) occurs.
- The presence of cusps generate more horizontal forces during function.
- Denture bases need frequent refitting to keep the occlusion stable and balanced.

**B. Semianatomic Teeth (Low Cusp or Modified Cusp Teeth)**

Indications
- Well formed ridges which offer good support and retention to dentures.
- When balanced occlusion is planned.
- Patients with mild discrepancies in jaw relations.

Advantages
- Balanced occlusion can be obtained easily.
- Better chewing efficiency compared to non anatomic teeth.
- Better esthetics when compared to non anatomic teeth.
- Balanced occlusion is not lost when settling occurs.
- Generate less horizontal forces during function when compared to anatomic teeth.

Disadvantages
- Less esthetic when compared to anatomic teeth.
- Less chewing efficiency when compared to anatomic teeth.

**C. Non Anatomic Teeth (Cuspless Teeth)**

Indications
- Patients with flat and serverely resorbed ridges.
- Patients with crossbite tooth relations.
- Patients with large discrepancy between centric jaw relation and centric occlusion.
- Patients with poor neuromuscular control.
- When balanced occlusion is not planned.
- Patients with deleterious habits such as bruxism.

Advantages
- Quick arrangement of teeth.
- Wide range of posterior teeth positions possible.
- No lateral stresses on mucosa with para function.
- Easier to use for patients with uncoordinated closures, in cases of Parkinsonia, dyskinesias and stroke.
- Freedom of occlusal movement from centric to eccentric positions.
- Prevents destruction of tissue and preserves integrity of residual ridges.

Disadvantages
- Less chewing efficiency.
- Less esthetic.
- Difficult to balance.

**D. Special Forms of Teeth**
i. Inverted cusp teeth should be used when poor resistance to lateral movement of dentures is anticipated.
ii. Flat teeth with compensating curves.
iii. Combinations of anatomic and non anatomic teeth for lingualized occlusion (upper anatomic and lower non anatomic teeth).
iv. Crossbite teeth.
v. Metal insert teeth (vitallium occlusal posteriors).

## III. SELECTION OF TEETH BASED ON TYPE OF MATERIAL

- Based on the type of material used, teeth are classified as

**A. Acrylic Teeth**
a. Conventional acrylic resin teeth

Indications
- When opposing arch consists of natural teeth.
- When opposing dentition has gold crowns or inlays.
- In cases where less interarch space available for tooth placement and require trimming of teeth.

Advantages
- They can be ground very thin to fit it into available space in cases of less inter arch space.
- They do not abrade the opposing natural teeth and gold crowns or inlays.
- They bond chemically to acrylic denture bases.
- The occlusal and facial surfaces of teeth are easily polished.
- They can be easily reshaped for esthetic purposes.

- They do not chip and have softer impact sounds.
- They cause less trauma to denture bearing area.

*Disadvantages*
- They wear with time which is clinically significant.
- They are subject to abrasion with inappropriate scrubbing or cleaning.
- Loss of occlusal vertical dimension due to wear.
- Loss of comminuting (masticatory) efficiency over a period of time.
- Stains and discolour with time.
- They may have to be replaced in 5 to 7 years because of excessive occlusal wear.
- Rebasing is difficult as it is difficult to remove acrylic teeth.

b. Interpenetrating polymer network (IPN) acrylic resin teeth.
- To overcome the drawbacks of conventional acrylic resin teeth like excessive wear, the interpenetrating polymer network (IPN) acrylic resin teeth were developed.
- This tooth material is a non filled, highly cross linked copolymer with an interpenetrating polymer network.
- Advantages of IPN acrylic resin teeth over conventional acrylic resin teeth are:
  - More harder
  - More abrasion resistant
  - More stain resistant
  - More heat resistant
- Hence, IPN acrylic resin teeth are preferred over conventional acrylic resin teeth because of improved properties and same indications.

### B. Porcelain Teeth

*Indications*
- When opposing arch does not contain natural teeth or gold crowns or inlays.
- In cases where more interarch space is available for tooth placement and do not require trimming of teeth.
- In cases with well formed ridges.
- When esthetics is major concern of the patient.

*Advantages*
- Wear is clinically insignificant over a long period of time.
- No significant loss of vertical dimension due to occlusal wear.
- Maintains comminuting (masticatory) efficiency over a long period of time.
- Provides better esthetics.
- Does not stain or discolour over a long period of time.
- Rebasing can be done easily as porcelain teeth are mechanically bond to acrylic denture base with the help of pins or channels within the teeth.

*Disadvantages*
- Difficult to grind and adjust in cases of less interarch space.
- Abrades opposing natural teeth or gold crowns or inlays.
- They cannot be chemically bond to acrylic denture bases, hence bond strength is less.
- They are brittle material, hence chipping or fracture occurs occasionally.
- They have sharp impact sound, making clicking noise.
- Causes more trauma to denture bearing area.

### C. Composite Teeth
- They bond chemically to acrylic denture bases, more esthetic and have greater wear resistance than conventional acrylic resin teeth.
- Hence, as with IPN acrylic resin teeth, viivoset teeth (composition teeth) can be used as substitute for conventional acrylic resin teeth.

### D. Porcelain Acrylic Combination Scheme
- The main disadvantages of porcelain teeth is that they produce clicking noise in function. To overcome this, a porcelain acrylic combination scheme was propsed. On this scheme, porcelain posterior teeth oppose the acrylic posterior teeth. This reduces the clicking sound as acrylic teeth act as cushion and absorbs stresses produced when porcelain teeth occlude with acrylic teeth.

### E. Acrylic Teeth with Amalgam Inserts
- Amalgam inserts also known as amalgam stops are placed in acrylic teeth to reduce the wear of resin teeth when porcelain teeth are placed in opposing arch (combination scheme). Cavities are prepared in the acrylic resin teeth on occlusal surfaces and amalgam is condensed into prepared cavities. Amalgam is shaped by moving the opposing teeth cusps over the amalgam, when it is still in curvable stage, in a programmed articulator or directly in patients mouth. The occlusion developed in this way is known as functionally generated occlusion.

F. **Acrylic Teeth with Gold Occlusal Surface**
- To reduce the wear of acrylic teeth when opposed by natural teeth or gold restorations or porcelain teeth, the acrylic teeth are modified with gold occlusal surface.
- The occlusal surfaces of acrylic teeth are prepared for gold restoration, wax patterns made and casted with gold. The final gold castings are cemented to prepared acrylic teeth to obtain the acrylic teeth with gold occlusal surface.

# 10 Occlusion

Occlusion—though the word looks complex, it has got a simple meaning, i.e. 'contact'. This chapter outlines you in brief about its concepts in a simple way.

## DEFINITION

- The relationship between the occlusal surfaces of the maxillary and mandibular teeth when they are in contact—GPT.
- Occlusion is a static position when the jaws are centrically or eccentrically related. Hanau used the term "articulation" to define the contacting of teeth as the mandible moved to and fro from centric relation and eccentric relation. Articulation is a dynamic movement.

## OBJECTIVES

1. Should provide for maximum intercuspation of the teeth with the condyles in centric relation.
2. Should incorporate in the occlusion those factors which reduce vertical stresses on denture bearing area.
3. Should provide for horizontal movement of the mandible from the centric related intercuspal position until those teeth most capable of bearing horizontal load come into function.
4. Should minimize harmful lateral forces.
5. Should be designed to facilitate chewing efficiency.
6. Should be designed to provide stability and retention to the dentures.
7. Should not traumatize the oral supporting structures and should preserve the alveolar bone and soft tissue.
8. Should maintain comfort and well being of the patient.

## CLASSIFICATION

- Based on occlusal relationship of posterior teeth, Angle classified occlusion as follows.

## CLASS I

- The mesiobuccal cusp of the mandibular permanent first molar occludes in the embrasure area between the maxillary second premolar and first molar.

- The mesiobuccal cusp of the maxillary permanent first molar falls in the buccal groove of the permanent mandibular first molar.
- The mesiobuccal cusp of the maxillary permanent first molar is situated in the central fossa area of the mandibular permanent first molar.

## CLASS II

- The mesiobuccal cusp of the mandibular permanent first molar with the central fossa area of the maxillary permanent first molar.
- The distobuccal cusp of the maxillary permanent first molar occludes in the buccal groove of the mandibular first molar.
- The distolingual cusp of the maxillary permanent first molar occludes in the central fossa area of the mandibular first molar.

## CLASS III

- The distobuccal cusp of the mandibular permanent first molar is situated in the embrassure area between the maxillary second molar and maxillary first molar.
- The mesiobuccal cusp of the maxillary first molar occludes in the embrassure between the mandibular first and second permanent molars.
- The mesiobuccal cusp of maxillary first permanent molar is occluded in mesial pit of mandibular permanent second molar.

## THEORIES OF OCCLUSION

1. **Bonwills Theory of Occlusion**
   - According to Bonwills theory of occlusion, the teeth move in relation to each other as guided by the condylar and the incisal guidances. It is also known as theory of equilateral triangle in which, the distance between the condyles is equal to the distance between the condyle and the midpoint of the mandibular incisors. Each side of equilateral triangle measures about 4 inches.
2. **Conical Theory of Occlusion**
   - It is proposed by RE Hall. According to this theory, mandibular teeth move over the surfaces of the maxillary teeth as over the surface of a cone, generating an angle of 45 degrees with the central axis of the cone tipped at 45 degrees to the occlusal plane.
3. **Spherical Theory of Occlusion**
   - According to spherical theory of occlusion, mandibular teeth move over the surface of the maxillary teeth as over a surface of sphere with a diameter of 8 inches. The centre of the sphere located in the region of glabella. The surface of sphere passes through the glenoid fossa and articulating eminences.

## REQUIREMENTS OF COMPLETE DENTURE OCCLUSION

1. Stability of occlusion at centric relation position and in an area forward and lateral to it.
2. Balanced occlusal contact bilaterally for all eccentric mandibular movements.
3. Unlocking the cusps mesiodistally to allow for gradual but inevitable setting of the bases due to tissue deformation and bone resorption.
4. Control of horizontal force by buccolingual cusp height reduction according to residual ridge resistance from and interarch distance.
5. Functional lever balance by favourable tooth to ridge crest position.
6. Anterior incisal clearence during all posterior masticatory function and during bruxing activity.
7. Sharp ridges or cusps and generous slice ways to shear and shred with the minimum of force necessary.
8. Cutting, penetrating and shearing efficiency of occlusal surfaces.
9. Minimum occlusal contact areas for reduced pressure in comminuting food (lingual contact occlusion).

## TYPES OF OCCLUSION IN NATURAL DENTITION

1. Bilaterally balanced occlusion.
2. Canine guided occlusion.
3. Group function or unilateral balanced occlusion.
4. Mutually protected occlusion.

### 1. BILATERALLY BALANCED OCCLUSION

- In this type of occlusion there is bilateral, simultaneous, anterior and posterior occlusal contact of teeth in centric and all eccentric positions. This type of occlusion in natural dentition occurs in very few people.

### 2. CANINE GUIDED OCCLUSION

- Canine guided occlusion is a form of mutually protected occlusion in which the vertical and horizontal overlap of the canine teeth disengage the posterior teeth in the excursive movements of the mandible.

### 3. GROUP FUNCTION (UNILATERAL BALANCED OCCLUSION)

- In this type of occlusion there is unilateral, anterior and posterior occlusal contact of teeth in lateral movements on the working side (side towards which mandible moves) and disengagement of teeth on the balancing side. Thus simultaneous contact of teeth on working side act as a group to distribute occlusal forces.

## MUTUALLY PROTECTED OCCLUSION

- It is a type of occlusion that occurs most commonly in natural dentition in which one or group of teeth protects the other teeth during various mandibular movements. The posterior teeth protects the anterior teeth by disengaging the anterior teeth in maximum intercuspation. The anterior teeth protects the posterior teeth by disengaging posterior teeth on both sides during protrusive movements of mandible, i.e. when mandibular and maxillary anterior teeth come in edge to edge to relation. This is called as Christensens phenomenon. Canines on the working side protects all the other teeth by disengaging all the teeth on both sides except canines on working side. This is called as canine guided occlusion as explained above. Thus canine guided occlusion is a type of mutually protected occlusion.

## TYPES OF OCCLUSAL CONCEPTS IN COMPLETE DENTURE OCCLUSION

1. Balanced occlusion.
2. Non balanced occlusion.
   a. Spherical concept of occlusion.
   b. Organic concept of occlusion.
   c. Neurocentric concept of occlusion.
3. Lingualized occlusion.

## BALANCED OCCLUSION

### DEFINITION

- Balanced occlusion is the bilateral, simultaneous, anterior and posterior occlusal contact of teeth in centric and eccentric positions—GPT.

### AIM

- In the case of balanced occlusion, the aim is to achieve even contacts between all maxillary and mandibular teeth on the working side (i.e., the side towards which mandible moves) during lateral movements. At the same time, there should be multiple contacts between the mandibular and maxillary teeth on the balancing side (i.e., the side from which mandible moves) which should not destabilise the denture. There should also be simultaneous anterior and posterior contacts during protrusive movements of mandible.

## NEED FOR BALANCED OCCLUSION IN COMPLETE DENTURES

- In natural dentition or in unbalanced occlusion when the mandible is protruded so that upper and lower anteriors come in contact with each other there will be disocclusion or gap between the upper and lower posterior teeth. This is called as the Christensen's phenomenon. If same occlusion is provided in complete dentures results in instability of dentures, i.e. maxillary dentures will be displaced downwards in posterior region and mandibular dentures will be displaced upwards in the posterior region. To prevent this, simultaneous contacts of all teeth should be provided during protrusive movements in complete dentures.
- Similarly during lateral movements of mandible in natural dentition, the canines on working side contact each other and remaining teeth on working side and all teeth on balancing side will be dis occluded resulting in spaces or gap between the opposite teeth. If the same occlusion is provided in complete dentures results in instability of dentures and uneven distribution of forces to underlying structures. The upper denture will be displaced downwards on balancing side and lower denture will be displaced upwards on balancing side. To prevent this simultaneous contact of all teeth should be provided in complete dentures during lateral movements of mandible.
- In natural dention, the occlusal surfaces of opposite teeth glide along each other during movement from centric occlusion to eccentric occlusion. Any obstruction to this movement in complete dentures due to occlusal or cuspal interferences of opposite teeth results in instability of denture. Hence, occlusal interferences should be avoided to achieve balanced occlusion in complete dentures.

### Advantages

1. Enhances retention and stability of complete dentures.
2. Forces are distributed equally all over the denture bearing area resulting in reduced resorption of alveolar bone.
3. Patient is more comfortable in performing various mandibular movements.

### Disadvantages

- According to famous statement "Enter bolus, exit balance" by Shephered, balanced occlusion is not possible during mastication. That is, when the food is in mouth (enter bolus) there will be simultaneous disocclusion of teeth and loss of balance of dentures. Hence, some authors argue that it is not necessary to provide balanced occlusion in complete denture fabrication.

## FACTORS AFFECTING BALANCED OCCLUSION— (HANAU'S QUINT)

- According to Hanau, there are five factors which affect the balanced occlusion. Hence these five factors are also known as Hanau's quint.
  1. Condylar guidance
  2. Incisal guidance
  3. Plane of occlusion
  4. Cuspal inclination
  5. Compensating curves.

### 1. CONDYLAR GUIDANCE

- It is defined as "mandibular guidance generated by condyle and articulate disc traversing the contour of the glenoid fossa—GPT.
- Glenoid fossa guides the condyle during mandibular movements. Thus the slope of the glenoid fossa which determines the path of movement of condyle is called as the condylar guidance. It is the posterior determinant of mandibular movement.
- Slope of glenoid fossa is 'S' shaped, hence condyle moves along a 'S' shaped path.
- Condylar guidance has two components
  a. Horizontal condylar guidance
  b. Lateral condylar guidance
- Horizontal condylar guidance helps in guiding the mandible during protrusive movements.
- Lateral condylar guidance helps in guiding the mandible during side ward and lateral movements of mandible.
- The condylar path should be determined on the patient and set on the instrument so that the patients temperomandibular joint is in harmony with the occlusion as programmed on the articulator.
- Horizontal condylar guidance of patient is programmed in the articulator with the help of protrusive jaw relation records.
- Lateral condylar guidance of patient is programmed in the articulator with the help of lateral jaw relation records or by using Hanau's formula in the case of a Hanau articulator.

  Hanau's formula - $L = \dfrac{H}{8} + 12$

  $L \rightarrow$ lateral condylar guidance
  $H \rightarrow$ horizontal inclination

- Among all factors affecting balanced occlusion, condylar guidance cannot be controlled or altered by dentist. It is unique for each patient. Remaining factors can be controlled or altered by dentist.

### 2. INCISAL GUIDANCE

- It is defined as "the influence of the contacting surfaces of mandibular and maxillary anterior teeth during mandibular movements"—GPT.
- During protrusive movements of mandible, the incisal edge of the lower anteriors slide along the slopes of the lingual surfaces of the upper anterior teeth before reaching edge to edge contact. Thus the lingual surface of maxillary anteriors guide the mandible during protrusive movement and is called as the incisal guidance.
- It is usually expressed in degrees of angulation from the horizontal by a line drawn in the sagittal plane between the incisal edges of upper and lower incisor teeth when closed in centric occlusion. It is called as the incisal guide angle.
- Incisal guidance is determined under the control of dentist in fabrication of complete dentures.
- For complete dentures the incisal guidance should be as flat as esthetics and phonetics will permit. If the incisal guidance is steep, it requires steep cusps, steep occlusal plane or a steep compensating curve to obtain occlusal balance, which may result in instability of dentures due to steep inclined planes.
- If anterior tooth arrangement requires more vertical overlap, an equal amount of compensating horizontal overlap should be given to reduce the incisal guidance (incisal guide angle) there by rendering stability to the dentures. So, in complete dentures, less vertical overlap and more horizontal overlap of anterior teeth results in shallow incisal guide angle, which is necessary for stability of complete dentures.

### 3. PLANE OF OCCLUSION

- It is the average plane established by the incisal and occlusal surfaces of the teeth. Generally, it is not a plane but represents the planar mean of the curvature of these surfaces.
- Plane of occlusion is established anteriorly by the height of lower canine and posteriorly by the height of retromolar pad. It is also related to alatragus line or campers line. In complete denture fabrication, plane of occlusion should be parallel to alatragus line or campers line.
- Although plane of occlusion is determined and controlled by dentist during complete denture fabrication, it should not be altered more as it can cause serious functional problems.

### 4. CUSPAL INCLINATION

- It is the angle by the average slope of a cusp with the cusp plane measured mesiodistally or buccolingually—GPT.

- Cusps on teeth or the inclination of cuspless teeth play an important role in balanced occlusion. Cuspal inclination is determined by the angles of the cuspal slopes to the horizontal plane.
- Cuspal inclinations modify the effect of the plane of occlusion and compensating curves. Cuspal inclines should not be too steep as it can increase lateral forces. Usually, the mesiodistal cusp heights that interdigitate lock the occlusion so that reposition of the teeth due to settling of the base cannot take place. To avoid this problem, it is advocated that all mesiodistal cups heights be eliminated in anatomic type teeth.

### 5. COMPENSATING CURVES

- It is defined as the anteroposterior curvature (in the median plane) and the mediolateral curvature in the frontal plane in the alignment of the occluding surfaces and incisal edges of the artificial teeth that are used to develop balanced occlusion—GPT.
- Compensating curves are the most important determinants of balanced occlusion in complete dentures. They are the artificial curves introduced into the complete dentures to achieve balanced occlusion.
- They are called as compensating curves because they compensate for the space formed between the upper and lower occlusal surfaces of posterior teeth during protrusive lateral movements of the mandible. That is they compensate for the Christensens phenomenon occurring in natural dentition, so that upper and lower occlusal surfaces of posterior teeth occlude with each other and there won't be any space between them during protrusive and lateral movements of mandible, there by providing stability and balanced occlusion for artificial dentures.
- Compensating curves are the counter parts of natural curves existing in natural dentition. So, it is necessary to know about curves in natural dentition before knowing about compensating curves.

### Curves in Natural Dentition
1. Antero posterior curve - curve of Spee
2. Mediolateral curves - curve of Monson
   - curve of Wilson

*Curve of Spee (Fig. 2.10.1)*
- It is defined as the anatomic curve established by the occlusal alignment of the teeth, as projected onto the median plane, begining with the cusp tip of the mandibular canine and following the buccal cusp tips of the premolar and molar teeth, continuing through the anterior border of the mandibular ramus, ending with the anterior most portion of the mandibular condyle—GPT.

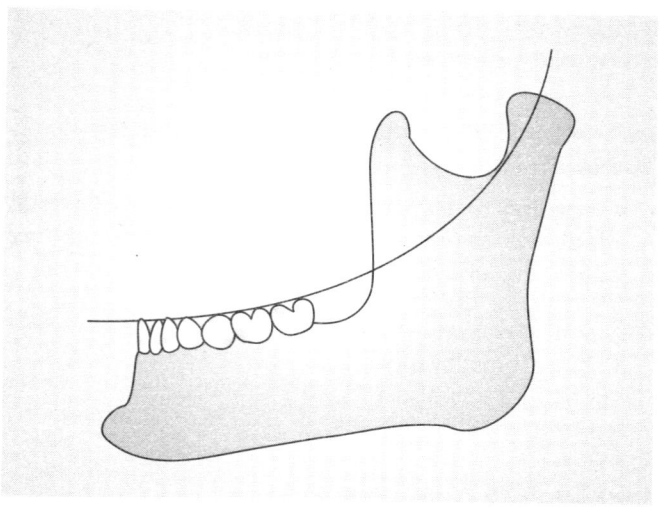

Fig. 2.10.1

*Curve of Monson*
- It is defined as the curve of occlusion in which each cusp and incisal edge touches or conforms to a segment of a sphere of 8 inches in diameter with its center in the region of glabella—GPT.
- It is a proposed ideal artificial curve based on Monson's spherical theory of occlusion.

*Curve of Wilson (Fig. 2.10.2)*
- It is a mediolateral curve that contacts the buccal and lingual cusp tips on each side of the arch. It results from lingual inclination of mandibular molar teeth, making the lingual cusps lower than the buccal cusps. Consequently, the buccal cusps maxillary molars are placed higher than the palatal cusps resulting in buccal inclination of maxillary molar teeth.
- In natural dentition this curve helps in resisting the masticatory loads better.

### CURVES IN ARTIFICIAL DENTITION

1. **Anteroposterior Compensating Curve (or) Compensating Curve for Curve of Spee**
   - It begins at the distal marginal ridge of the first posterior replacement tooth (which is usually the second premolar) and continues through the second molar. The amount of curvature developed is dependent on the steepness of the condylar guidance.

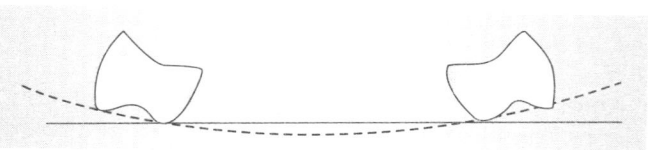

Fig. 2.10.2

- It is incorporated into the artificial occlusion by raising distal portions of the first and second molars to conform to a curve. The antero posterior curve is developed to provide the needed tooth structure for balancing contacts in the protrusive movement.
- This curve compensates for the spacing that occurs between upper and lower posterior teeth during protrusive movements of the mandible.

2. **Mediolateral Compensating Curve**
   - It is needed to provide the needed tooth structure during lateral movements of mandible. It compensates for the wedge-like opening formed when the mandible is moved laterally to the opposite side.
   
   A. **Compensating Curve for Monson Curve**
   - This curve runs across the buccal and palatal cusps of maxillary molars.
   - The artificial teeth should be set following this curve in order to obtain lateral balance of occlusion.
   
   B. **Compensating Curve for Curve of Wilson**
   - This curve is obtained by tilting the maxillary molars such that the buccal cusps are higher than the palatal cusps. Subsequently, the mandibular molars are tilted lingually which results in lateral balance of occlusion.
   - This curve runs opposite to the direction of Monson curve and hence also called as antimonson curve.

3. **Pleasure Curve**
   - It is defined as the helicoidal curve of occlusion that when viewed in the frontal plane conforms to a curve that is convex superiorly except for the last molars which reverses that pattern—GPT.
   - It was proposed by Max pleasure in order to provide balanced occlusion and improve stability of the dentures.

4. **Reverse Curve** (Fig. 2.10.3)
   - This is not a compensating curve. It is given for the maxillary first premolar by raising the palatal cusp higher than the buccal cusp.

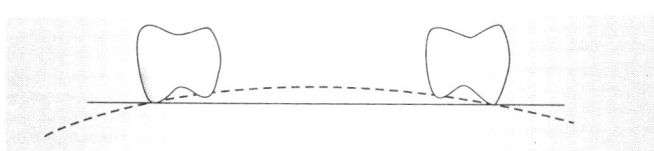

Fig. 2.10.3

## Differences between Natural occlusion and complete denture occlusion

| Natural occlusion | Artificial occlusion |
|---|---|
| 1. The roots of natural teeth are surrounded by periodontal tissues and firmly anchored to the bone. | 1. In complete artificial occlusion, all the teeth are embedded in denture bases seated on slippery soft tissues (oral mucosa). |
| 2. In natural dentition the teeth receive individual pressures of occlusion and can move independently. They can migrate to adjust to occlusal pressures. | 2. In complete dentures, artificial teeth move as a single unit along with denture base over the supporting structures. |
| 3. The presence of periodontal ligament surrounding each tooth helps in proprioception and also acts as cushion to absorb some of the forces directed towards the bone. | 3. Proprioception and cushion like effect is lost due to absence of periodontal ligament. |
| 4. Malocclusion of natural teeth may be uneventful for years. | 4. Malocclusion on artificial teeth evokes an immediate response and involves all of the teeth and denture base. |
| 5. Non vertical forces on natural teeth (lateral forces) during function effect only teeth involved and are usually well tolerated. | 5. Non vertical forces (lateral forces) on complete dentures during function effect all the teeth on the denture base. |
| 6. Incising with natural teeth does not affect the posterior teeth. | 6. Incising with artificial teeth effects all the teeth on the denture base. |
| 7. In natural teeth, bilateral balance is rarely found; if present it is considered as balancing side interference. | 7. In complete dentures, bilateral balance is generally considered necessary for stability of dentures. |
| 8. Due to more favourable leverage and power, the second molar is considered as favourable area for masticating hard bits in natural dentition. | 8. If heavy masticatory forces are applied in second molar area of complete dentures results in tipping and instability of dentures. |
| 9. Neuromuscular co-ordination is normal in natural dentition. | 9. Neuromuscular co-ordination is reduced. |
| 10. They take up masticating loads of 44 pounds (20 kg). | 10. They take up masticatory loads of 13–16 pounds (6–8 kg). |
| 11. Area of support in each jaw is 45 cm$^2$. | 11. Area of support in maxillary arch is 22.96 cm$^2$ and in mandibular arch is 12.25 cm$^2$. |
| 12. Resorption of bone is compensated by opposition of bone and thickness of bone is maintained. | 12. Bone undergoes continuous resorption resulting reduced thickness of bone. It results in looseness of dentures over period of time. |
| 13. Neutral zone is the area where teeth are placed such that forces of buccal musculature are compensated by the forces of lingual musculature. In natural dentition, neutral zone is created by muscular forces. | 13. Neutral zone is created by dentist. |
| 14. In natural dentition, centric occlusion is slightly (2–3 mm) infront of centric relation in 90% of individuals and centric occlusion coincides with centric relation in 10% of individuals | 14. In artificial dention or in complete dentures, the centric occlusion and centric relation coincides. |

# Articulators

**CHAPTER 11**

Articulators form the next key role in fabrication of CD after the dental casts and models as they simulate patient's TMJ and jaws. This chapter describes about articulators in detail.

## DEFINITION

An Articulator may be defined as a mechanical instrument that represents the temporomandibular joints and jaws to which the maxillary and mandibular casts may be attached to simulate some or all mandibular movements—GPT

## OBJECTIVES

1. It should hold opposing casts in a predetermined fixed relationship
2. It should open and close
3. It should be able to produce border and intra-border movements of the teeth similar to those in the mouth
4. It should develop a prosthesis that will be harmonious in the oral cavity

## USES

1. Mounting of dental casts for diagnosis, treatment planning and patient education
2. To plan dental procedures that involve positions, contours and relationships of both natural and artificial teeth as they relate to each other
3. To aid in fabrication of dental restorations and lost dental parts
4. To arrange artificial teeth for complete and removable partial dentures
5. To correct and modify completed restorations

## REQUIREMENTS OF AN ARTICULATOR (ACCORDING TO WINKLER)

### A. Minimal Articulator Requirements

1. The articulator must accurately maintain the correct horizontal and vertical relationships of patient casts
2. The patient casts must be easily removable and attachable to the articulator without losing their correct horizontal and vertical relationship

3. The articulator should have an incisal guide pin with a positive stop that should be adjustable and calibrated
4. The articulator should accept a face bow transfer utilizing an anterior reference point
5. The articulator should be able to open and close in a hinge like fashion
6. The construction of articulator should be accurate, rigid and of a non corrosive material
7. The design of articulator should be such that there is adequate distance between the upper and lower members and that vision is not obscured from the rear
8. The articulator should be stable on the laboratory bench and not too bulky and heavy

**B. Additional Articulator Requirements**

These are required in cases of denture fabricated with balanced occlusion
1. The condylar guides should allow lateral and protrusive movements
2. Condylar guides should be adjustable horizontally
3. The articulator should have provisions for adjustment of Bennett movement
4. The incisal guide table should be customizable.

## CLASSIFICATION

### I. BASED ON THE INSTRUMENTS FUNCTION

It was presented at the International Prosthodontic Workshop on Complete Denture Occlusion at the University of Michigan in 1972.

**A. Class – I**
Simple holding instruments capable of accepting a single static registration. Vertical motion is possible but only for convenience
*E.g.* J. B Gariot's Hinge Articulator

**B. Class – II**
Instruments that permit horizontal as well as vertical motion but do not orient the motion to the temporomandibular joint via a face bow transfer
1. **Class – II A**
   Eccentric motion permitted is based on average or arbitrary values
   *E.g.* Grittman articulator (1899) – Based on Bonewills theory; Gysi simplex articulator (1914)
2. **Class – II B**
   Eccentric motion permitted is based on theories of arbitrary motion
   *E.g.* maxilla mandibular instrument (Monson's Instrument-1918) – Based on Monson's spherical theory of occlusion
3. **Class – II C**
   Eccentric motion permitted is determined by the patient using engraving methods
   *E.g.* House articulator (1927)

**C. CLASS – III**
Instruments that simulate condylar pathways by using average or mechanical equivalents for all or parts of the motion. These instruments allow for joint orientation of the casts via a face bow transfer
1. **Class – III A**
   Instruments that accept a static protrusive registration and use equivalents for the rest of the motion
   *E.g.* Hanau model H (1923); Dentatus (1944)
2. **Class – III B**
   Instruments that accept a static lateral protrusive registration and use equivalents for the rest of the motion
   *E.g.* Gys Trubyte articulator (1926); Kinoscope designed by Hanau (1927); Tripod type articulator by Stansberry (1928); Ney articulator by Depictro (1960); Hanau 130–21 by Richard Beu (1964); Teledyne articulator by Richard Beu (1975)

**D. CLASS – IV**
Instruments that will accept three dimensional dynamic registrations. These instruments allow for joint orientation of casts via face bow transfer.
1. **Class – IV A**
   The condylar paths are formed by registrations engraved by the patient. These instruments do not allow for discriminating capability
   *E.g.* TMJ instrument by Kenneth Swanson (1965)
2. **Class – IV B**
   Instruments that have condylar paths that can be angled and customized either by selection from a variety of curvatures, by modifications or both
   *E.g.* Gnathoscope by Charles Stuart (1965); Denar articulator (D4A) by Niles Gurichet (1968); Simulator by Ernest Granger

### II. BASED ON THEORIES OF OCCLUSION

1. **Bonwills Theory of Occlusion**
   According to this theory, teeth move in relation to each other as guided by the condylar control and the incisal point. It is also known as the theory of equilateral triangle which has a 4 inch distance between the condyles and between each condyle and to the lower central incisor point.
   *E.g.* Bonwills articulator; Gysi simplex articulator
2. **Conical Theory of Occlusion**
   According to this theory, lower teeth move over the surfaces of upper teeth as over the surface of a cone, with a generating angle of 45 degrees and

the central axis of the cone tipped at 45 degree to the occlusal plane.
*E.g.* Hall automatic articulator

3. **Spherical Theory of Occlusion**
According to this theory, teeth move over the surface of the upper teeth as over the surface of a sphere with a diameter of 8 inches. The centre of the sphere is located in the region of the glabella and the surface of the sphere passes through the glenoid fossa along the articulating eminences or concentric with them. The upper member of the instrument moves anteroposteriorly and mediolaterally according to Monson's spherical theory.
*E.g.* Monson's maxilla mandibular instrument

### III. BASED ON INSTRUMENT DESIGN

1. **Arcon Type Articulator**
The term 'Arcon' was coined by Bergstroms
In Arcon type articulators the condyles are in the lower member and the condylar guides are curved and are on the upper member
*Advantage:* condyles move in a relationship to their condylar housing that is similar to the way the condyles move in relationship to the glenoid fossae in the skull. This makes easier visualization of condylar movements
*E.g.* Hanau arcon H2 (1977); Hanau radial shift articulator (1981); Hanau wide vwe; Whip-Mix articulator; Denar Mark II articulator

2. **Non-Arcon Type or Condylar Articulator**
They have condylar on the upper member and condylar guides in the lower member
*E.g.* Hanau H2 articulator.

### IV. BASED ON PLANE OF REFERENCE

1. **Campers Plane**
A plane established by the inferior border of the right or left ala of the nose and the superior border of the tragus of both ears
*E.g.* SS multiarticulator; Stratos articulator; Kavo articulator

2. **F H Plane (Frankfort Horizontal plane)**
A plane established by the lowest point in the margin of the right or left bony orbit and the highest point in the margin of the right or left bony auditory meatus
*E.g.* Hanau articulator, dentatus articulator, whip mix articulator, Denar mark-II articulator

### V. ACCORDING TO VARIOUS INVESTIGATORS

1. **According to Gills (1926), Boucher (1934), and Kingery (1934)**
Adjustable
Non adjustable.

2. **According to Beck (1962)**
Suspension instrument
Axis instrument
Tripod instrument

3. **According to Weinberg (1963)**
Arbitrary
Positional
Semiadjustable
Fully adjustable

4. **According to Possett (1968)**
Plane line
Mean value
Adjustable

5. **According to Sharry (1974)**
Simple
Hinge type
Fixed guide type
Adjustable

6. **According to Riliani (1980)**
Fully adjustable
Semi adjustable
Non adjustable

7. **According to Thomas**
Arbitrary
Positional
Functional

8. **According to Heartwell**

**Class I:** These instruments receive and reproduce three dimensional graphic tracings (pantograms). *E.g.* Stuart gnathologic computer, TMJ stereographic, Denar D5A, Hanau modular system, SAM-2

**Class II:** These instruments will not receive three dimensional graphic recording

*Type 1 (Hinge):* Twin stage occluder, Stephens articulator

*Type 2 (Arbitrary):* Verticulator, transgraph

*Type 3 (Average):* Dentatus, Hanau, Whip mix, Denar, Panadent

*Type 4 (Special):* Stansbery tripod, Kile Dentograph.

### Advantage

1. Better visualization of the casts and restorations in occlusion especially from the lingual side
2. Articulator acts as a patient in absence of patient and hence patient cooperation is not required
3. Chair side time is reduced
4. Patient appointment time is reduced
5. Saliva, tongue and cheek hindrances are eliminated
6. Refinement of occlusion can be done

## Disadvantage and Limitations

1. It is subjected to errors in tooling, metal fatigue and wear
2. It can simulate but cannot duplicate all the jaw movements
3. No provision to correct errors that are made during jaw relation records.

## PARTS OF MEAN VALUE ARTICULATOR

- It is a non adjustable articulator. It is designed using fixed dimensions, which are derived from the average distance between the incisal and condylar guidance of the population
- It is non arcon type articulator with condylar guidance in lower member and condylar rods in upper member

A. Upper member
- It is a triangular frame (equilateral triangle) with base of triangle placed posteriorly and apex anteriorly. Each side of triangle measures about 110 mm.

Parts
  i. **Condylar elements:** Two condylar elements are present—one on either side of base of triangle posteriorly. They articulate with condylar guidance of the lower member.
  ii. **Vertical rod:** Apex of upper member has provision for placement of vertical rod. It determines the anterior height of articulator. It should rest on center of incisal guide table during articulation
  iii. **Thumb screw:** Helps in fixing vertical rod to upper member
  iv. **Incisal pin:** Vertical rod has provision for placement of incisal pin. It guides in placement of anterior teeth during teeth arrangement. Incisal edge of maxillary central incisors at the midline should touch the tip of pin during articulation
  v. **Retentive pin:** Helps in retention of casts to the articulator

B. Lower member
- It is a 'L' shaped frame with a horizontal and vertical arm

  Parts
  i. **Horizontal arm:** It is triangular in shape and corresponds to the upper member
     a. *Incisal guide table*—present at the apex of the horizontal arm anteriorly. It helps in establishing the incisal guidance by maintaining incisal guide angle
     b. *Retentive pin*—helps in retention of casts to articulator
  ii. **Vertical arm:** It is triangular in shape and connects upper member to the lower member
     a. *Condylar guidance slots* – present on the upper portion of both vertical arms. They guide the movement of condylar elements
     b. *Horizontal rod* – it is present in vertical arm lower member. It should coincide with the plane of occlusion while articulation
     c. *Stabilizing rod.*

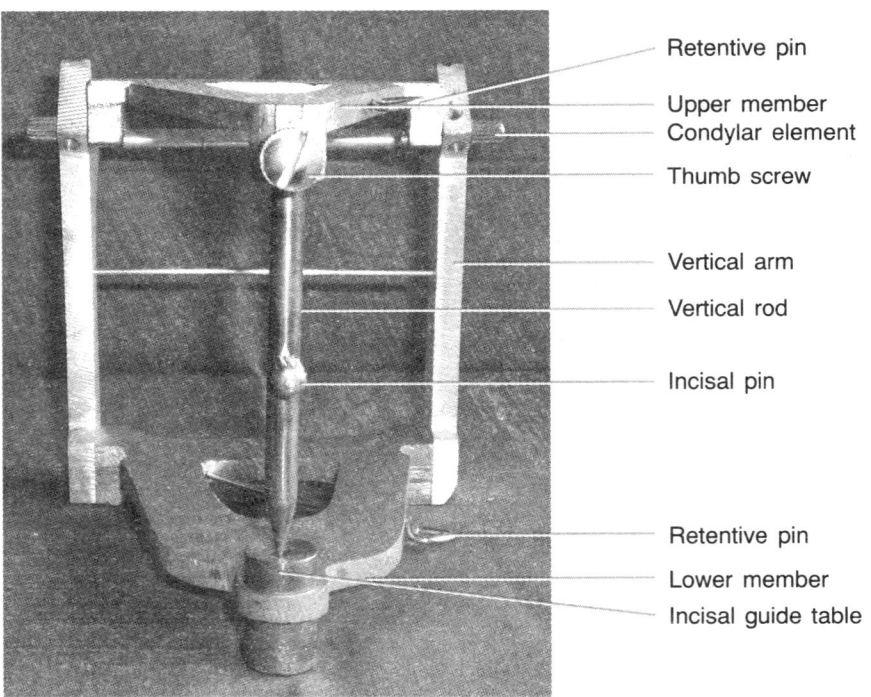

**Fig. 2.11.1:** Parts of mean value articular, front view

# Articulators

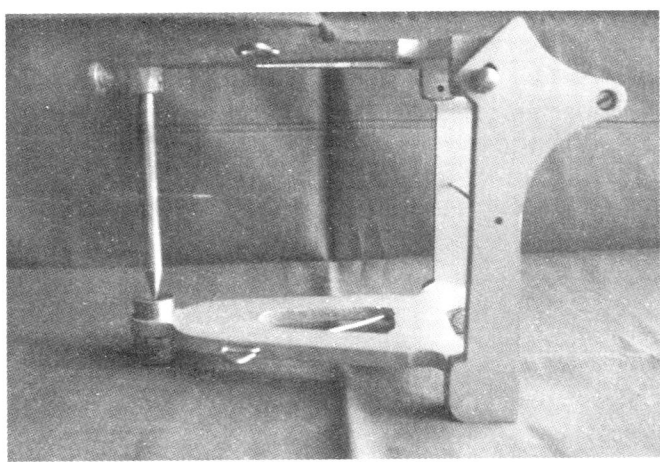

Fig. 2.11.2: Mean value articulator, side view

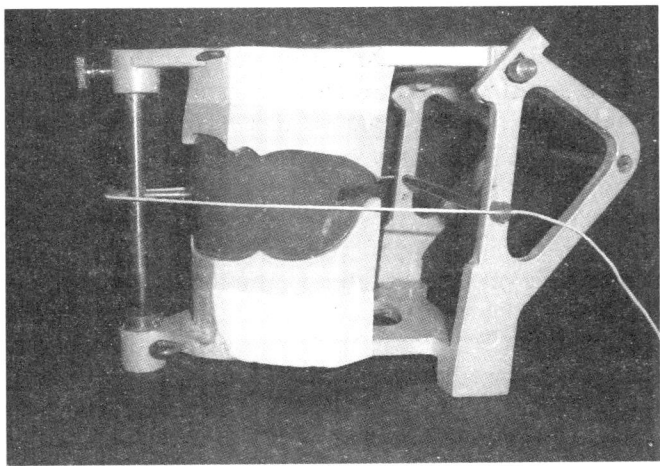

Fig. 2.11.4: Mean value articulator with thread relation, side view, mounted

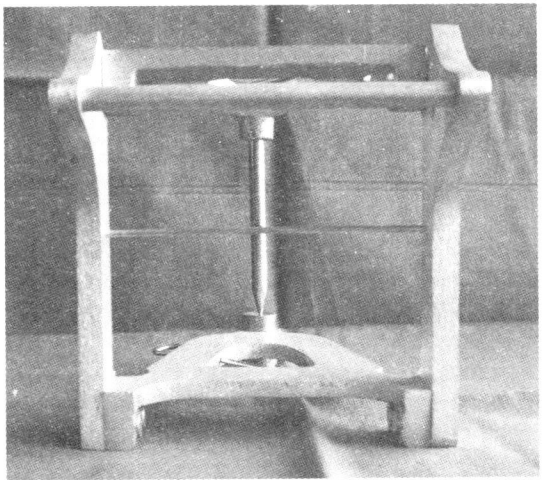

Fig. 2.11.3: Mean value articulator, posterior view

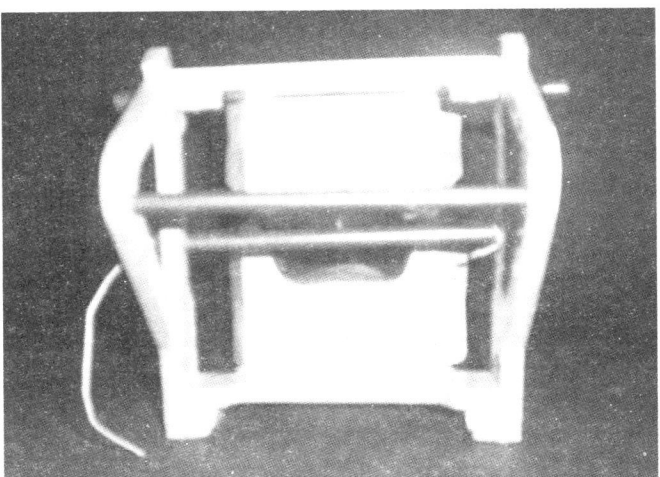

Fig. 2.11.5: Mean value articulator, posterior view, mounted

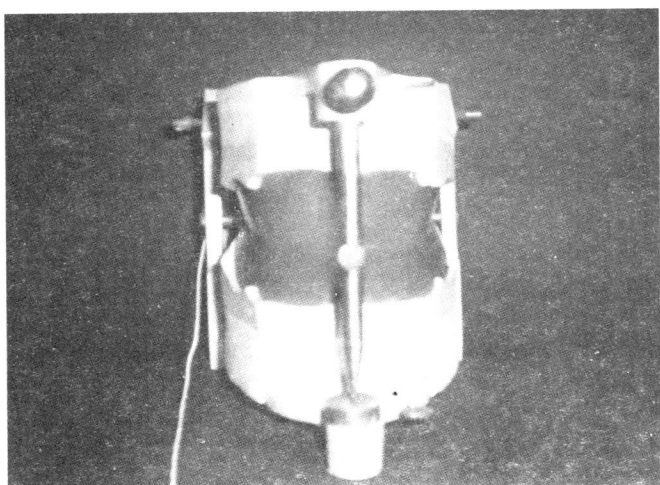

Fig. 2.11.6: Mean value articulator, front view, mounted

## GLOSSARY

*Adjustable articulator:* An articulator that allows some limited adjustment in the sagittal and horizontal planes to replicate recorded mandibular movements

*Anterior guide pin:* That component of an articulator, generally a rigid rod attached to one member, contacting the anterior guide table on the opposing member. It is used for the purpose of maintaining the established vertical separation. The anterior guide pin and table, together with the condylar elements, direct the movements of the articulators' separate members

*Anterior guide table:* That component of an articulator on which the anterior guide pin rests to maintain the occlusal vertical dimension and influence articulator movements. The guide tables influences the degree of separation of the casts in all relationships

*Arcon:* A contraction of the words "ARTICULATOR" and "CONDYLE," used to describe an articulator containing the condylar path elements within its upper member and the condylar elements within the lower member

*Arcon articulator:* An articulator that applies the arcon design; this instrument maintains anatomic guidelines by the use of condylar analogs in the mandibular element and fossae assemblies within the maxillary element

*Articulation:* (1) The place of union or junction between two or more bones of the skeleton—see CRANIOMANDIBULAR A., TEMPOROMANDIBULAR A. (2) in speech, the enunciation of words and sentences—see SPEECH A. (3) in dentistry, the static and dynamic contact relationship between the occlusal surfaces of the teeth during function

*Articulator:* A mechanical instrument that represents the temporomandibular joints and jaws, to which maxillary and mandibular casts may be attached to simulate some or all mandibular movements—usage: articulators are divisible into four classes.

*Class I articulator:* A simple holding instrument capable of accepting a single static registration; vertical motion is possible.

*Class II articulator:* An instrument that permits horizontal as well as vertical motion but does not orient the motion to the temporomandibular joints.

*Class III articulator:* An instrument that simulates condylar pathways by using averages or mechanical equivalents for all or part of the motion; these instruments allow for orientation of the casts relative to the joints and may be arcon or nonarcon instruments

*Class IV articulator:* An instrument that will accept three dimensional dynamic registrations; these instruments allow for orientation of the casts to the temporomandibular joints and simulation of mandibular movements

*Average value articulator:* An articulator that is fabricated to permit motion based on mean mandibular movements—called also Class III articulator

*Condylar articulator:* An articulator whose condylar path components are part of the lower member and whose condylar replica components are part of the upper member—called also nonarcon articulator

*Condylar guidance:*
Mandibular guidance generated by the condyle and articular disc traversing the contour of the glenoid fossae 2 condylar guidance

The mechanical form located in the upper posterior region of an articulator that controls movement of its mobile member condylar guide assembly

The components of an articulator that guide movement of the condylar analogues condylar guide inclination

The angle formed by the inclination of a condylar guide control surface of an articulator and a specified reference plane

*Fully adjustable gnathologic articulator:* An articulator that allows replication of three dimensional movement plus timing of recorded mandibular motion— called also Class IV articulator

*Incisal guidance:* (1) the influence of the contacting surfaces of the mandibular and maxillary anterior teeth on mandibular movements (2) the influences of the contacting surfaces of the guide pin and guide table on articulator movements

*Incisal guide:* The part of an articulator that maintains the incisal guide angle (GPT-4)

*Incisal guide angle:* (1) anatomically, the angle formed by the intersection of the plane of occlusion and a line within the sagittal plane determined by the incisal edges of the maxillary and mandibular central incisors when the teeth are in maximum intercuspation 2: on an articulator, that angle formed, in the sagittal plane, between the plane of reference and the slope of the anterior guide table, as viewed in the sagittal plane

*Incisal guide pin:* see ANTERIOR GUIDE PIN

*Incisal guide table:* See ANTERIOR GUIDE TABLE

*Nonadjustable articulator:* An articulator that does not allow adjustment to replicate mandibular movements

*Nonarcon articulator:* (1) any articulator which broadly replicates the three dimensional motions of the left and right condylar compartments (2) any articulator design in which the condylar element (analog) is not part of the lower member of the articulator and may be used to simulate the three dimensional motions of the left and right condylar compartments

*Semi-adjustable articulator:* An articulator that allows adjustment to replicate average mandibular movements—called also Class III articulator

# Teeth Arrangement

**CHAPTER 12**

Teeth arrangement—an important step where the three primary objectives of a prosthesis are to be fulfilled, i.e. mastication, phonetics and esthetics. Dentist should be aware of all the concepts and procedures in arranging the teeth.

### DEFINITION

- Teeth arrangement can be defined as placement of teeth on trial denture bases for aesthetics, phonetics and function.

### OBJECTIVE

1. To provide a comfortable and atraumatic occlusion.
2. To assist in preparing food for deglutition.
3. To impart a pleasing and natural appearance.
4. To assist in speech.

### GUIDELINES FOR TEETH ARRANGEMENT

#### A. Anterior Teeth

a. *Frontal view*
   1. Parallel to interpupillary line.
   2. Incisal edge of maxillary incisors should be 1 to 2 mm below maxillary lip at rest.
   3. No bulging should be evident the nostrils.
   4. Philtrum should be restored if possible.
   5. Full vermilion border of lip should be seen.
   6. Maxillary incisal edges should follow the line of the lower lip in smiling.

b. *Sagittal view*
   1. Upper lip should be everted and not fallen in.
   2. Tooth support of the lip is by 2/3 of the incisal labial surface of the anteriors.

c. *Horizontal view*
   1. Central incisor should be 8 to 10 mm anterior to the midpoint of the incisive papilla.
   2. Canines are on a line drawn perpendicular to the midline of the palate, through the center of the incisive papilla.

#### B. Posterior Teeth

a. *Frontal view*
   1. Maxillary posteriors (premolars) should be placed buccally enough so as to avoid too large a dark buccal corridor upon smiling, but not to eliminate it.

2. The occlusogingival length of the maxillary first premolar tooth should be long enough so that denture base material is not obvious or smiling.
3. The occlusal surface of the mandibular first bicuspid should never be superior to the corner of the mouth when the mouth is open only sufficiently to receive food.
4. Posterior plane of occlusion should not drop down posteriorly or maxillary posterior teeth will show too much during smiling.

b. *Sagittal view*
1. Posterior plane of occlusion should be parallel to the ala-tragus line.
2. Posterior plane of occlusion should be at a level between 1/3 to 2/3 the height of the retromolar pad.

c. *Horizontal view*
1. Lower buccal cusps or central fossae should be placed over the crest of the ridge.

## GUIDELINES ON THE CAST

- Guidelines are to be drawn on the maxillary and mandibular casts to determine the positions of the artificial teeth.

### A. Maxillary cast

1. Place a ruler parallel to the anterior border of the incisal papilla and make a line on the either side of the margin of the cast parallel to this border. This line helps in anterior placement of teeth.
2. Draw a line along the mid palatal suture, bisecting the incisive papilla. This line guides the median line-compare this line with the median line that was made on the maxillary occlusal rim.
3. When the canine eminences are present on the cast, the most distal extent is recorded with a line on the cast. When the eminences are not visible on the cast use the points that were recorded at the corners of the mouth using the maxillary occlusal rim as reference. The six maxillary anterior teeth occupy the space between the distal of the right canine eminence and the distal of the left canine eminence.

### B. Mandibular Cast

1. A line is drawn parallel to the frontal plane, bisecting the residual ridge. The direction of the resorption of the residual ridge must be considered when this line is placed. It guides in anterior placement of mandibular teeth.
2. Mark a point that designates the distal of the mandibular canine. When the canine eminences are not visible on the cast, use the points that were recorded at the corners of the mouth using the mandibular occlusal rim as reference. Mark a point at the center of retromolar pad. Draw a line that follows the crest of the residual ridge from the canine point to a point that bisects the retro molar pad. (By joining the two points). This line guides the buccolingual placement of mandibular posterior teeth.
3. Divide the retromolar pad into 3 equal parts, i.e. upper 1/3rd, middle 1/3rd, lower 1/3rd anterioposteriorly. The junction of upper and middle third is used to determine the vertical height of the mandibular molars.

## ANDREWS SIX KEYS TO NORMAL OCCLUSION

- Lawrence F Andrews studied 120 casts of non orthodontic patients with normal occlusion for 4 years (1960–64). He identified 6 key characteristics and suggested that for normal occlusion to exist these six characteristics had to be present. These 6 keys should be followed while teeth arrangement.

### Key I

*Molar Relationship*

- The distal surface of the distal marginal ridge of the upper first permanent molar contacts and occludes with the mesial surface of the mesial marginal ridge of the lower second molar.
- The mesiobuccal cusp of the upper first permanent molar falls within the groove between the mesial and middle cusps of the lower first permanent molar.
- The mesiolingual cusp of the upper first molar seats in the central fossa of the lower first molar.

### Key II

*Crown Inclination (mesiodistal "tip")*

- In normally occluded teeth, the gingival portion of the long axis (the line bisecting the clinical crown mesio distally or the line passing through the most prominent part of the labial or buccal surface of a tooth) of each crown is distal to the occlusal portion of that axis. The degree of tip varies with each tooth type.

### Key III

*Crown Inclination (labiolingual or buccolingual torque)*

- Crown inclination is the angle between a line 90 degrees to the occlusal plane and a line tangent to the middle of the labial or buccal surface of the clinical crown.

- The crowns of the maxillary incisors are so placed that the incisal portion of the labial surface is labial to the gingival portion of the clinical crown.
- In all other crowns, the occlusal portion of the labial or buccal surface is lingual to the gingival portion.
- In the maxillary molars the lingual crown inclination is slightly more pronounced as compared to the cuspids and bicuspids.
- In the mandibular posterior teeth the lingual inclination progressively increases.

### Key IV

*Absence of Rotations*

- Teeth should be free of undesirable rotations.
- If rotated, a molar or bicuspid occupies more space than it would normally.
- A rotated incisor can occupy less space than normal.

### Key V

*Tight Contacts*

- In the absence of such abnormalities as genuine tooth size discrepancies, contact points should be tight.

### Key VI

*Flat Curve of Spee*

- A flat occlusal plane is a must for stability of occlusion.
- It is measured from the most prominent cusp of the lower second molar to the lower central incisor, no curve deeper than 1.5 mm is acceptable from a stand point of stability.

## PRINCIPLES OF TEETH ARRANGEMENT

### A. Maxillary Teeth

1. Central incisor
   *Front view*—(mesiodistal angulation)
   The long axis of the tooth inclines slightly to the mesial side or perpendicular to the horizontal plane.
   *Side view*—(labiolingual inclination)
   The long axis of tooth inclines labially by about 15°.
   *Occlusal plane*—(glass plate relation / horizontal plane). The incisal edge is in contact with the occlusal plane (Figs 2.12.1 and 2.12.2).

2. Lateral incisor
   *Front view*
   The long axis of tooth slopes more towards mesial side when compared to central incisor.

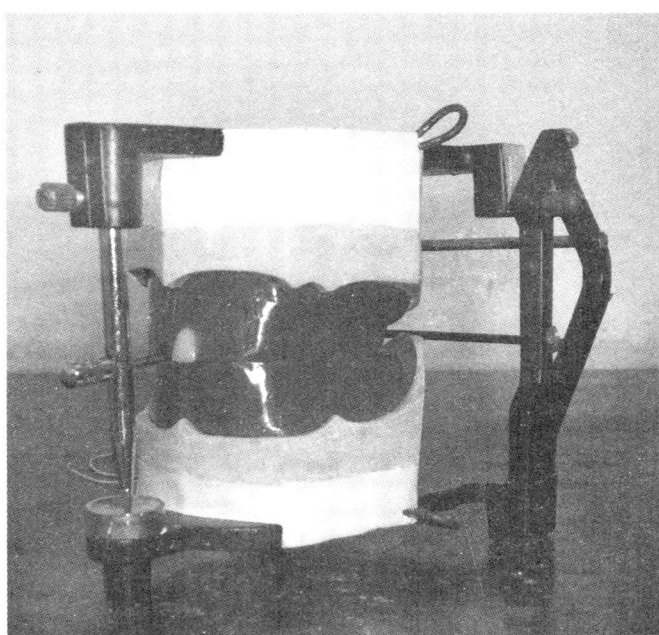

**Fig. 2.12.1:** Arrangement of maxillary central incisor-in articulator relation, labial view

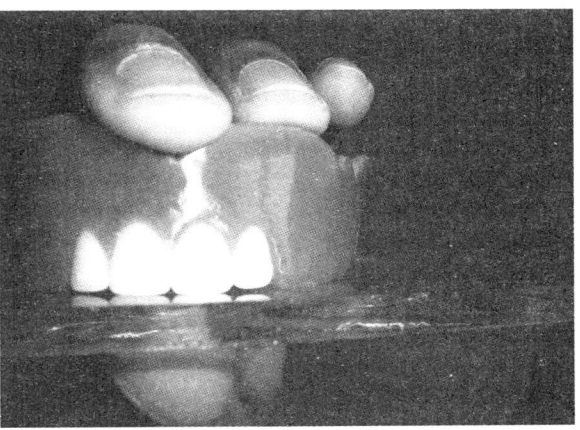

**Fig. 2.12.2:** Arrangement of maxillary CI and LI, in glass plate relation

*Side view*
The long axis of tooth inclines labially by about 20°
Occlusal plane
The incisal edge is about 1mm short of the occlusal plane (Figs 2.12.2 and 2.12.3).

3. Canine
   *Front view*
   The long axis of canine is parallel to the vertical axis. (straight without inclination). Mesial surface of canine is more visible than distal surface.
   *Side view*
   The long axis is parallel to the vertical axis. It means there is no labiolingual inclination. Hence, cervical

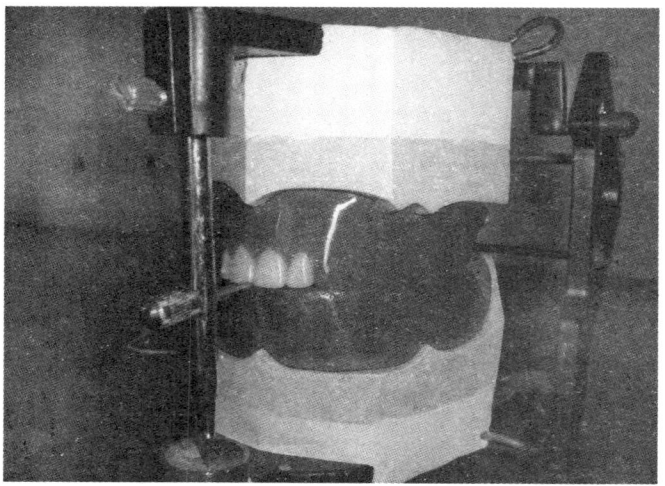

**Fig. 2.12.3:** Arrangement of maxillary central and lateral incisors, in articulator relation, labial view

portion of labial surface of canine appears more prominent.

*Occlusal plane*

The cusp tip of canine is in contact with the occlusal plane (Figs 2.12.4 to 2.12.8).

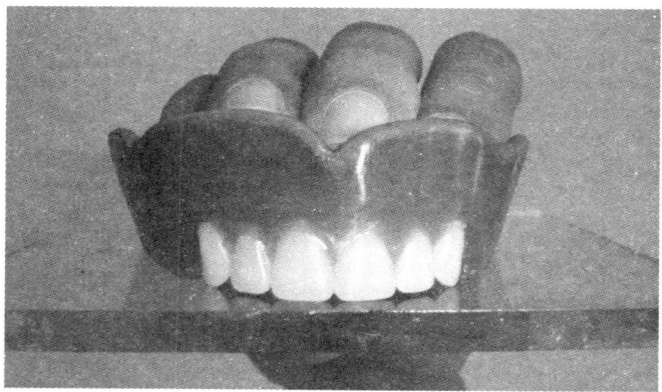

**Fig. 2.12.4:** Management of maxillary canine, in glass plate relation, front view

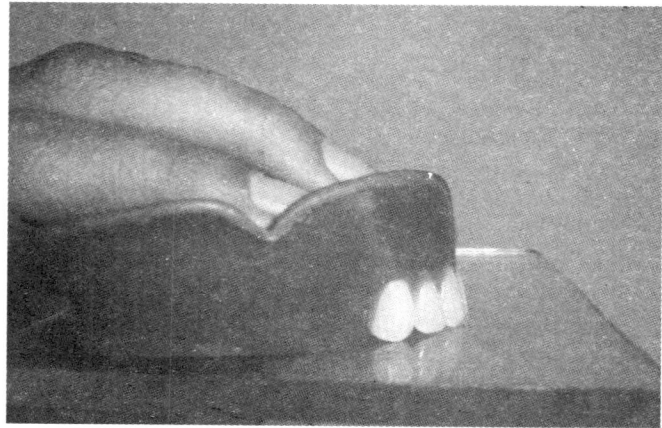

**Fig. 2.12.5:** Arrangement of maxillary canine, in glass plate relation, side view

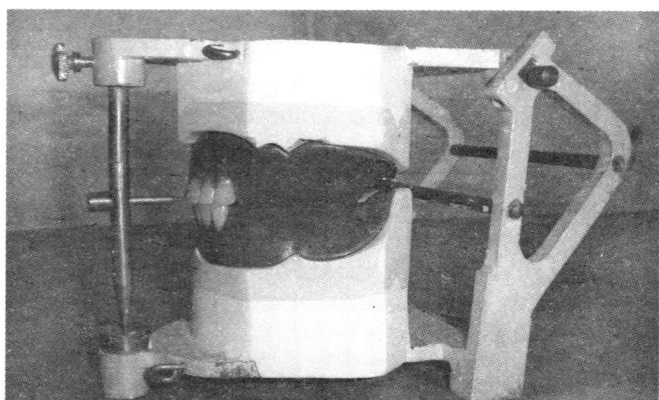

**Fig. 2.12.6:** Arrangement of maxillary canine, in articulator relation, view labial

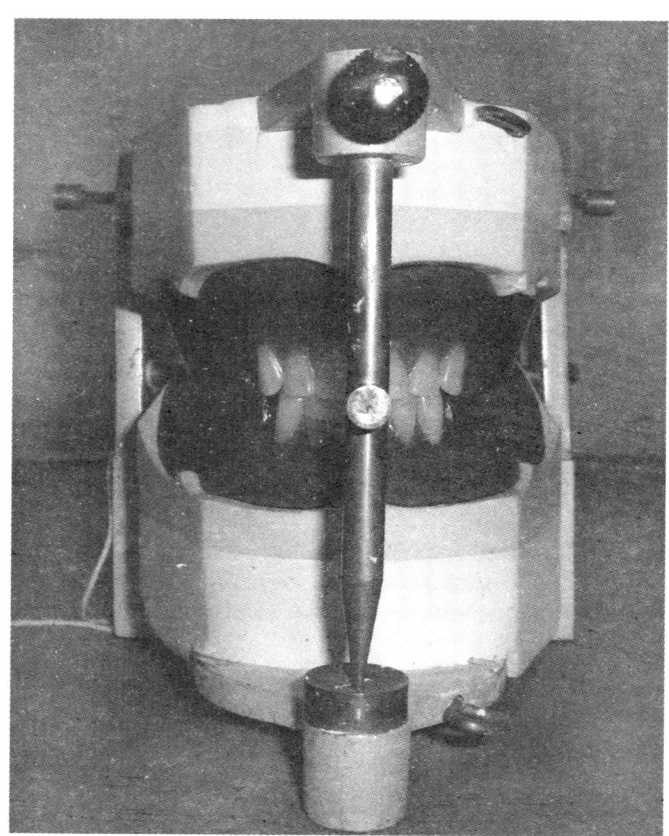

**Fig. 2.12.7:** Arrangement of maxillary canine, in articulator relation labial view

4. *First premolar*

*Front view*

Long axis of tooth is parallel to the vertical axis.

*Side view*

Long axis of tooth has slight lingual inclination.

*Occlusal plane*

Buccal cusp of first premolar is in contact with occlusal plane.

Palatal cusp of first premolar is about 1 mm short of occlusal plane (Figs 2.12.9 to 2.12.11).

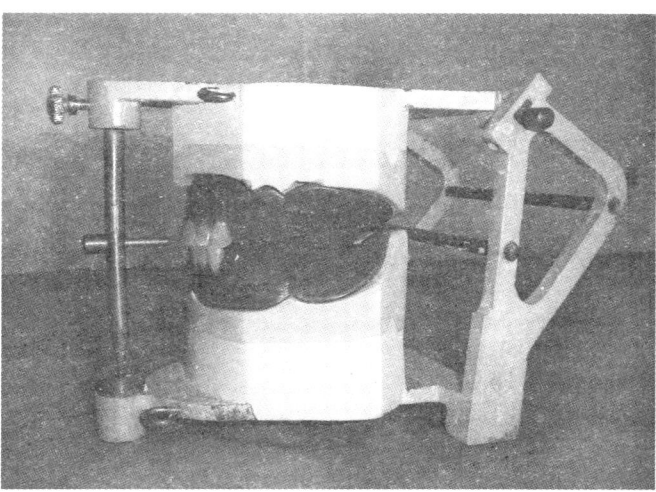

Fig. 2.12.8: Arrangement of maxillary canine, in articulator relation labial view

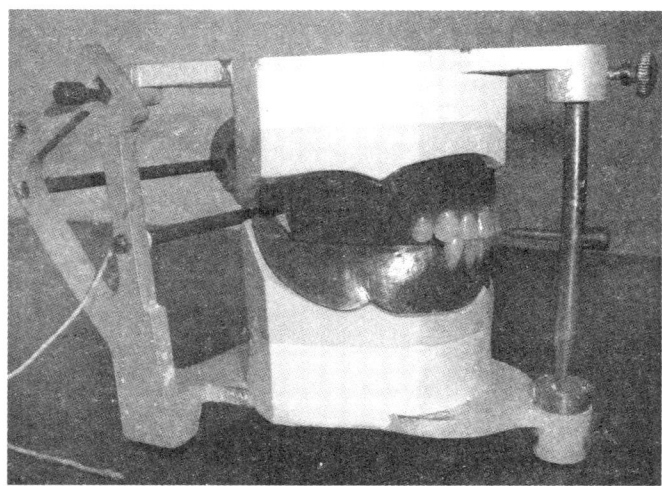

Fig. 2.12.11: Arrangement of maxillary first premolar, in articulator relation, view labial

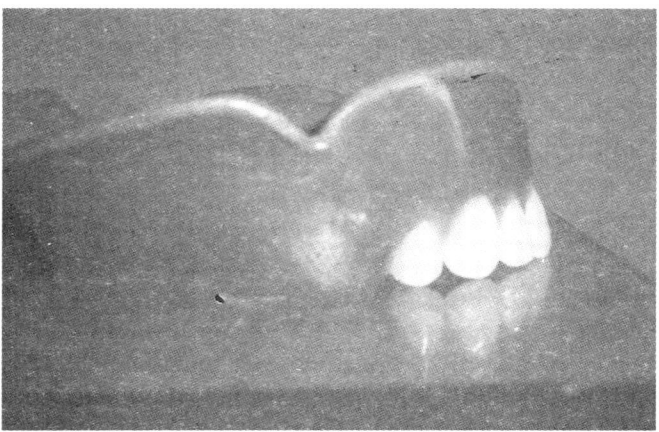

Fig. 2.12.9: Arrangement of maxillary first premolar, in glass plate relation, side view

5. *Second premolar*
   *Front view*
   The long axis of tooth is parallel with the vertical axis.
   *Side view*
   The long axis of tooth is parallel with the vertical axis.
   *Occlusal plane*
   Both buccal and palatal cusps of second premolar are in contact with the occlusal plane (Figs 2.12.12 and 2.12.13).
6. *First molar*
   *Front view*

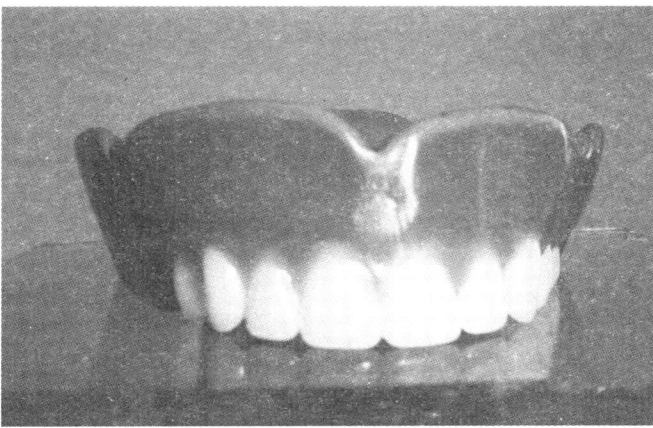

Fig. 2.12.10: Arrangement of maxillary first premolar, in glass plate relation, front view

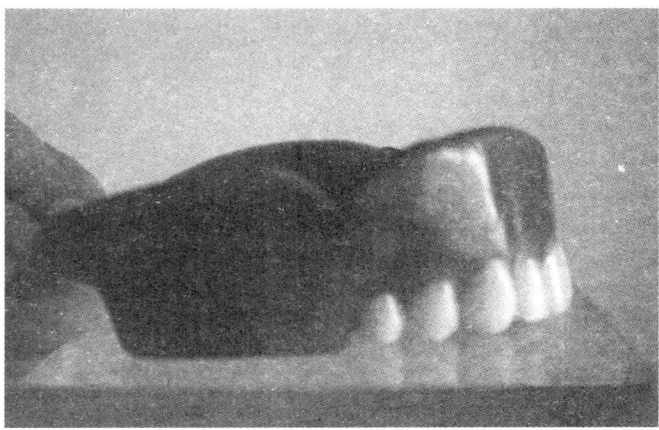

Fig. 2.12.12: Arrangement of maxillary second premolar, in glass plate relation, side view

The long axis of tooth inclines distally
*Side view*
The long axis tooth inclines buccally
*Occlusal plane*
Only mesiopalatal cusp of first molar is in contact with the occlusal plane (Figs 2.12.14 and 2.12.15).

7. *Second molar*
*Front view*
The long axis of tooth inclines more distally when compared to first molar.
*Side view*
The long axis of tooth inclines more buccally when compared to first molar.
*Occlusal plane*

All four cusps are clear of the occlusal plane, but the mesiopalatal cusp is nearest to occlusal plane (Figs 2.12.16 and 2.12.17).

## B. MANDIBULAR TEETH

1. *Central incisor*
*Front view*
The long axis of tooth inclines slightly mesially.
*Side view*
The long axis of tooth is inclined labially.
*Occlusal plane*
The incisal edge is about 2 mm above the occlusal plane although the amount depends on the

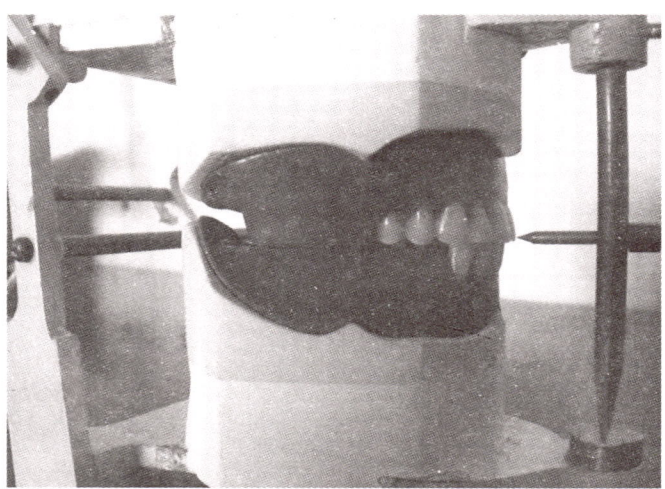

**Fig. 2.12.13:** Arrangement of maxillary second premolar, in articulator relation labial view

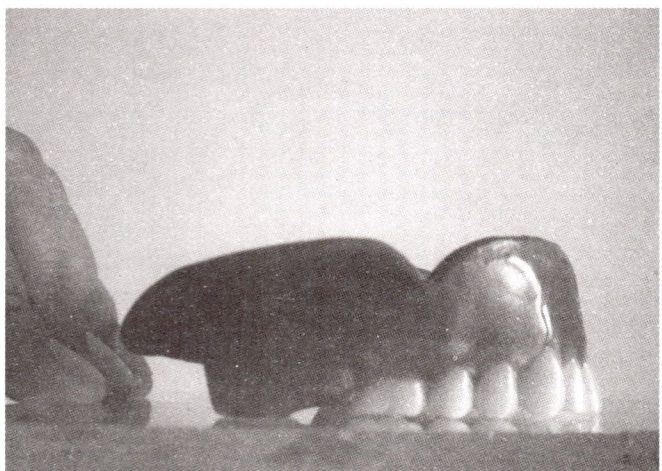

**Fig. 2.12.15:** Arrangement of maxillary first molar, in articulator relation, view labial

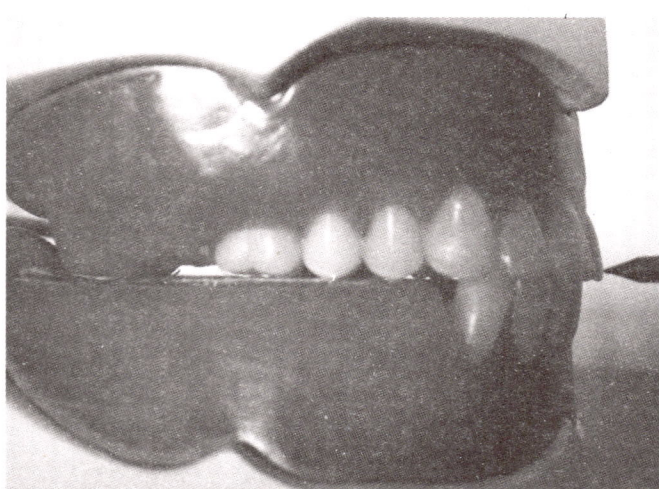

**Fig. 2.12.14:** Arrangement of maxillary first molar, in glass plate relation, side view

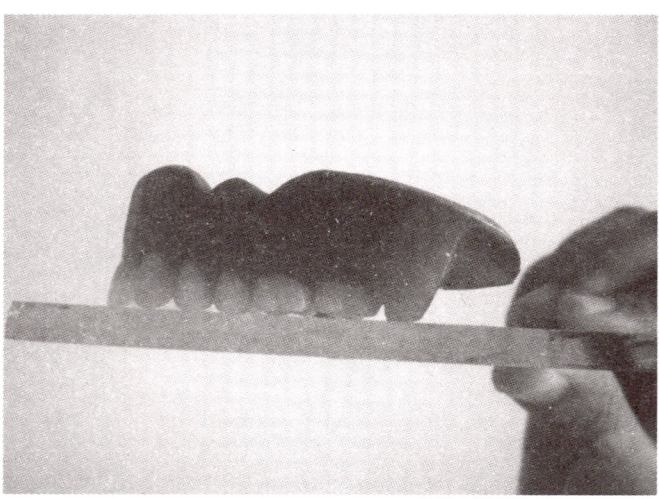

**Fig. 2.12.16:** Arrangement of maxillary second molar, in glass plate relation, side view

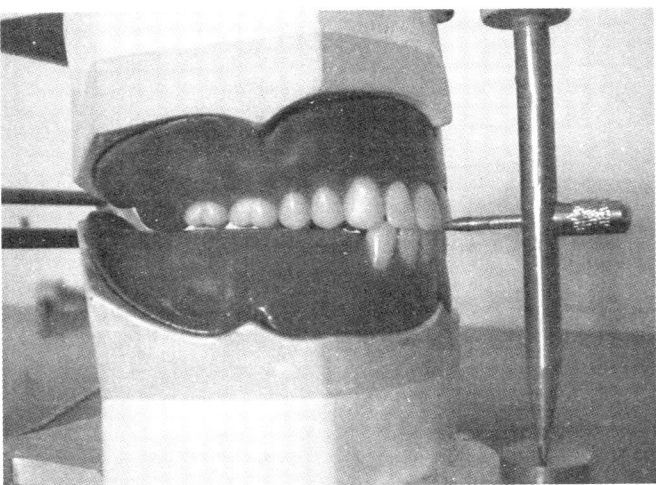

**Fig. 2.12.17:** Arrangement of maxillary second molar, in articulatory relation labial view

overjet.
2. *Lateral incisor*
   *Front view*
   The long axis of tooth inclines mesially.
   *Side view*
   The long axis of tooth slopes labially when viewed from side but not so steeply as the central incisor.
   *Occlusal plane*
   The incisal edge is about 2 mm above the occlusal plane.
3. *Canine*
   *Front view*
   The long axis of tooth is very slightly inclined mesially.
   *Side view*
   The long axis of tooth is very slightly inclined lingually.
   *Occlusal plane*
   The canine cusp tip is slightly more than 2 mm above the occlusal plane (Figs 2.12.18 to 2.12.21).
4. *First premolar*
   *Front view*
   The long axis of tooth is parallel to the vertical axis.
   *Side view*
   The long axis of tooth is parallel to the vertical axis.
   *Occlusal plane*
   The lingual cusp of first premolar is below the occlusal plane and the buccal cusp is about 2 mm above the occlusal plane as it contacts the mesial marginal ridge of the upper first premolar (Figs 2.12.22 and 2.12.23).
5. *Second premolar*
   *Front view*
   The long axis of tooth is parallel to the vertical axis.
   *Side view*
   The long axis of tooth is parallel to the vertical axis.
   *Occlusal plane*
   Both lingual and buccal cusp are about 2 mm above

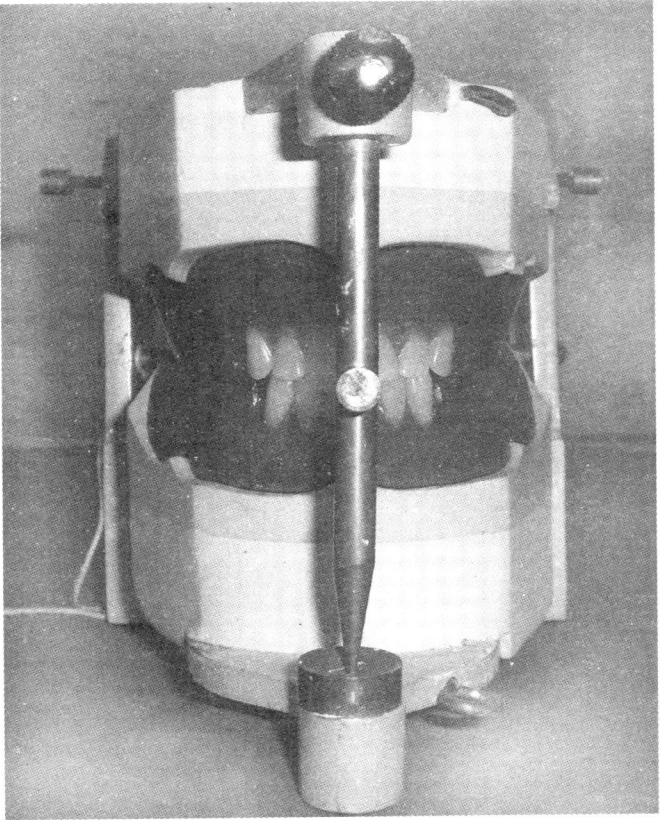

**Fig. 2.12.18:** Arrangement of maxillary canine, in articulator relation, labial view

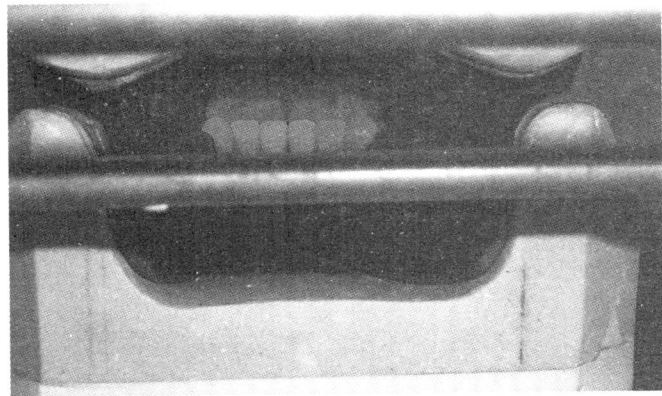

**Fig. 2.12.19:** Arrangement of mandibular anteriors, in relation to articulator, lingual view

the occlusal plane, the buccal cusp contacting the fossa between the two upper premolars (Figs 2.12.24 and 2.12.25).

6. *First molar*
   *Front view*
   The long axis of tooth leans mesially.
   *Side view*

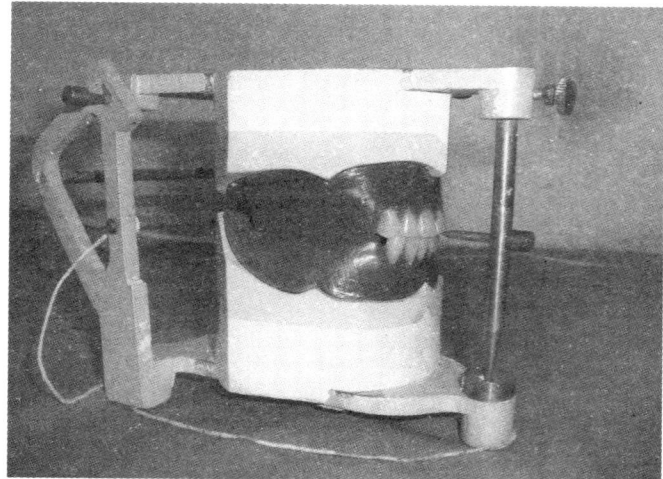

**Fig. 2.12.20:** Arrangement of mandibular and maxillary anteriors, in relation to articulator, labial view

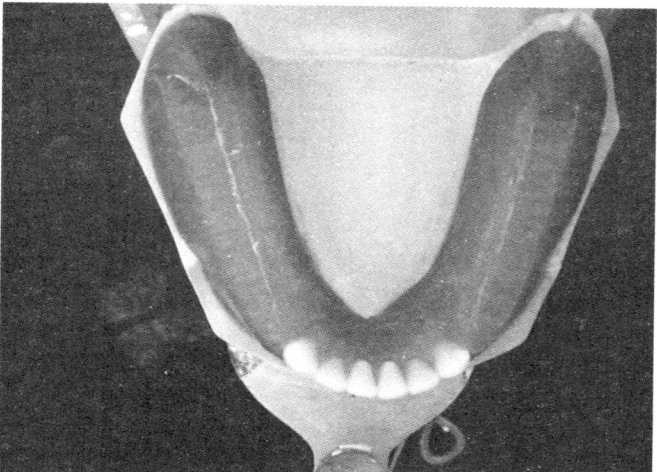

**Fig. 2.12.21:** Arrangement of mandibular anteriors in articulator relation, top view

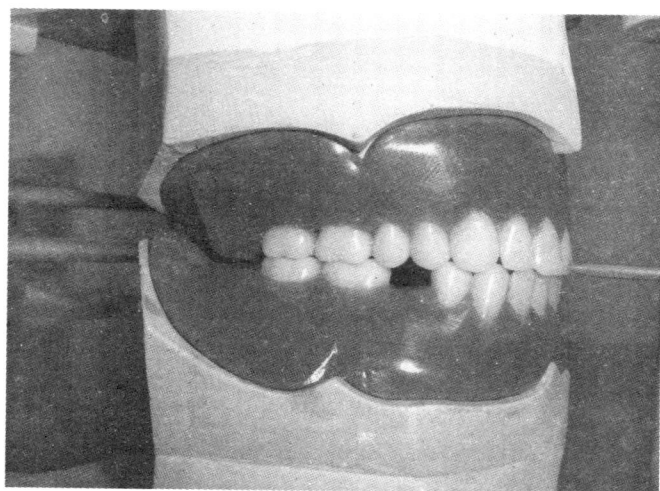

**Fig. 2.12.22:** Arrangement of mandibular first premolar, in articulator relation, view labial

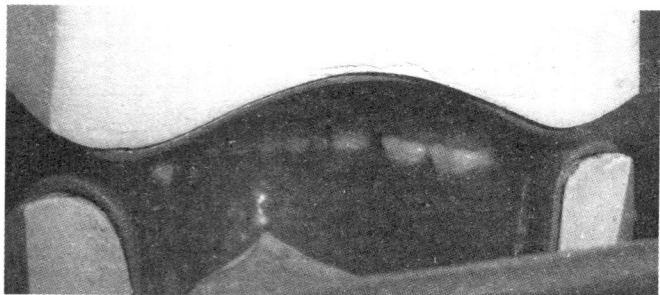

**Fig. 2.12.23:** Arrangement of mandibular first premolar, in articulator relation, lingual view

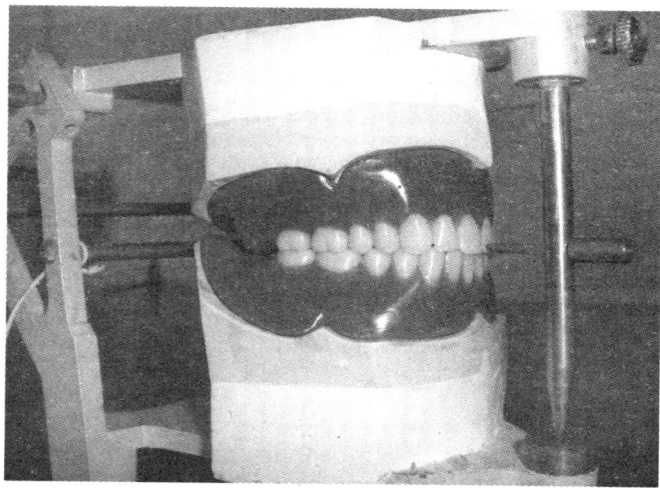

**Fig. 2.12.24:** Arrangement of mandibular second premolar, in articulator relation, labial view

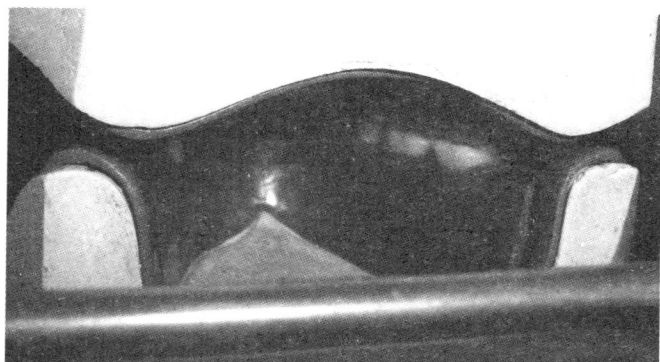

**Fig. 2.12.25:** Arrangement of mandibular second premolar, in articulator relation, lingual view

The long axis of tooth inclines lingually.

*Occlusal plane*

- All the cusps are at higher level above the occlusal plane than those of second premolar.
- The buccal cusps are at higher level than the lingual cusps and distal cusps are at higher level than mesial cusps.
- The mesiobuccal cusp occludes in the fossa between upper second premolar and first molar

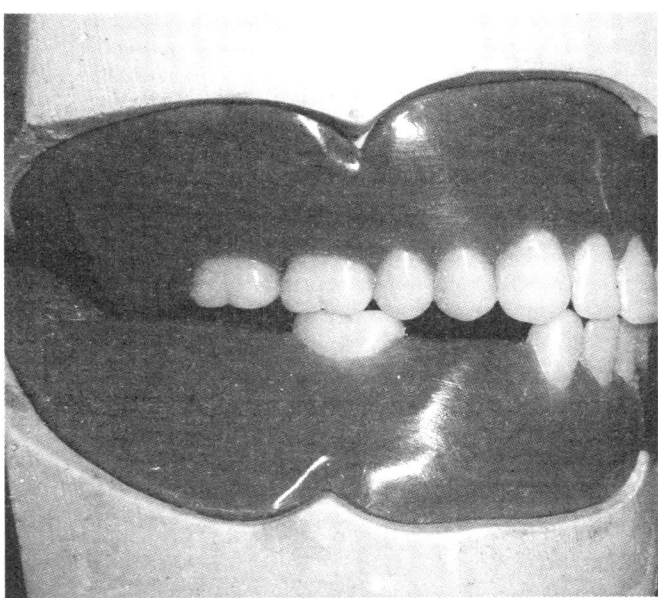

**Fig. 2.12.26:** Arrangement of mandibular second premolar, in articulator relation, labial view

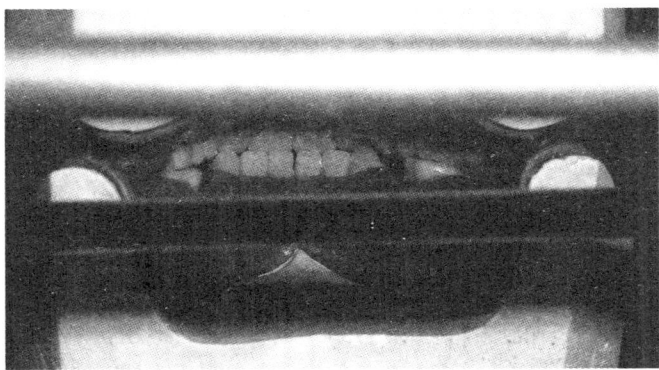

**Fig. 2.12.28:** Arrangement of mandibular first molar, in articulatory relation, lingual view

occlusal plane than those of the first molar.
- The buccal cusps are at higher level than lingual cusps and the distal cusps are at higher level than mesial cusps.
- The mesiobuccal cusp contacts the fossa between the two upper molars (Figs 2.12.29 and 2.12.30).

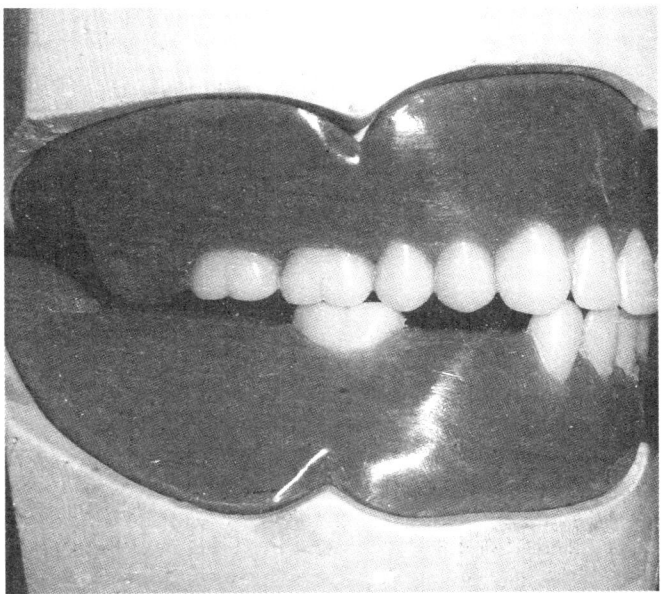

**Fig. 2.12.27:** Arrangement of maxillary, first molar, in articulator relation, labial view

(Figs 2.12.26 to 2.12.28).

7. *Second molar*
   *Front view*
   The mesial inclination of long axis of tooth is more pronounced when compared to first molar.
   *Side view*
   The lingual inclination of long axis of tooth is slightly more pronounced when compared to first molar.
   *Occlusal plane*
   - All the cusps are at a higher level above the

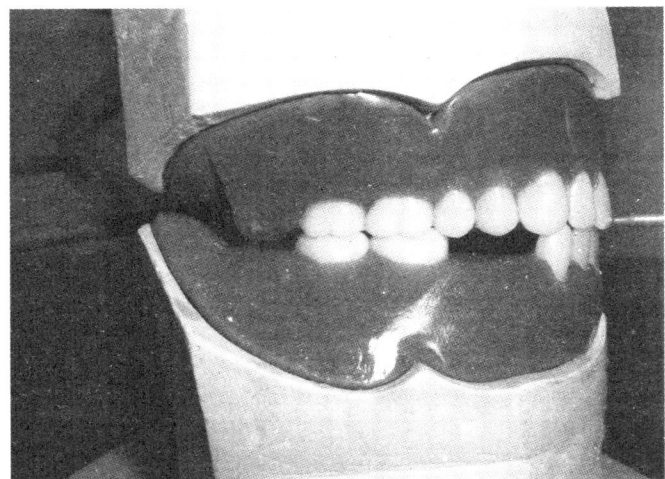

**Fig. 2.12.29:** Arrangement of mandibular second molar, in articulator relation, labial view

## THE ORDER OF TEETH ARRANGEMENT

### A. ANTERIOR TEETH

1. Left maxillary central incisor.
2. Right maxillary central incisor.

*Note:* It is helpful to set both central incisors and thus establish the midline before setting the lateral and canine.

3. Left maxillary lateral incisor.
4. Left maxillary canine.
5. Right maxillary lateral incisor.
6. Right maxillary canine.

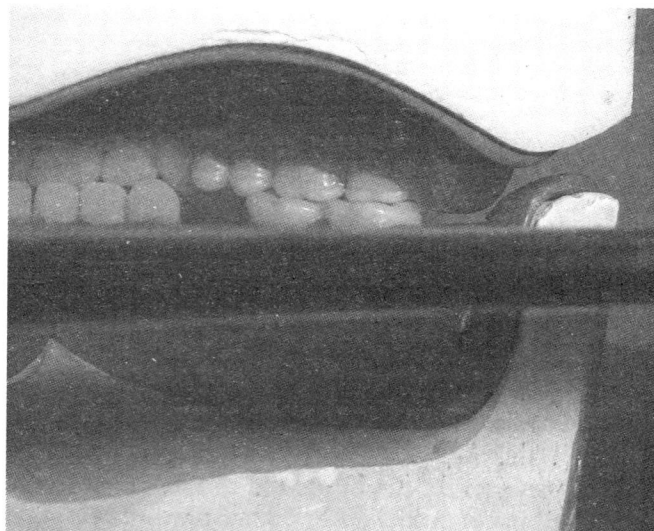

Fig. 2.12.30: Arrangement of mandibular second molar, in articulator relation, lingual view

7. Left mandibular central incisor.
8. Right mandibular central incisor.
9. Left mandibular lateral incisor.
10. Left mandibular canine.
11. Right mandibular lateral incisor.
12. Right mandibular canine.

B. POSTERIOR TEETH

- If due to lack of space, only three posterior teeth are to be arranged on either side, then it is more convenient to drop the first premolar and place the second premolar and the first and second molars into the available space. Eliminating the first premolar is a logical choice because this tooth has less occlusal surface for the mastication of food.
- In arrangement of posterior teeth, either maxillary or mandibular teeth can be arranged first.
- It is recommended to arrange mandibular posterior teeth first and then arrange maxillary posterior teeth. It is because lower ridge and its surrounding structures offer reliable landmarks for setting the lower posterior teeth and also arranging mandibular posteriors before maxillary posteriors provides better control of the orientation of the plane of occlusion both mediolaterally and superoinferiorly.
  i. If mandibular posteriors are arranged first then order to follow is:
    1. Mandibular left first premolar.
    2. Mandibular left second premolar.

*Note:* In the ideal situation, the mandibular first and second premolars, with their central grooves, are positioned on a line from the canine tip to 1 to 2 mm below the top of retromolar pad.

3. Maxillary left first premolar.
4. Maxillary left second premolar.
5. Mandibular left first molar.

*Note:* In the positioning of the mandibular first molar, the central groove is placed on the canine to retromolar pad reference line.

6. Maxillary left first molar.
7. Mandibular left second molar.
8. Maxillary left second molar.
9. Mandibular right first premolar.
10. Mandibular right second premolar.

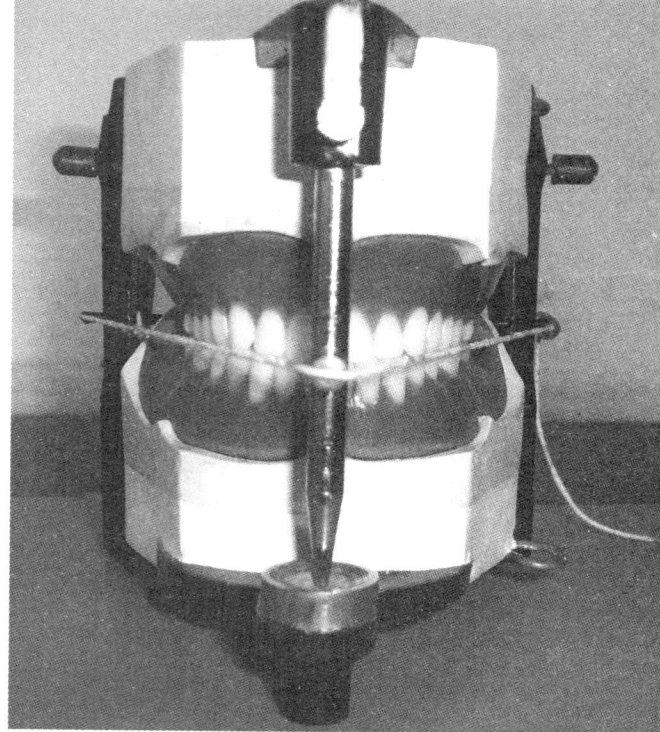

Fig. 2.12.31: Teeth arrangement completed, labial view

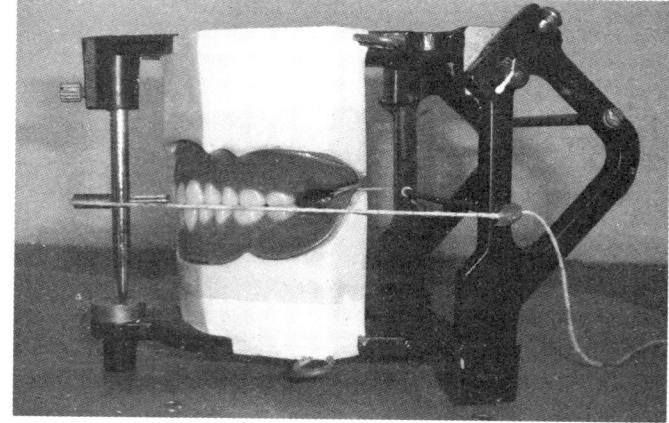

Fig. 2.12.32: Teeth arrangement completed, left side view

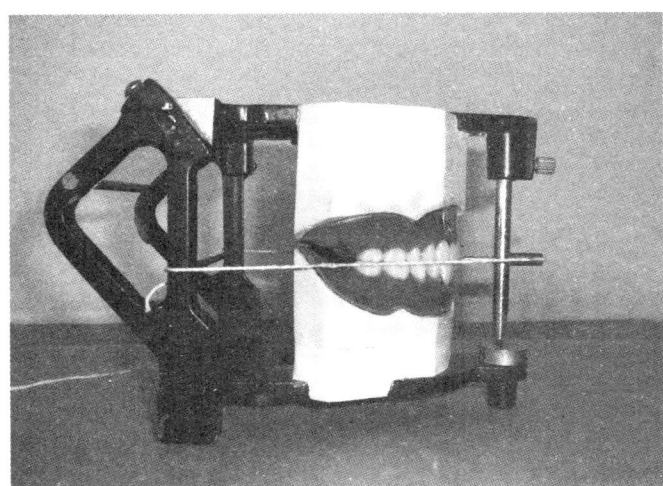

Fig. 2.12.33: Teeth arrangement completed, right side view

11. Maxillary right first premolar.
12. Maxillary right second premolar.
13. Mandibular right first molar.
14. Maxillary right first molar.
15. Mandibular right second molar.
16. Maxillary right second molar.

ii. If mandibular posteriors are arranged first then order to follow is
1. Maxillary left first premolar.
2. Maxillary left second premolar.
3. Maxillary left first molar.
4. Maxillary left second molar.

*Note:* During positioning of teeth from maxillary first premolar to second molar, the maxillary lingual cusps are aligned with the reference line that has been scribed on the mandibular wax occlusal rim from the mandibular canine tip to the middle of the retromolar pad.

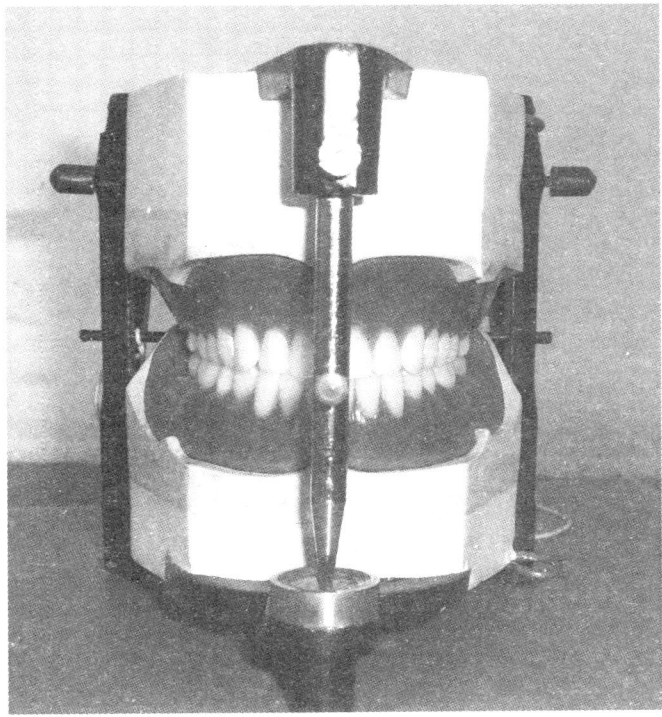

Fig. 2.12.34: Completed teeth setting, front view

5. Mandibular left first molar.
6. Mandibular left second molar.
7. Mandibular left second premolar.
8. Mandibular left first premolar.
9. Maxillary right first premolar.
10. Maxillary right second premolar.
11. Maxillary right first molar.
12. Maxillary right second molar.
13. Mandibular right first molar.
14. Mandibular right second molar.
15. Mandibulr right second premolar.
16. Mandibular right first premolar (Figs 2.12.31 to 2.12.34).

# CHAPTER 13

# Try-in Procedures

This is the last but one clinical step where the dentist should be more careful as he/she cannot modify anything once the procedure is crossed this step. He/she has to take all approvals from the patient and preferably their attendants also. This chapter mentions about the steps to be carried out in this appointment.

## PURPOSE

The main objective should be to compare the general tooth and arch position with the way the teeth might have grown. Wax sometimes camouflages the relationship so that errors can be overlooked.

While still on the articulator, the maxillary trial denture should be removed from the cast and mandibular teeth are compared with the maxillary cast to see if the relationships are logical. Then the mandibular denture is removed and the maxillary trial denture is checked against the mandibular cast. Inter alveolar distance should be observed to see if the technician has changed the vertical opening.

The mandibular denture should now be placed into the mouth and patient instructed to let the tongue tightly touch the inside of the denture to maintain the lingual seal. Subsequently, the patient should practice this tongue position and also train the tongue to be less active when first learning to chew.

The fit and extension of the mandibular denture should be checked. Under extension as well as over extension should be detected. The trial denture should have good stability and the dorsum of the tongue usually should be slightly above the occlusal surfaces of the posterior of teeth.

There is failure to verify jaw records during try-in in the patients having problem with muscles control. These patients usually have signs and symptoms of muscle splinting and of subclinical edema in the temporomandibular joint.

## INSTRUMENTS AND MATERIALS

- Patient's chart
- Gloves, mask and eye protection for patient and student/dentist
- Articulator with trial dentures graded by one of the prosthodontic faculty prior to patient appointment
- Water bath heated to 140 degrees F (60 degrees C)
- Hanau torch and matches

- Mouthwash
- Interocclusal recording media
- Spatulas, wax
- Buffalo Knife
- Straight hand piece
- Assortment of acrylic burs and stones
- Baseplate wax, pink, two sheets
- Mirrors (mouth and hand).

## PROCEDURES TO BE DONE DURING TRY-IN

1. Verifying the Jaw Relation Record
   - Centric relation
   - Physiologic rest position
   - Occlusal vertical dimension
2. Esthetics
3. Phonetics
   - Its not the speech sound itself that is critical but the interrelationships of the tongue, teeth, denture base, and the lips.
   - Make sure the trail bases are cleaned, free of extra wax, of the appropriate thickness and stable or the phonetics will be difficult to judge.
   - Valves for modifying the flow of air to produce speech sounds:
     - Labial*
     - Labiodental*
     - Dental and alveolar (anterior)*
     - Palatal*
     - Velar (posterior)
     *affected by tooth position

## LABIAL SOUNDS

- Sounds are b, p, and m which are made at the lips
- Insufficient support of the lips by the teeth and denture base can cause these sounds to be defective

## LABIODENTAL SOUNDS

- f and v are made between the maxillary incisors and the labiolingual center to the posterior third of the lower lip
- For correct positioning, the incisal edges should touch the wet-dry line during the f and v production

## DENTAL AND ALVEOLAR SOUNDS

- Dental sounds th (this, that, these, those) are made with the tip of the tongue extending slightly between the maxillary and mandibular anterior teeth.
- The palate of the denture base that is too thick in the area of the rugae will also cause problems with speech
- With the silibant sounds a phrase such as "I went to church to see the judge" will test the position of the teeth
- If this phrase is not clear there is an error in the horizontal and vertical overlap of the anterior teeth
- This test will not tell you which are incorrect—the maxillary or mandibular anterior teeth.
- S sounds can be considered dental and alveolar speech sounds.
- If the space is too small a whistle will result, if too broad and thin an sh will result as a lisp.
- Adjust the palate of the denture as necessary to correct this sound.
- Mississippi, sixty-six, See Sally by the seashore.

## ALVEOLAR SOUNDS

- Alveolar sounds such as t, d, n, s, and z are made by contact of the tip of the tongue with the anterior most part of the palate or the lingual side of the anterior teeth.
- Silibants (s, z, sh, zh, ch, and j) are alveolar sounds.
- The maxillary and mandibular incisors should approach end to end but not touch.

# CHAPTER 14
# Waxing and Carving

The polished surfaces of dentures influence retentive quality and esthetic values of the denture. The polished surfaces are developed by contouring the wax. The wax surfaces around the teeth are known as the "art portion" of the polished surfaces. It should imitate the form of the tissues around the natural teeth for esthetic reasons. The form of the denture bases between the teeth and the border should be shaped in such a manner as to aid retention by the mechanical directional forces of the muscles and tissues.

## REQUIREMENTS

1. They should duplicate the covered soft tissues as accurately as possible.
2. Labial and buccal fullness of the maxillary and mandibular dentures should be present.
3. Notches should be provided to accommodate the mucous membrane attachment both in size and direction.
4. The contour of the denture flanges should be compatible with the shape of the cheeks and lips.
5. The contour of the lingual flange of the mandibular dentures should have the least possible amount of bulk, except at the border. This thickness is under the narrower portion of the tongue and it greatly enhances the seal of contacting the mucolingual fold.
6. The palatal section of the maxillary dentures should be nearly a reproduction of the patient's palate, rugae included.

## WAXING

Waxing is defined as *the contouring of the wax base of the trial denture into the desired form.*

## CARVING

Carving is defined as *restoring the anatomic forms of the lost tissues.*

## FESTOOING

Festooning is defined as *carrying in the base material of a denture that simulates the contour of the natural tissues that are being replaced by a denture.*

## MAXILLARY DENTURE BASE CONTOUR

### Waxing

Place strips of base plate wax along the facial surface of the trial denture so that they extend from the gingival third of the teeth to the edge of the cast with a hot plate spatula, lute the strips to the underlying wax at ¼ inch intervals and melt the wax in contact with necks of the teeth. Allow sufficient thickness of wax in border areas for rounded margins. The palatal surfaces of the maxillary dentures should be waxed to a uniform thickness of 2.5 mm. The wax pattern should be made of uniform thickness throughout of main portion of the denture.

## Carving

After the wax has cooled, start contouring different areas, to a shape as they look in natural tissues.

### Gingival Margins

The gingival margins have a scalloped appearance. Gingival margins are carved at an angle of 45 degree to the tooth surface.

The level of exposure depends on the age of the patient. Older patients have more receded gums.

### Gingival Bulge

Gingival bulge is convex band of gingival tissue running immediately apical to the facial gingival margin.

It is about 2 to 3 mm wide anteriorly, barely visible in the premolar region and 5 to 6 mm wide in the molar region.

### Interdental Papilla

The interdental papilla is convex is shape both mesio distally and occlusogingivally. It extends up to the contact point of two adjacent teeth.

Interdental papilla vary with the age of the patient. Care should be taken not to remove excess wax inter proximally as this can result in food lodgement.

### Gingival Groove

Gingival groove is shallow groove carved about 1 to 1.5 mm apical to the gingival margin on the facial side.

### Peripheral Roll

The borders of the dentures should be well rounded and should completely fill the sulcus inorder to obtain a good seal. The buccal and lingual borders are known as the peripheral roll.

### Root Prominences

The canine has the most prominent root followed by that of central incisor, lateral incisor and premolars. All root eminences should blend into the peripheral roll, between each root projection is a shallow triangular depression. The apex of these interadicular fassae point towards and extend 1.5 to 2 mm short of the interdental papilla.

### Canine Fossa

A shallow concavity is carved distal to the canine eminence. This is necessary for normal facial expression.

### Buccal Flange

Between the gingival bulge and peripheral roll, the buccal flange should be made slightly concave. This helps to accommodate the buccinators muscle.

### Palatal Surface

The palate is given a uniform thickness of 2.5 mm. Excess bulk here can interfere with tongue function and speech.

Maximum space should be given for tongue. Laterally the palatal slope is continuous with the palatal surface of the teeth.

### Rugae

The rugae duplicated especially if they were present in the previous denture.

### Stippling

Stippling refers to the orange peel like appearance of the attached gingiva. This can be observed in the mouth after drying the gums

Stippling is done by pressing the tips of a bristle brush into the softened wax.

Stippling is more prominent between the roots.

## MANDIBULAR DENTURE BASE CONTOUR

The gingival features like gingival bulge, groove, stippling, etc. are similar to that of maxillary. Root prominences are given for the premolars and the anterior teeth. The canine eminence is most prominent followed by lateral and central incisors.

### Buccal Flanges

The areas between the gingival bulge and peripheral, roll is made slightly concave to accommodate the buccinators and aid in retention.

The premolar region should never incline buccally, buccal placement of the premolars or buccal inclination of the hinge can cause displacement of the denture by the modiolus.

### Lingual Flange

The anterior and middle part of the lingual flange slopes towards the tongue; it may be made slightly concave.

Care should be taken to avoid making a deep depression immediately below the teeth, as it can cause displacement of the denture during tongue functions. The retromylohyoid portion of the flange slopes away from the tongue, blending into the retromylohyoid fossa.

### Polishing

Carving of the work is followed by polishing. Prior to polishing excess wax on the tooth surface should be removed. Wax is smoothened by gentle flaming using an alcohol, followed by immediate cooling in chilled water.

After the preliminary arrangement of artificial teeth is done, the final occlusion is developed and corrected on the articulator. It is essential that the accuracy of the jaw relation records made with the occlusal rims be tested, perfected if incorrect, and then verified to be correct. It is essential that the movements of the articular simulate mandibular position or movements of the patient within the range of normal adjusted that they approximate the condylar guiding factors within the temporomandibular joints. These adjustments of the condylar elements of the articular are made by means of interocclusal eccentric records.

# Processing of Dentures

**CHAPTER 15**

Once the try-in is over and the trial denture is considered satisfactory, then it is processed. The goal in processing a denture is to duplicate the recording base or trial denture into a hardened polished plastic material that will fit the mouth better than the trial base and yet will not introduce any new errors to the established esthetic and occlusal relationships. It generally involves replacing the trial base and the waxed portions with the final denture material. The most commonly used denture base material is heat cured methyl methacrylate resin. Other denture base materials used are auto polymerizing resin, light cured resin, type IV gold alloys and base metal alloys. Hence, in this chapter we will discuss the steps involved in Processing Dentures using heat cured methyl methacrylate resin as denture base material.

## STEPS IN DENTURE PROCESSING

1. Sealing the cast.
2. Separating the cast.
3. Investing the denture.
4. Wax elimination (dewaxing).
5. Mixing and packing of acrylic resin dough.
   a. Trial packing of acrylic resin
   b. Final closure and bench curing
6. Curing procedures.
   a. Processing cycles
   b. Bench cooling
7. Deflasking.
8. Remounting and selective grinding
9. Finishing and polishing.

### 1. Sealing the Cast

- Once the waxing and festooning is complete, the denture is sealed to the cast at its borders with molten wax.
- This maintains the position of the denture on the cast and also prevents plaster from getting under the trial denture (Figs 2.15.1 to 2.15.4).

### 2. Seperating the Cast

- Once the trial denture is sealed to the cast, the cast along with trial denture is separated from articulator by tapping with mallet over a plaster knife placed at the junction of cast and plaster mounting.
- The articulator with the mounting plaster is kept safely aside till the curing is complete for laboratory remounting of casts (Figs 2.15.5 and 2.15.6).

### 3. Investing the Denture

- Investing procedures which surround the denture with investing material to form a mold are also known as flasking procedures.

# 170 Pre-Clinical Prosthodontics

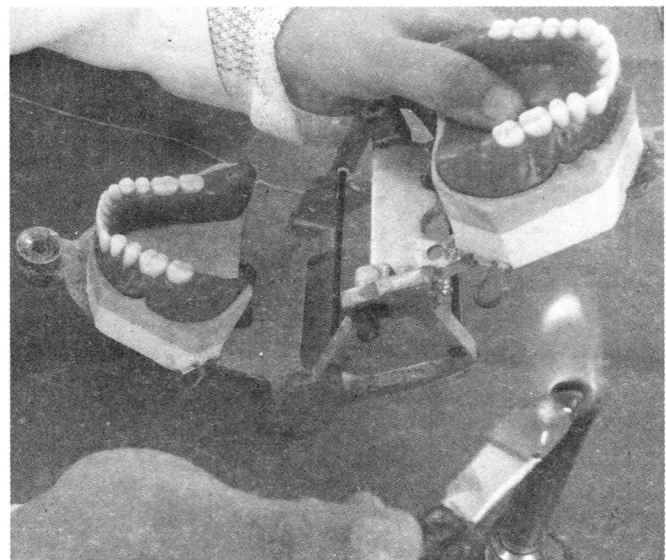

Fig. 2.15.1

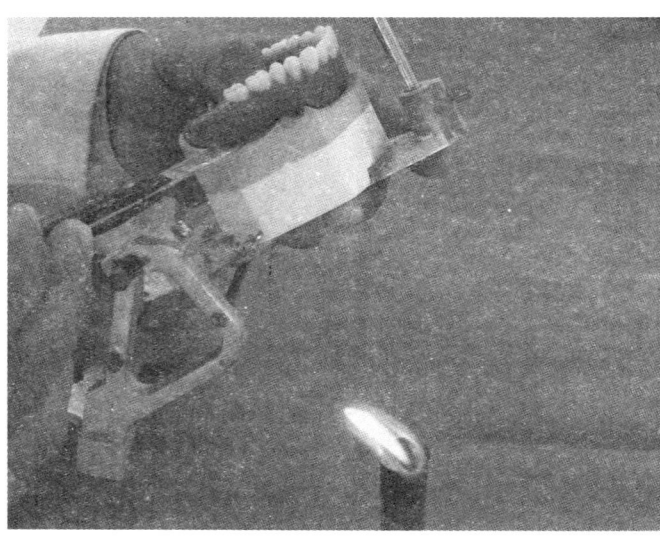

Fig. 2.15.2

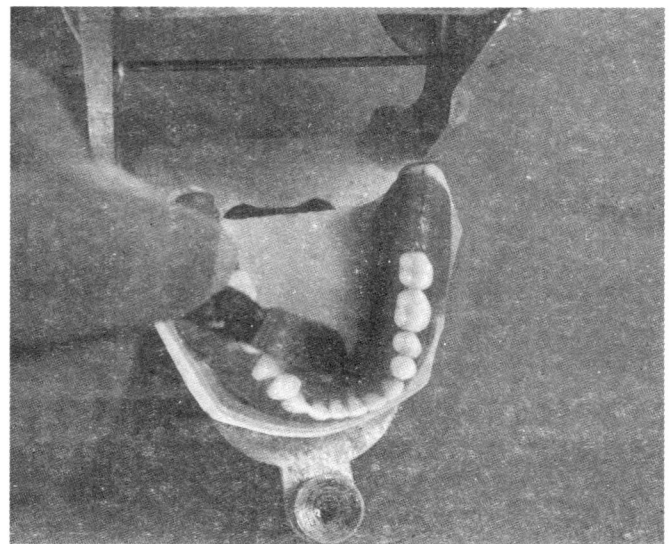

Fig. 2.15.3

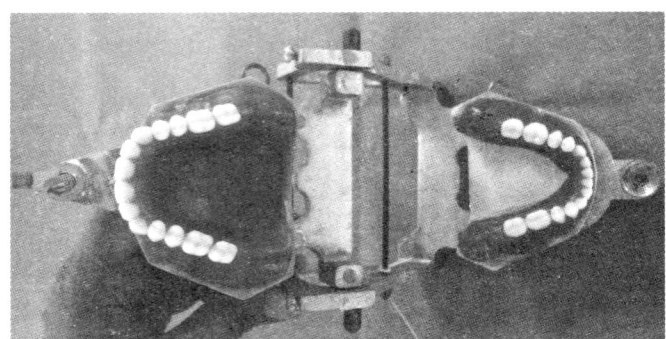

Fig. 2.15.4

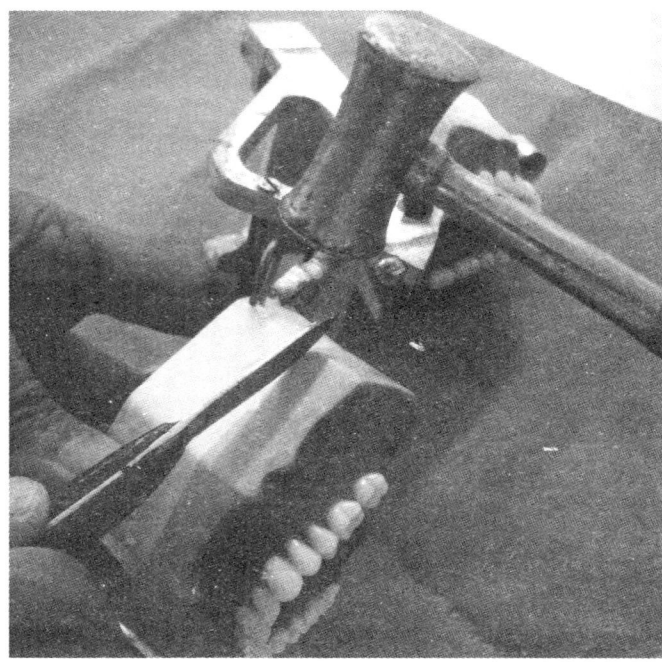

Fig. 2.15.5

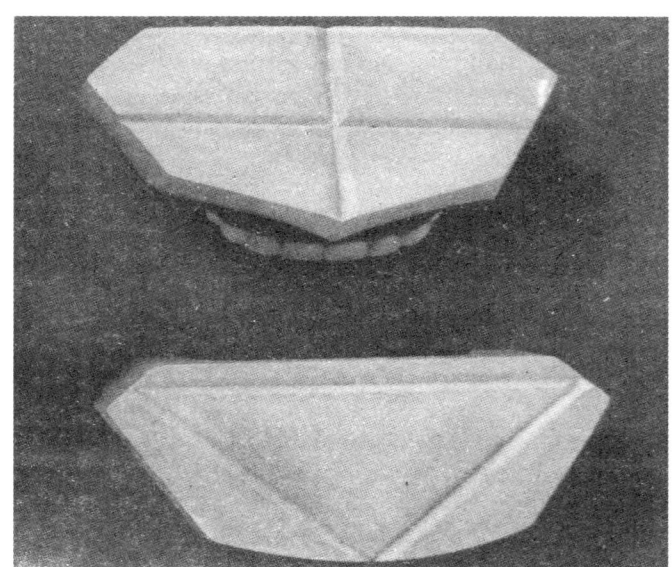

Fig. 2.15.6

- Flasking or investing is a procedure by which the trial denture is surrounded with dental plaster or dental stone in a metal flask.
- Flasking should be done using only dental stone which is 2½ to 3 times stronger than plaster, is more accurate and limits tooth movement better.
- There are mainly three types of techniques followed for investing or flasking procedures.
  a. Three pour technique
  b. Four pour technique
  c. Two pour technique

a. Three pour technique
  - In this technique, three mixes of dental stone are used.
    i. *Soaking the cast:* First cast is soaked in slurry water for few minutes before flasking (Fig. 2.15.7).
    ii. *Checking the fit of cast:* The fit of cast in the flask is checked and excess height of the cast is reduced by trimming the base of the cast (Fig. 2.15.8).

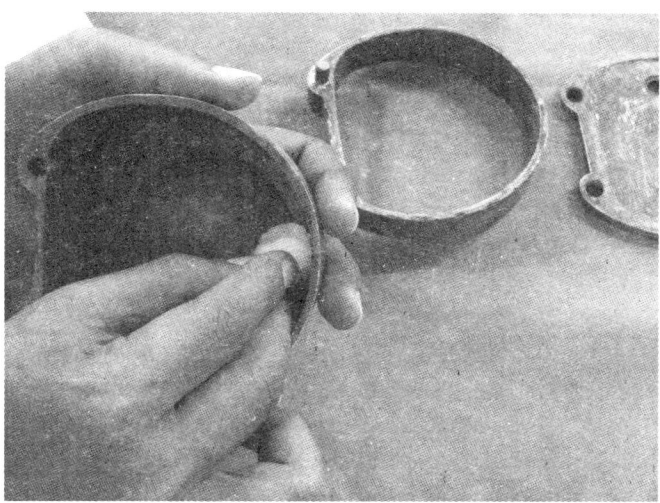

**Fig. 2.15.9**

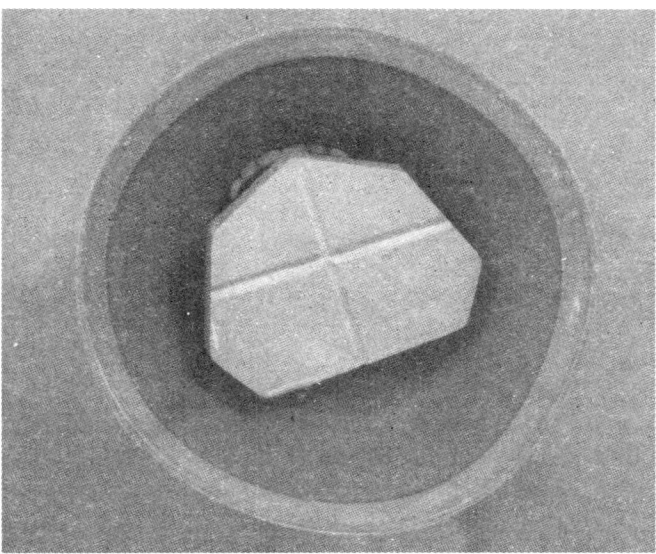

**Fig. 2.15.7**

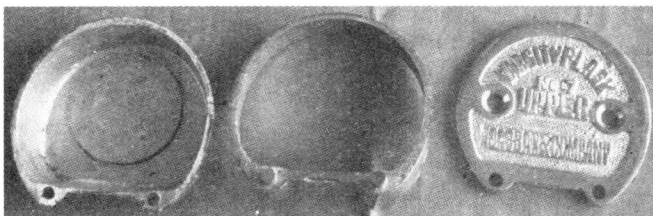

**Fig. 2.15.8**

  iii. *Lubricating the flask:* The inner surface of the flask is lubricated with petroleum jelly. This aids in easy and clean removal of dental stone from flask during deflasking procedures (Fig. 2.15.9).

  iv. *First pour of dental stone:* Each mix of dental stone should be weighed, the water measured (28 to 30 cc/100g), spatulated for at least 30 seconds and the mixing bowl held on a vibrator for 15 seconds to remove air bubbles. Separating medium is applied to the base and sides of the cast and allowed to dry, for easy retrieval of casts during deflasking procedures. Mixed dental stone is filled into the lowest portion of the flask and the cast along with the attached trial denture is settled into it. The first pour should be in level with the land area of the cast and the lower half of the flask. The stone is smoothened making sure that there are no undercuts. After each pour the dental stone is allowed to set for 20 minutes (Figs 2.15.10 to 2.15.19)

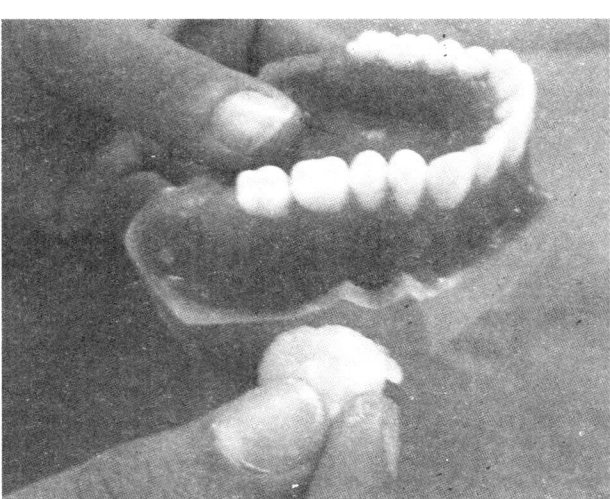

**Fig. 2.15.10**

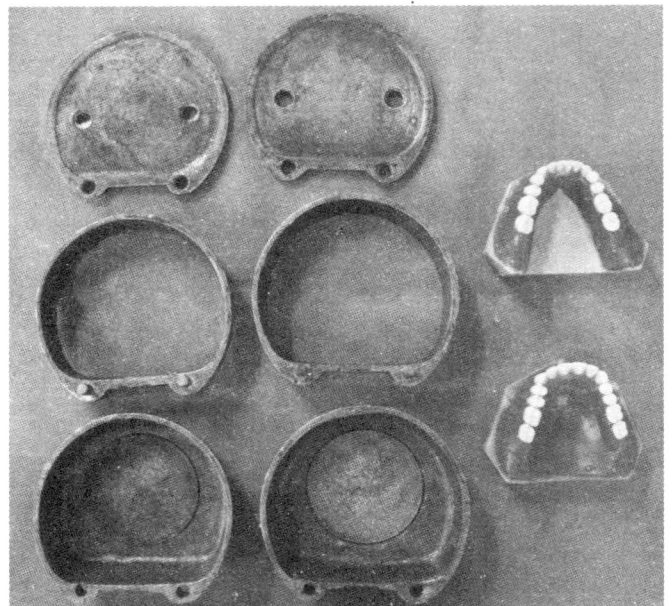

Fig. 2.15.11

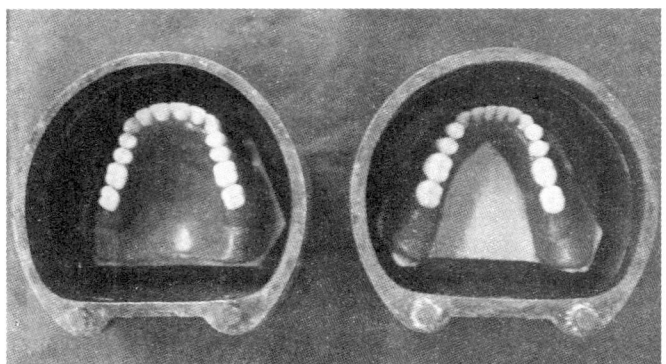

Fig. 2.15.12

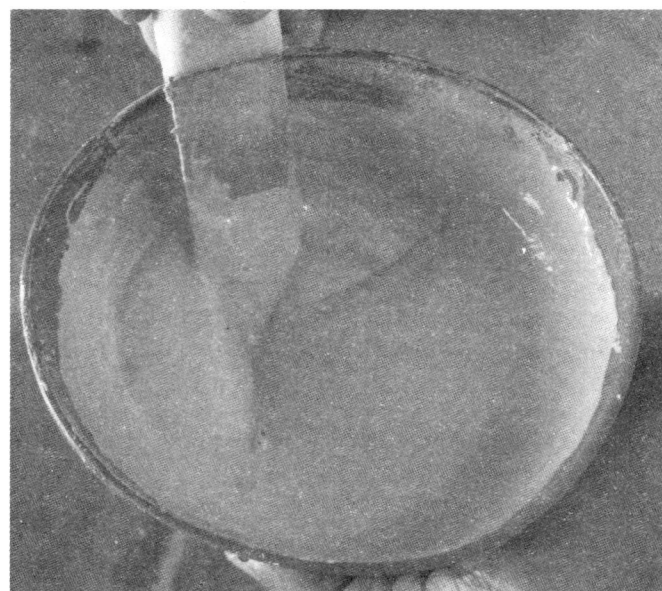

Fig. 2.15.13

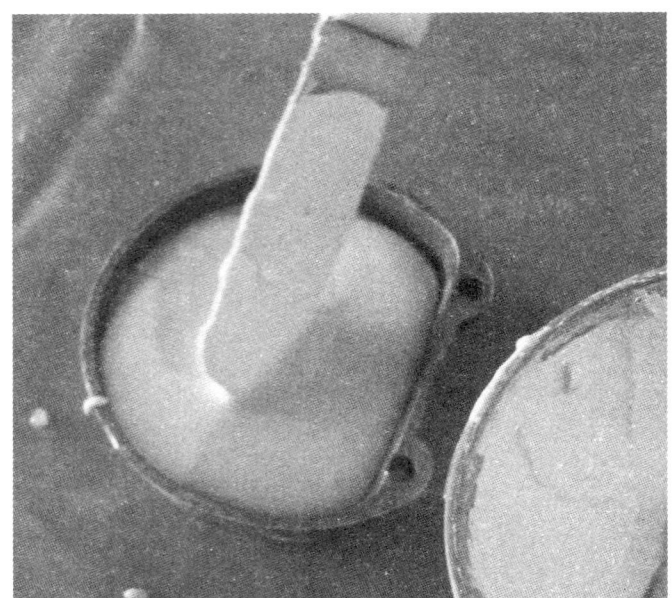

Fig. 2.15.14

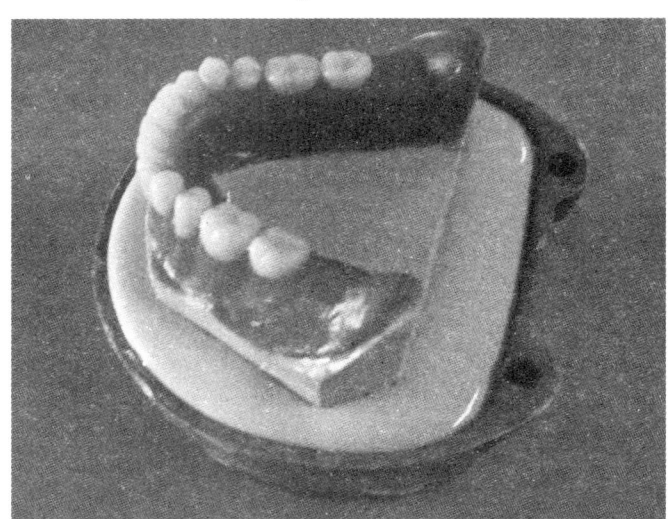

Fig. 2.15.15

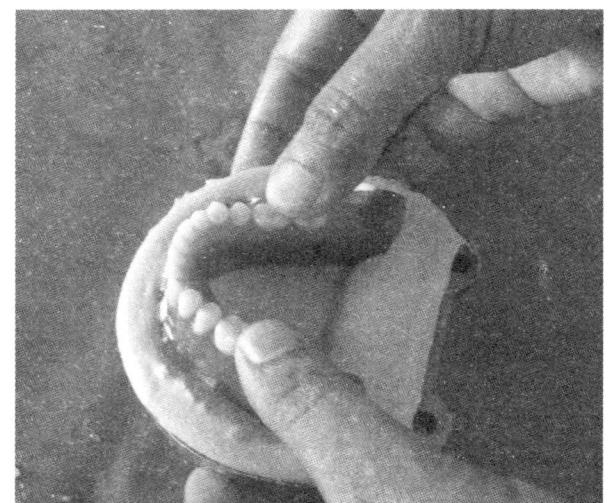

Fig. 2.15.16

## Processing of Dentures

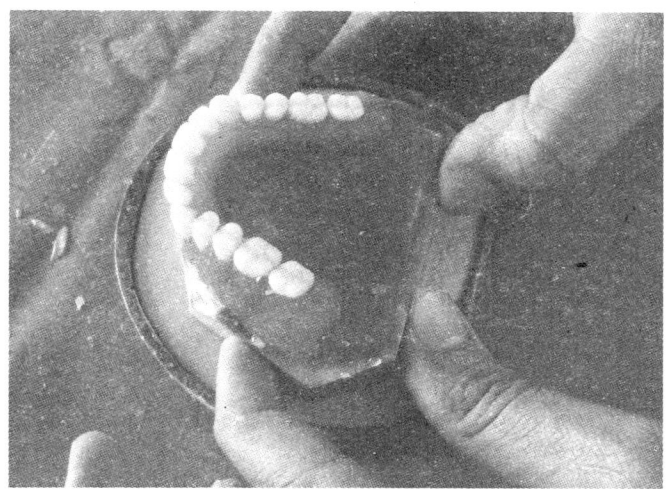

Fig. 2.15.17

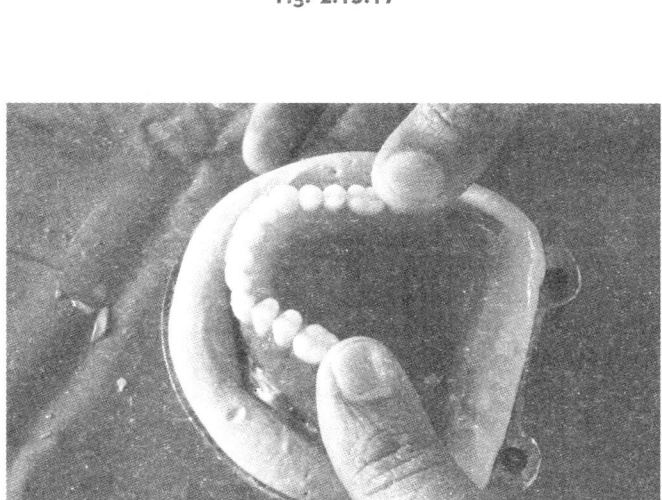

Fig. 2.15.18

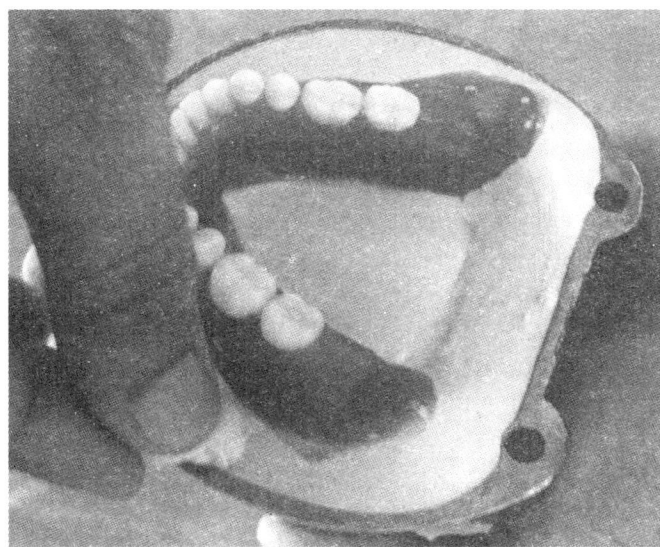

Fig. 2.15.19

v. *Second pour of dental stone:* After the first pour of dental stone is set; separating medium is applied over the dental stone and the cast. The upper half of the flask (without lid) is assembled over lower half and checked for proper closure. The two halves must meet exactly. The second mix of dental stone is poured into the assembled dental flask up to the level of occlusal and incisal edges of the teeth. Using a finger, remove the stone on the occlusal and incisal surfaces of teeth. The stone is smoothed making sure that there are no undercuts. Allow the second pour to set for 20 minutes (Figs 2.15.20 to 2.15.27).

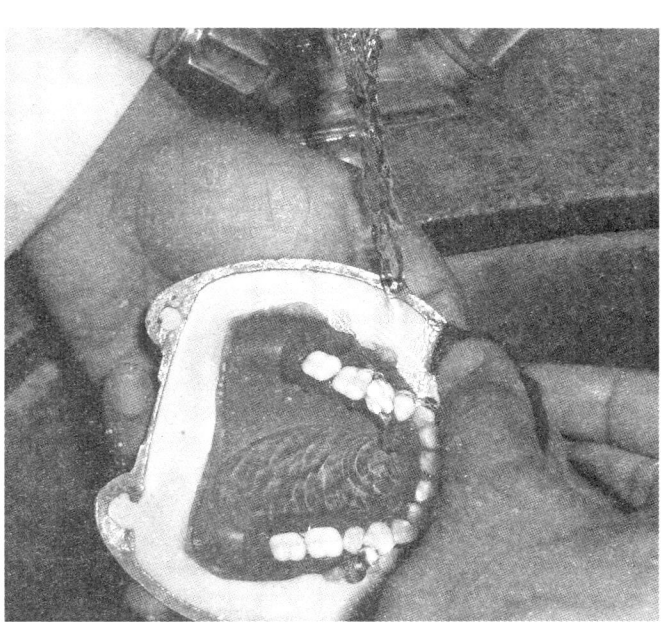

Fig. 2.15.20

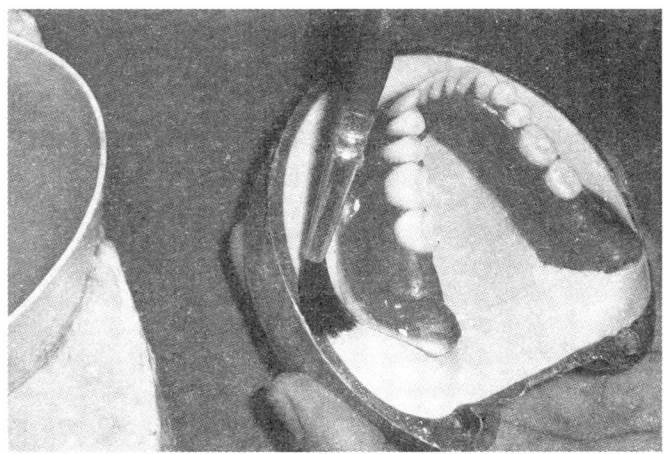

Fig. 2.15.21

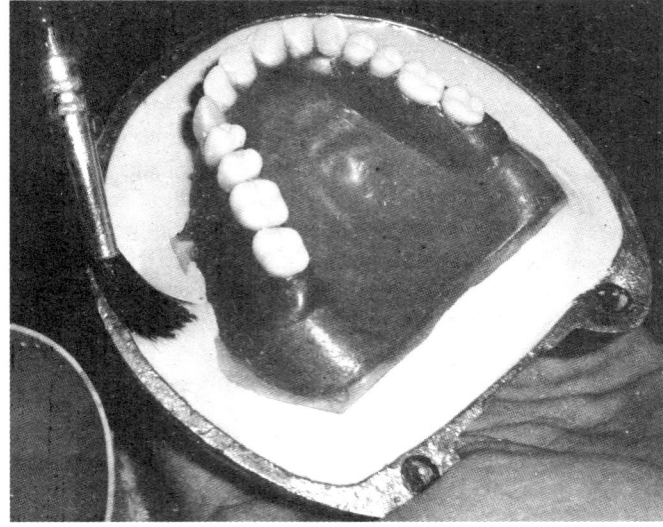

Fig. 2.15.22

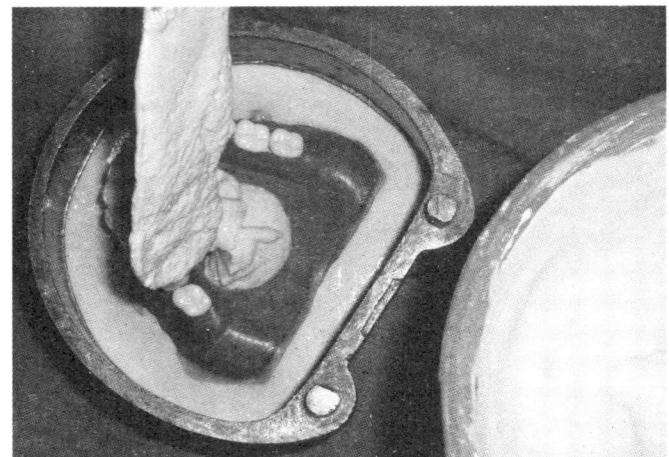

Fig. 2.15.25

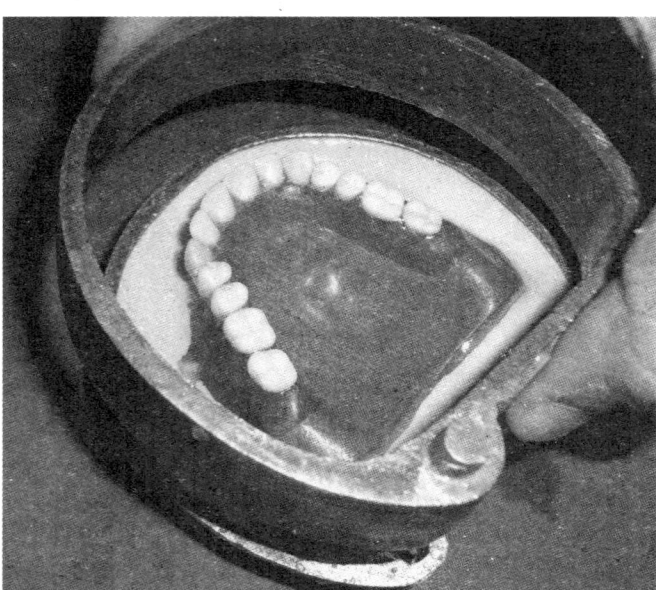

Fig. 2.15.23

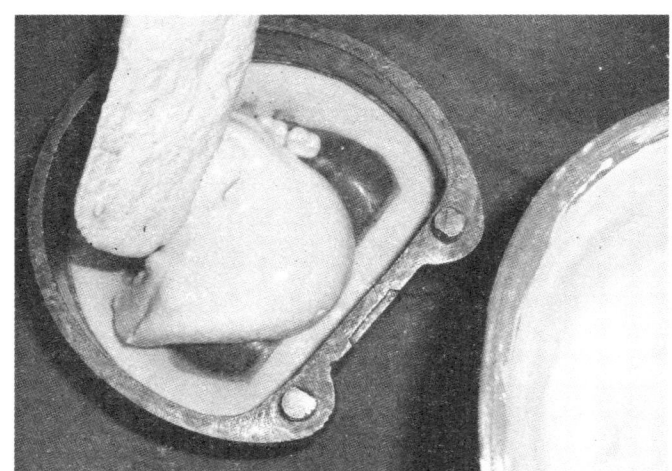

Fig. 2.15.26

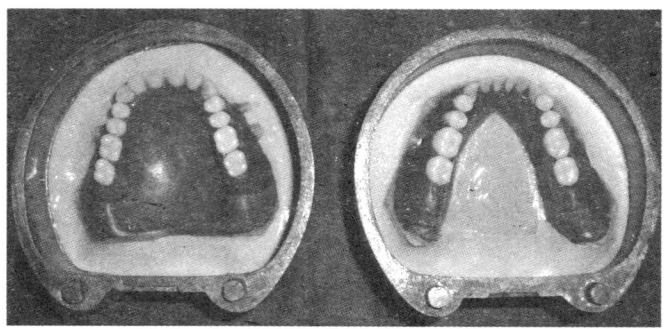

Fig. 2.15.24

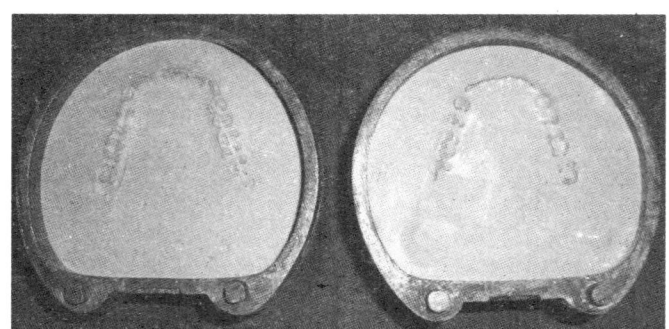

Fig. 2.15.27

vi. *Third pour of dental stone:* After the second pour of dental stone is set, separating medium is applied again over the dental stone and the third mix of dental stone is poured into remaining part of the denture flask, slightly excess oozing out to lock the lid of the flask to the upper half of the flask. After placing the lid over the flask, the flask is placed in a clamp and tightened using light pressure. Allow the third and final pour of dental stone to set for 20 minutes (Figs 2.15.28 to 2.15.35).

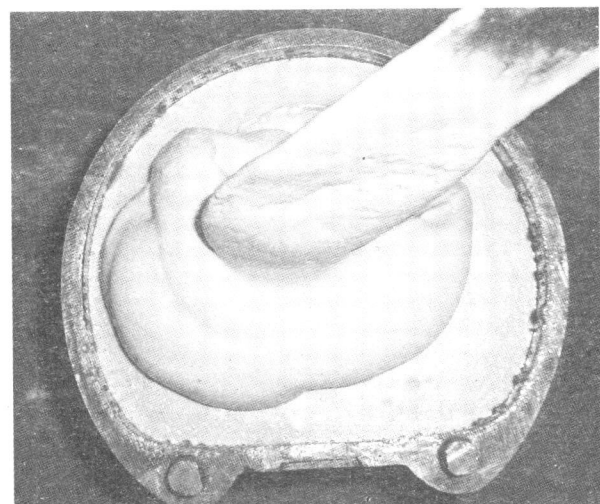

Fig. 2.15.30

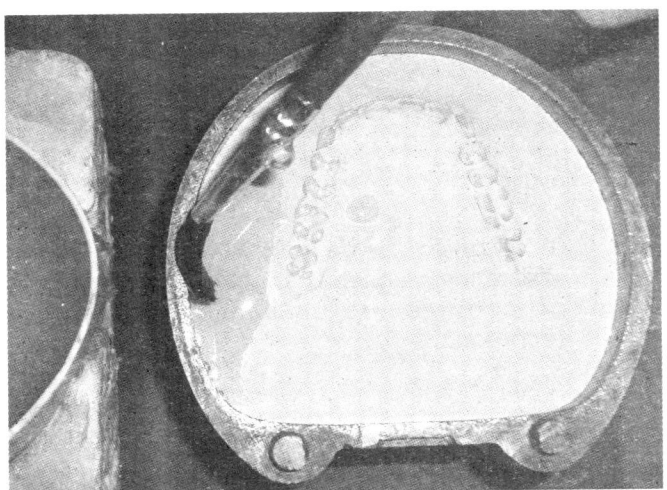

Fig. 2.15.28

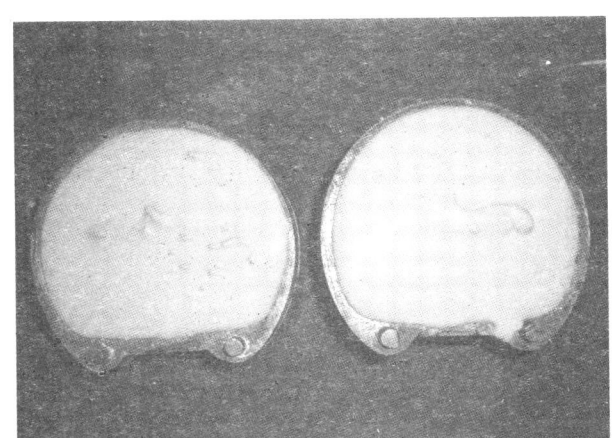

Fig. 2.15.31

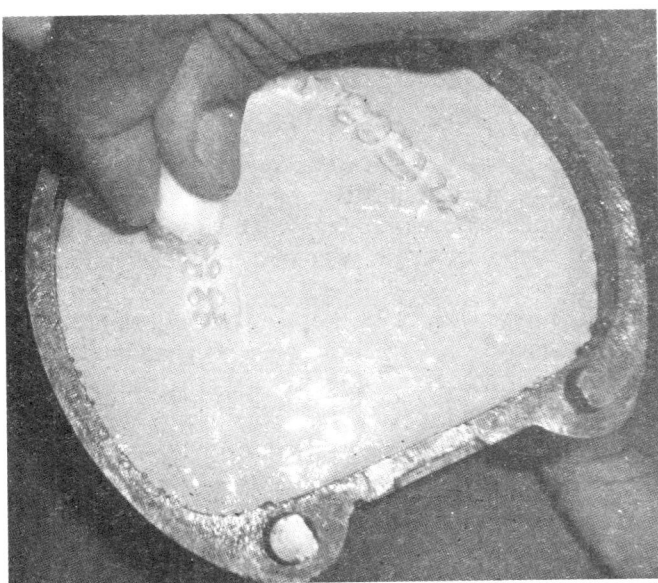

Fig. 2.15.29

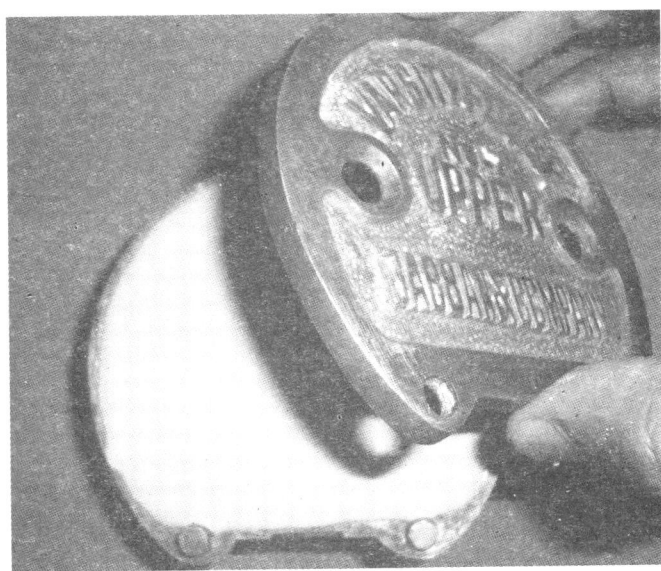

Fig. 2.15.32

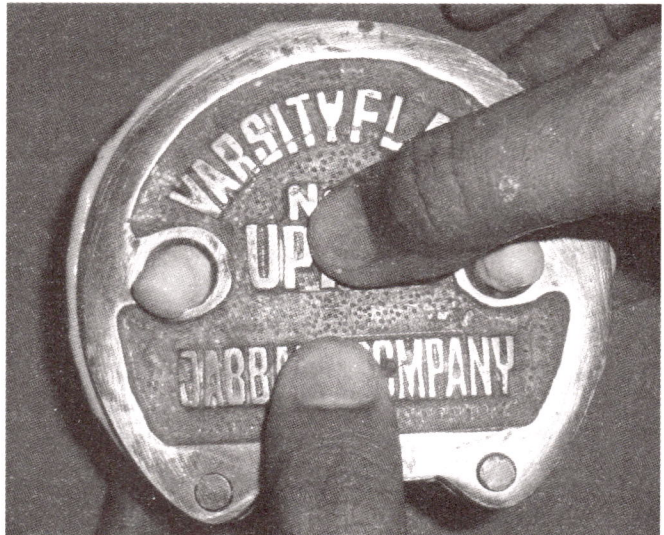

Fig. 2.15.33

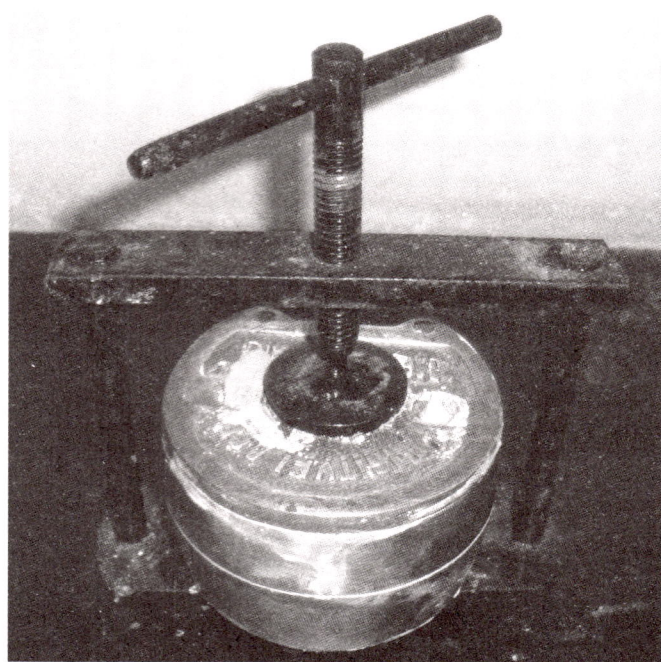

Fig. 2.15.35

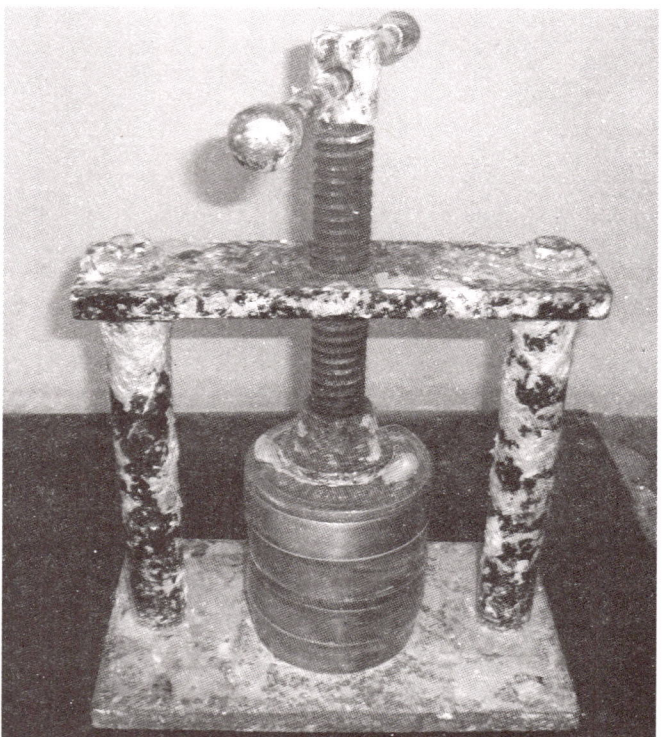

Fig. 2.15.34

### b. Four pour technique

- In this technique, four mixes of dental stone are used. It similar to tree pour technique except for a stone core. After the first pour of dental stone sets, a stone core is developed over the wax surfaces of the dentures. The core is about 2 to 4 mm in thickness and is ended 2 to 3 mm below the occlusal surfaces of the teeth. Grooves are placed in the stone core for retention of the next pour. Once the stone core sets, separating medium is applied. The rest of the procedures are similar to three pour technique.

### c. Two pour technique

- In this technique, only two mixes of dental stone are used. In the first pour, the cast is flasked in the lower half similar to the three pour technique. In the second pour, the rest of the flask is completely filled. Deflasking and recovery of denture is difficult, if the flasking of dentures is done using two pour technique.

### 4. Wax Elimination (Dewaxing)

- Wax elimination or de waxing is a process in which flasked trial denture along with clamp is placed in boiling water in order to chelate a mold space by eliminating the wax and temporary denture base.
- The flask should be kept in boiling water for a maximum of 3 to 5 minutes, so that the wax is not permitted to penetrate into the dental stone (Fig. 2.15.35).
- After 3 to 5 minutes, the flask is removed from boiling water and opened carefully. The softened wax and trial denture base are discarded. Flush the mold with clean boiling water to remove remaining traces of wax (Figs 2.15.36 to 2.15.43)

Processing of Dentures 177

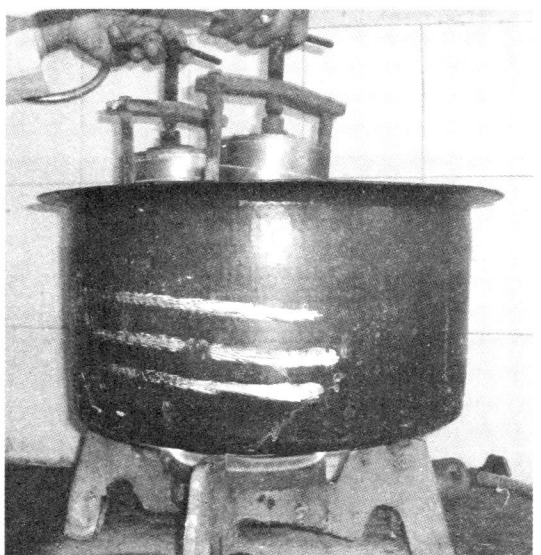

Fig. 2.15.36

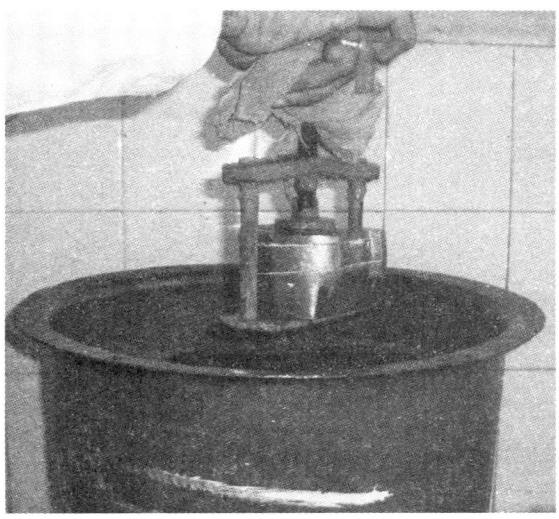

Fig. 2.15.37

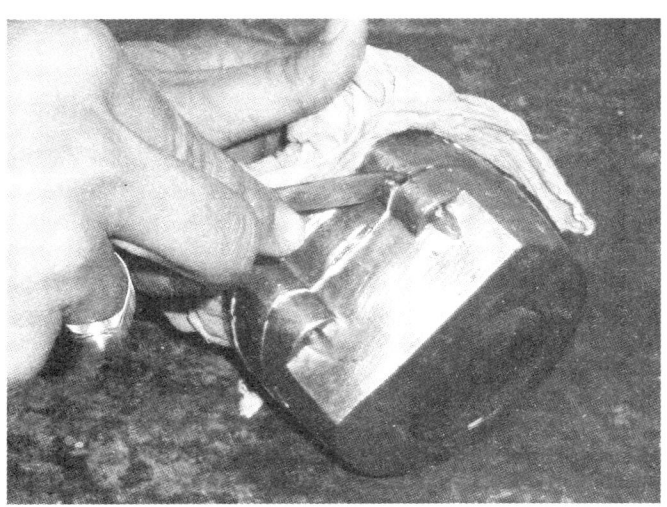

Fig. 2.15.38

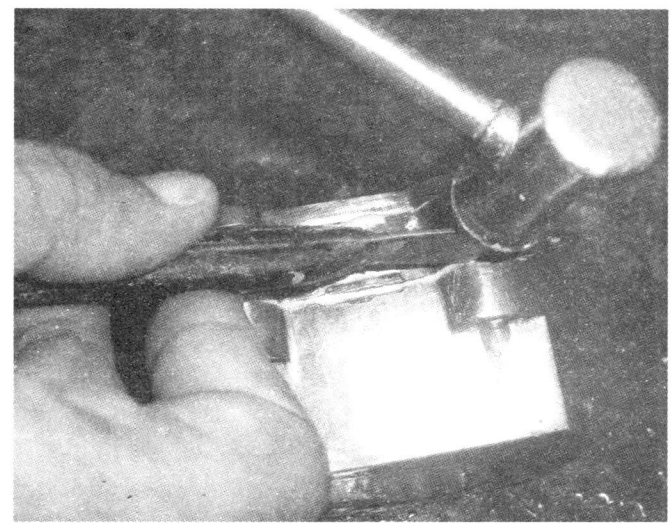

Fig. 2.15.39

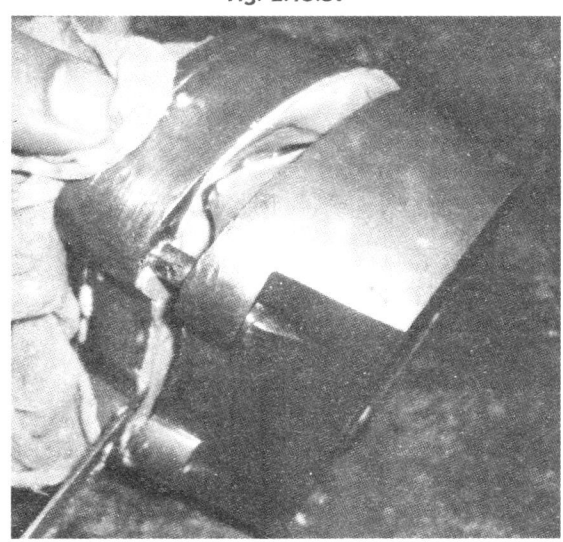

Fig. 2.15.40

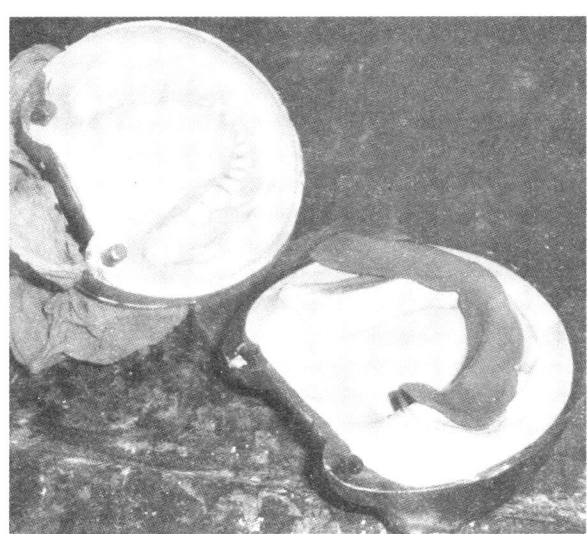

Fig. 2.15.41

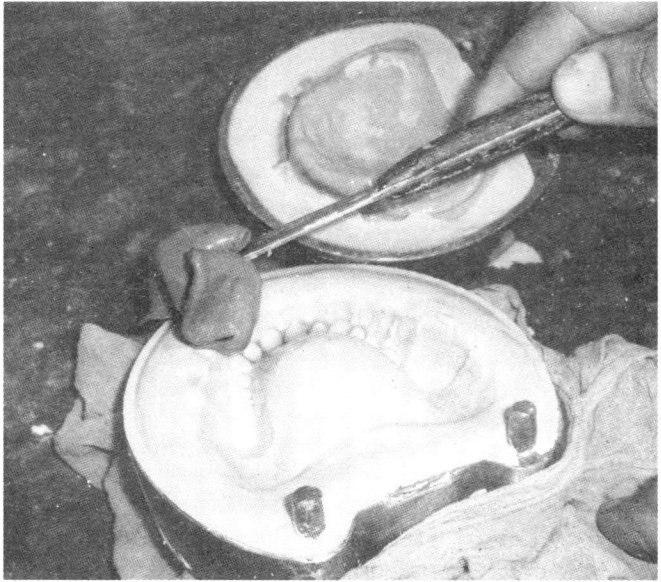

Fig. 2.15.42

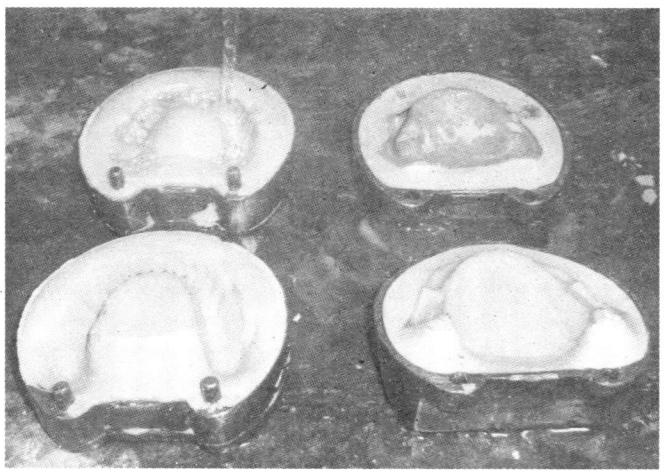

Fig. 2.15.43

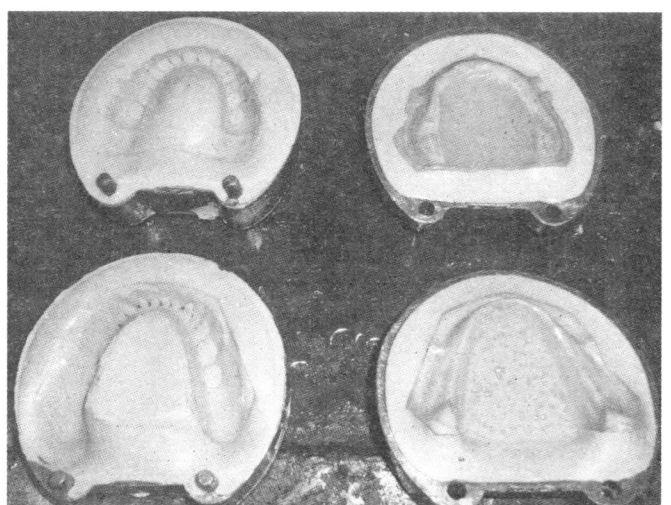

Fig. 2.15.44

- Next, a hot household detergent solution must be brushed on all inner flask surfaces, followed by a thorough clean hot water or steam rinse (Figs 2.15.45 to 2.15.47)

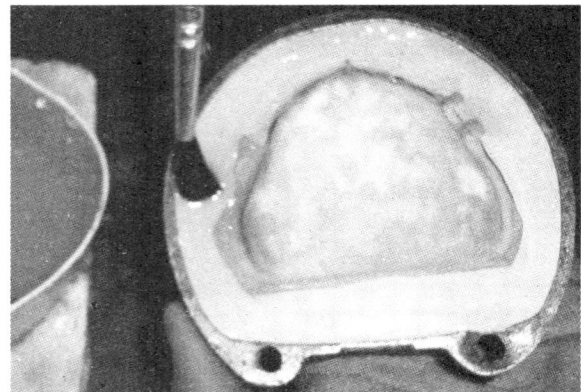

Fig. 2.15.45

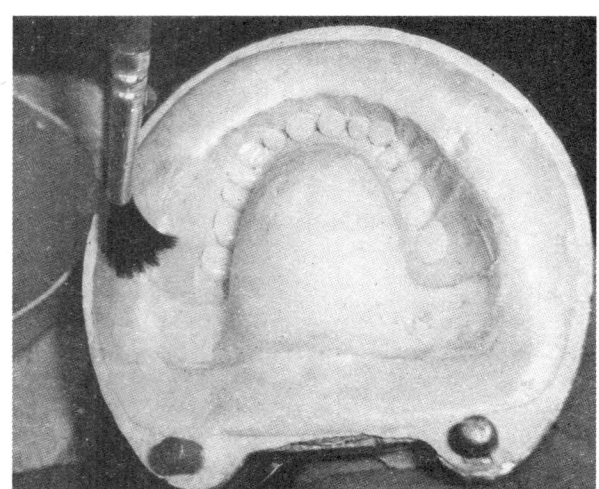

Fig. 2.15.46

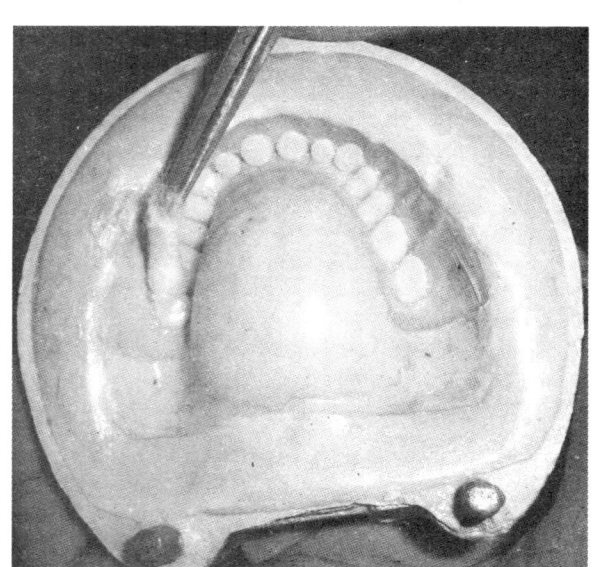

Fig. 2.15.47

- The use of three separate water tanks or two water tanks and a steam line is recommended. One tank is for wax removal, one is for detergent rinse, and contains pure clean water for the final rinse immediately prior to applying the separating medium. The separating medium (alginate tin foil substitute) should be applied over the dental stone casts while the flasks are warm and wet.

5. **Mixing and Packing of Acrylic Resin Dough**

   a. Trial packing of acrylic resin
      - Heat cure acrylic resin is mixed with a spatula in a clean porcelain jar (powder to liquid ratio should be 3:1) and the lid is closed to prevent evaporation of monomer. Once it reaches dough stage, it is removed from jar, formed into a roll and adapted into the mold space. No more than four to six flasks should be packed from one mix of resin dough, the fewer the better (Figs 2.15.48 to 2.15.56)

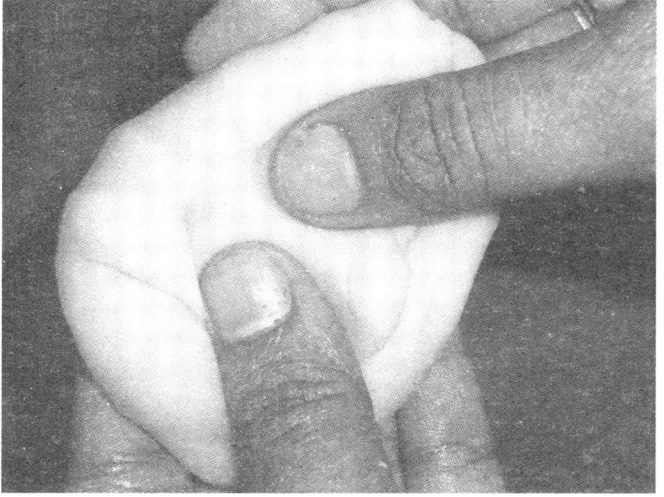

Fig. 2.15.50

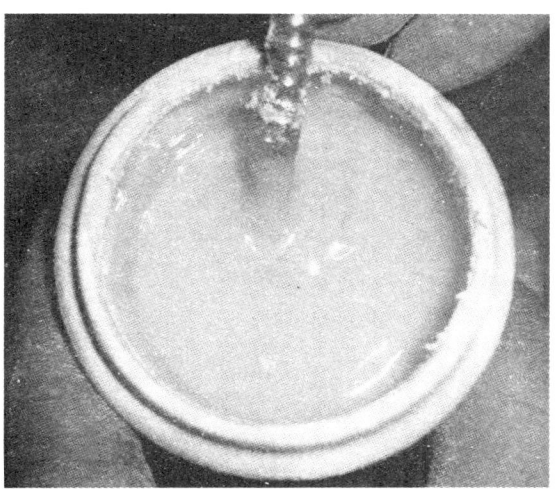

Fig. 2.15.48

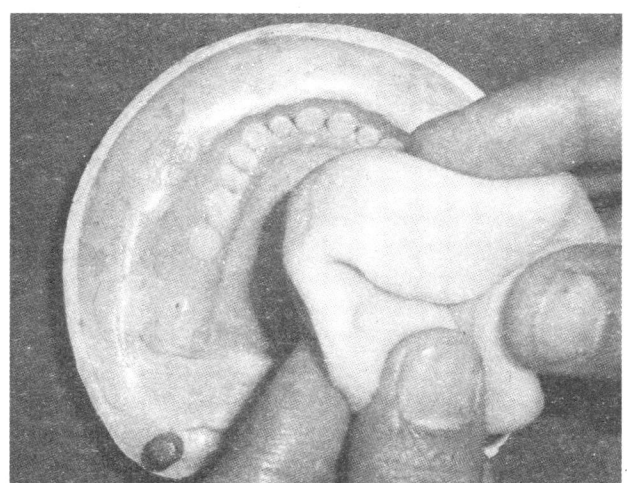

Fig. 2.15.51

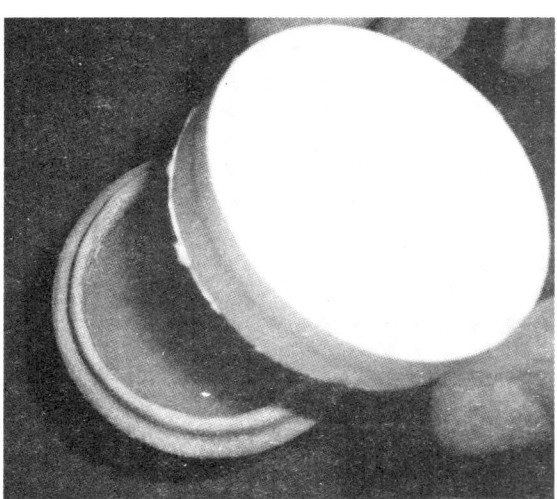

Fig. 2.15.49

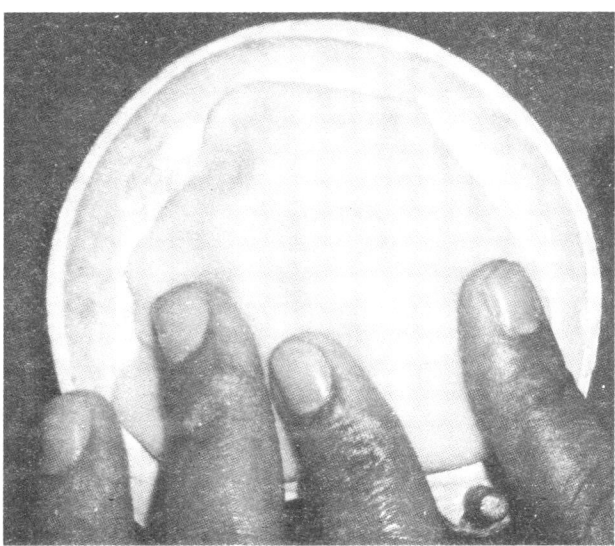

Fig. 2.15.52

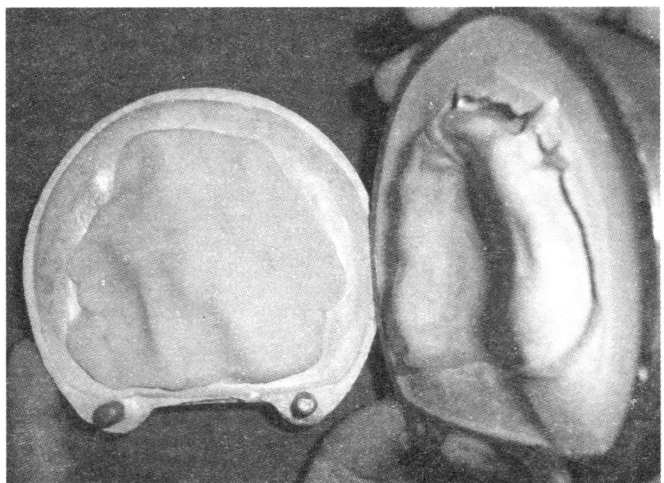

Fig. 2.15.53

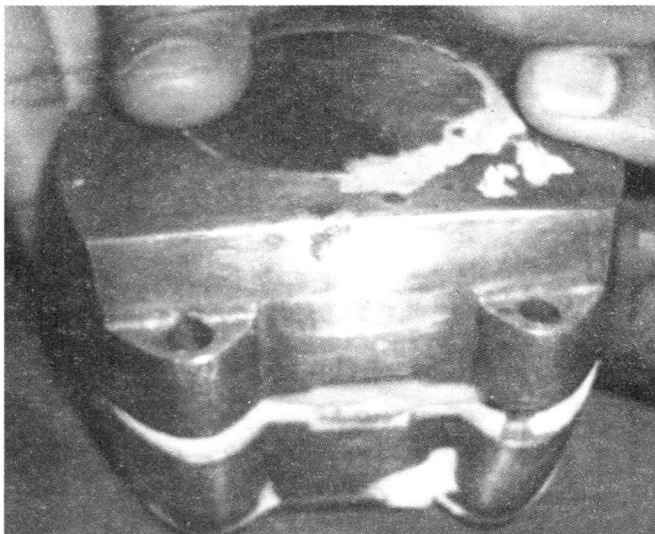

Fig. 2.15.54

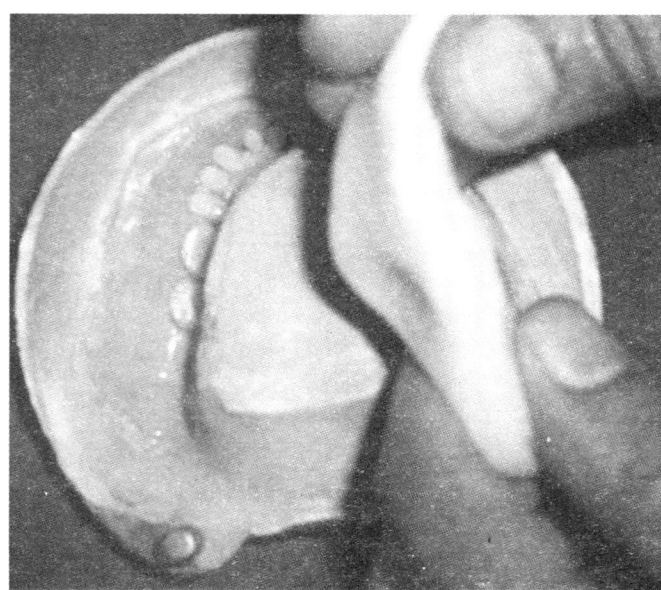

Fig. 2.15.55

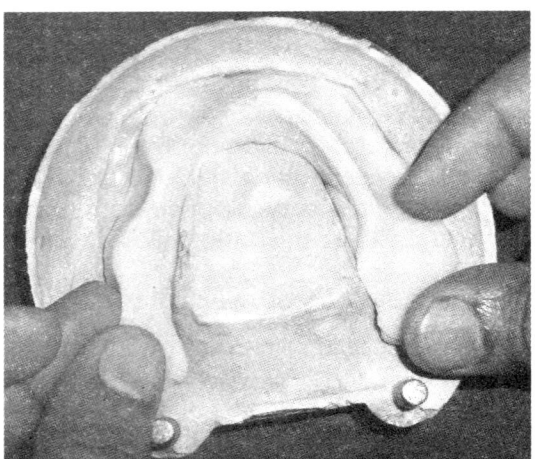

Fig. 2.15.56

- A plastic separating sheet is placed over the dough and the two halves of the flask are closed slowly by applying pressure. The pressure applied should always be increased gradually and steadily by placing it in hydraulic press. This allows the resin dough to flow and fill the mold better as well as improve its density (Figs 2.15.57 to 2.15.61).

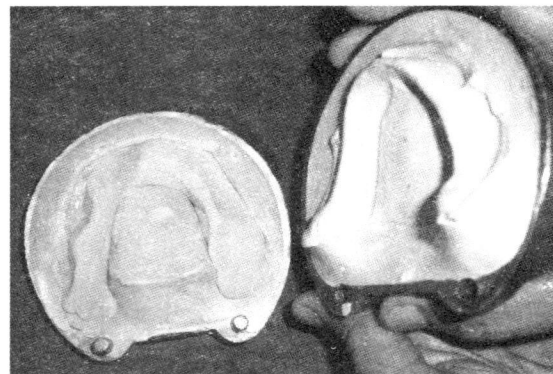

Fig. 2.15.57

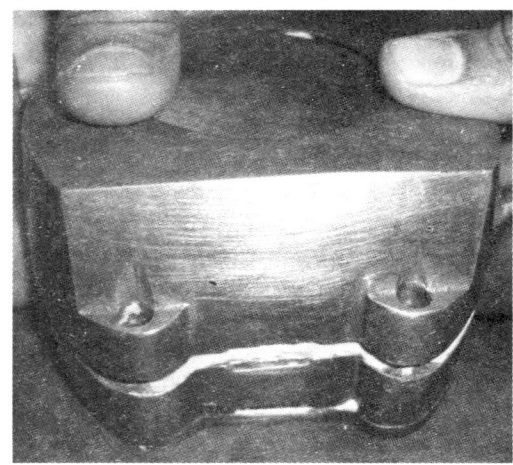

Fig. 2.15.58

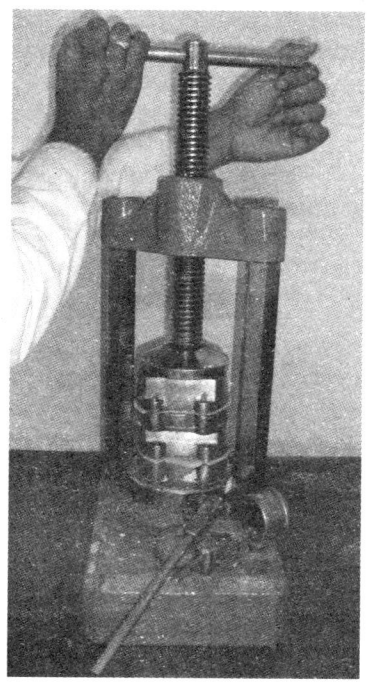

Fig. 2.15.59

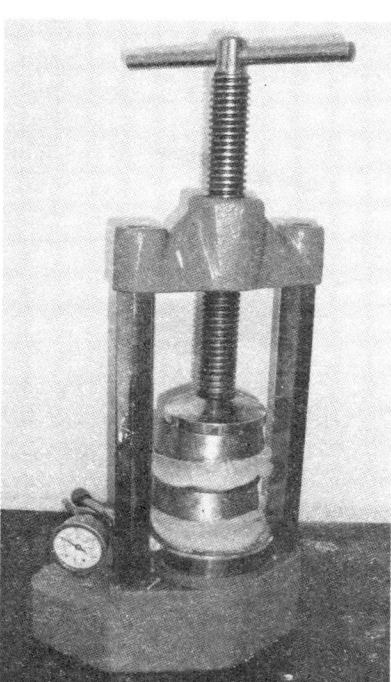

Fig. 2.15.60

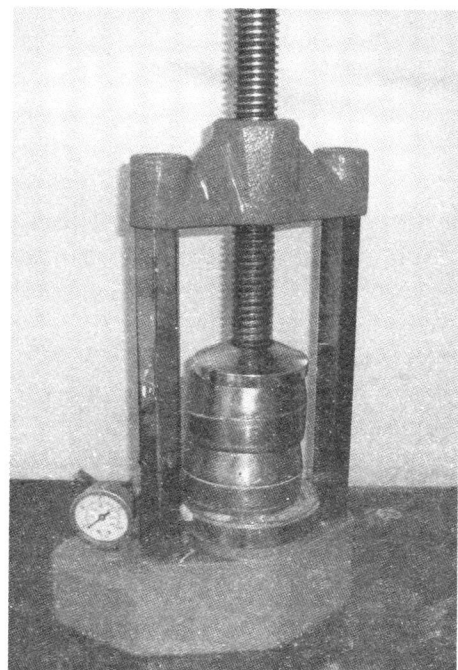

Fig. 2.15.61

- Separate the two halves of the flask, remove plastic sheet and trim off excess acrylic. Now again place the plastic sheet and close the two halves of flask. It is usually possible to have each mold properly compressed and filled after the third trial closure. The trial packing may be repeated until no more flash is formed.

b. Final closure and Bench cooling
  - In the final closure, the plastic separating sheet is removed and the flask is transferred to clamp. Never add excess resin dough prior to the final flask closure. It is better to remove three pea sized portions of dough immediately before the final closure. The addition of any excess resin prior to final flask closure causes greater tooth movement, greater opening of the vertical dimension and may fracture porcelain teeth (Fig. 2.15.62).
  - Ideally, the properly packed flasks should be allowed to stand for 30 to 60 minutes (bench cooling) before beginning the curing cycle. The bench curing allows better equalization of pressures and better monomer penetration.

6. Curing Procedures (Figs 2.15.63 to 2.15.65)
   a. Processing cycles
      i. *Short processing cycle:* The flask is kept in water at room temperature and the

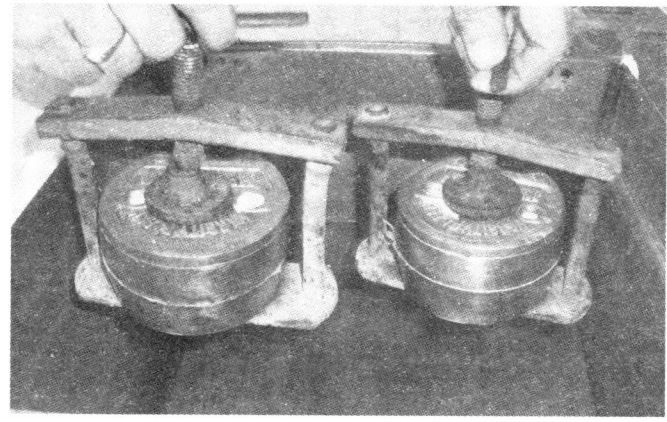

Fig. 2.15.62

temperature is raised to 74 °C (165 °F) and maintained for two hours. It is then brought to boil for one hour.

   ii. *Long processing cycle:* The flask is kept in water at room temperature and the temperature is raised to 74 °C (165 °F) and maintained for eight hours. In this technique boiling is not necessary. This technique is recommended for extremely thick dentures. It reduces the chances of porosity caused by boiling of monomer.

   b. Bench cooling
      - It is important to allow a minimum of one hour bench cooling out of water before deflasking

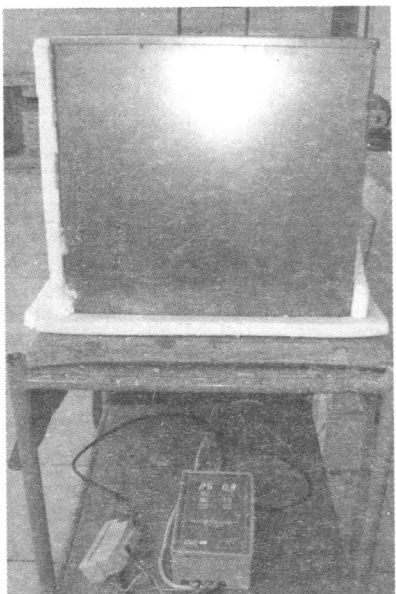

Fig. 2.15.63

to minimize internal stresses and subsequent warpage of the dentures. Frequently, with automatic processing units, the water has cooled by morning and deflasking can be done immediately if the water is luke warm or cooler. Cold-cured acrylic resin dentures should be allowed to cure in their flasks for 2½ hours at room temperature.

### 7. Deflasking

- Deflasking is a process by which the processed final denture is retrieved from the flask. The two halves of the flask are separated by inserting a strong wedge like instrument between the halves. The three pour technique facilitates easy separation of three layers. Dental stone is removed layer by layer, first upper layer, next middle layer and last the dental stone surrounding the base. Care should be taken to prevent the separation of the denture from the cast. This is necessary for the remount procedure (Figs 2.15.66 to 2.15.67).

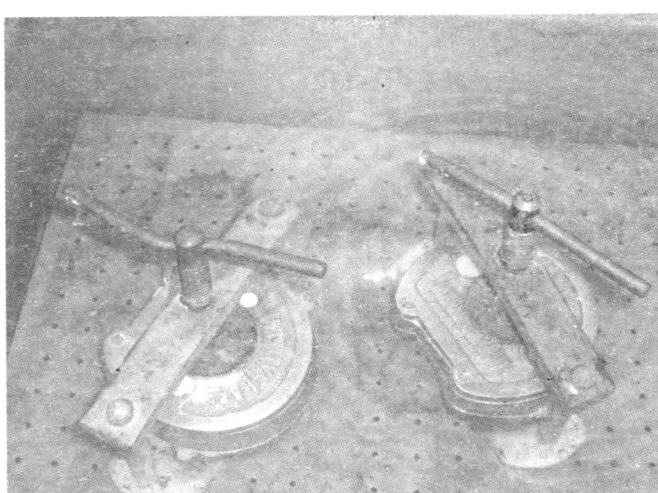

Fig. 2.15.64

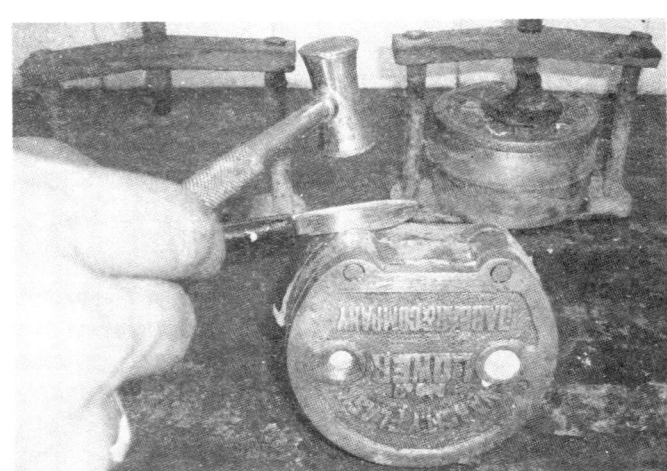

Fig. 2.15.66

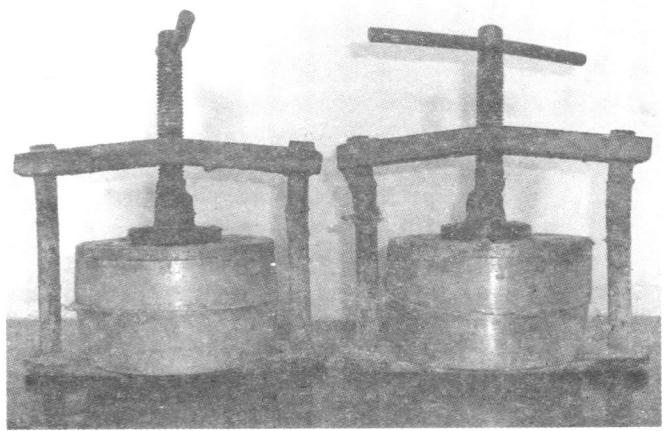

Fig. 2.15.65

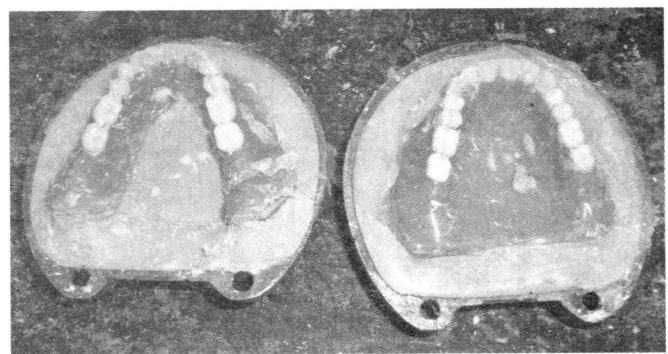

Fig. 2.15.67

## 8. Remounting and Selective Grinding

- Denture processing can often cause changes in the position of teeth as well as distortion of the resin. To correct these processing errors, remounting and selective grinding procedures are carried out.
- The casts are repositioned back on their plaster mounts in the articulator using the index grooves on the base of the cast as guide. They are secured to the mounting with sticky wax or cyanoacrylate glue.
- Articulating paper is placed between the opposing occlusal surfaces and occlusal prematurities are corrected following the selective grinding procedures, to obtain proper occlusion.

## 9. Finishing and Polishing

- Any plaster adhering to the denture is removed by shell blasting or by dissolving it in a suitable commercial gypsum solvent. The excess flash is trimmed off with a lathe mounted wheel, bur or arbor band. Dental stone present between gingival margins is removed with a chisel. Frenal notches are adjusted with a fissure bur. Finally before polishing, the denture is smoothed with sand paper attached to a mandrel, starting with a coarse paper and proceeding to fine sand paper.
- Polishing of denture is done with motorized wet rag wheel and pumice slurry. Resin teeth must be covered or protected during pumice and rag-wheel smoothing; otherwise teeth appear yellow because of loss of outer labial enamel shade. Gingival crevices should be polished with a brush wheel and an abundance of wet pumice. Final gloss is obtained with French chalk or other commercially available agents applied on a buff. Felt cones and dry rag wheels should not be used for polishing as they quickly generate lots of heat and cause warpage of denture. Once the finishing is completed, the denture is stored in water until the delivery of dentures to the patient (Figs 2.15.68 to 2.15.78).

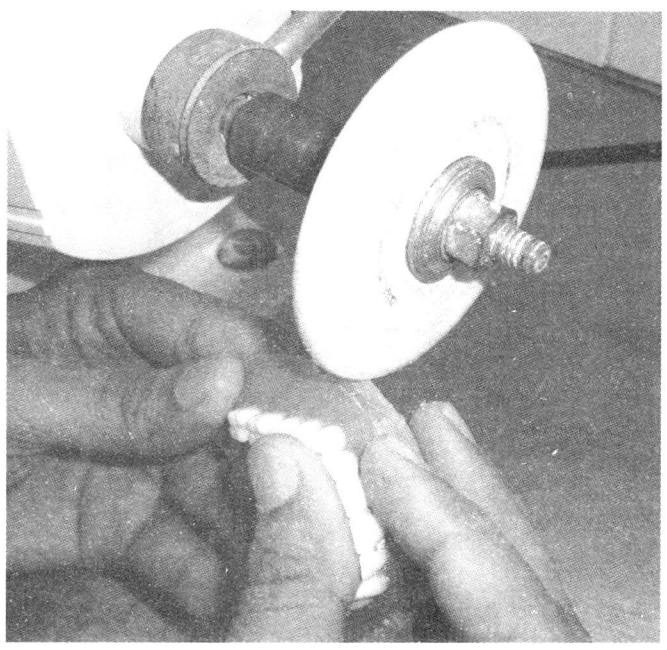

Fig. 2.15.69

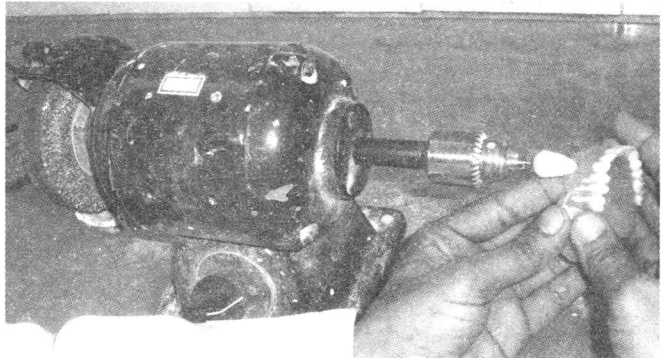

Fig. 2.15.70

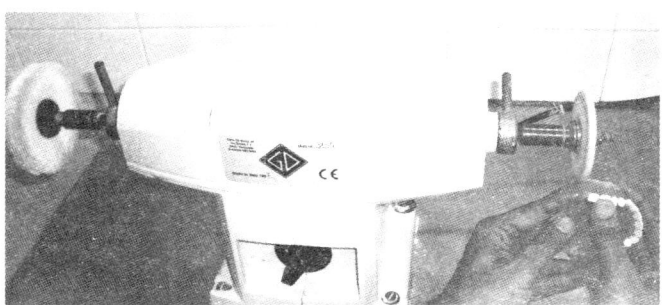

Fig. 2.15.68

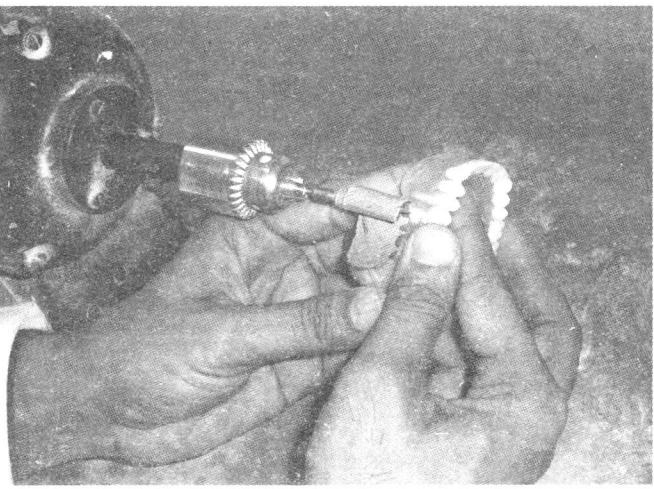

Fig. 2.15.71

### 184 Pre-Clinical Prosthodontics

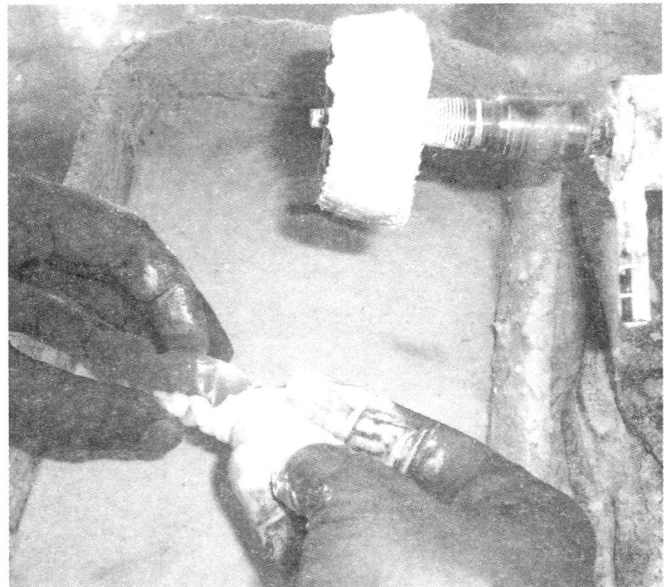

Fig. 2.15.72

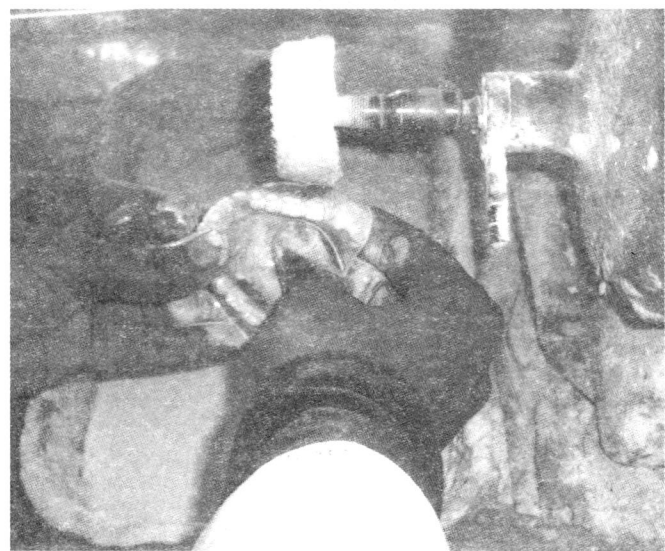

Fig. 2.15.73

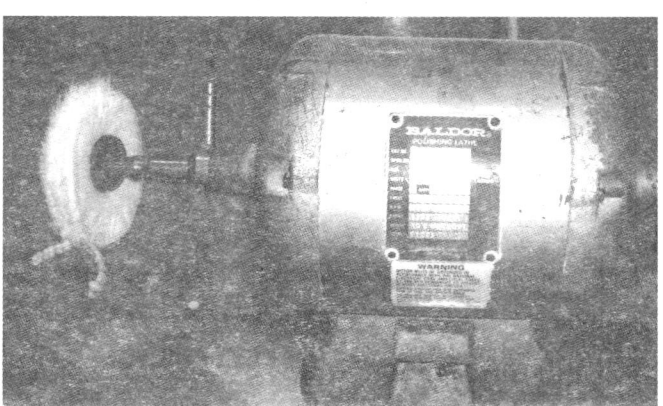

Fig. 2.15.74

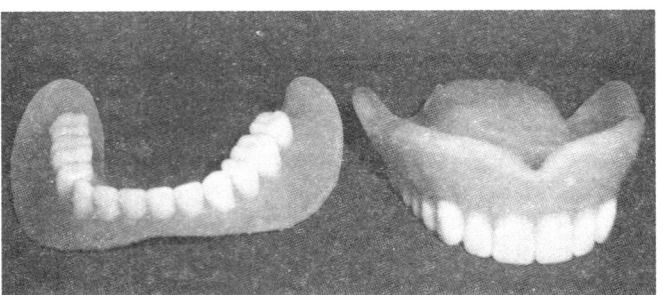

Fig. 2.15.75

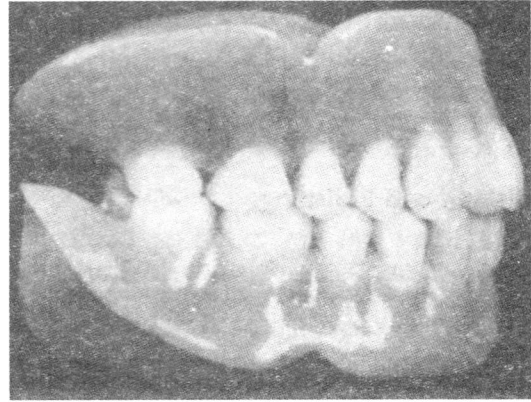

Fig. 2.15.76

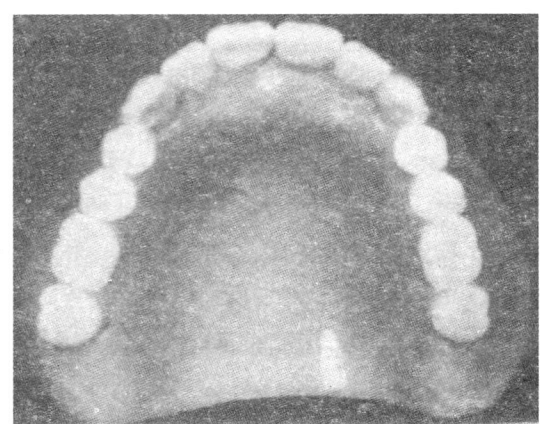

Fig. 2.15.77

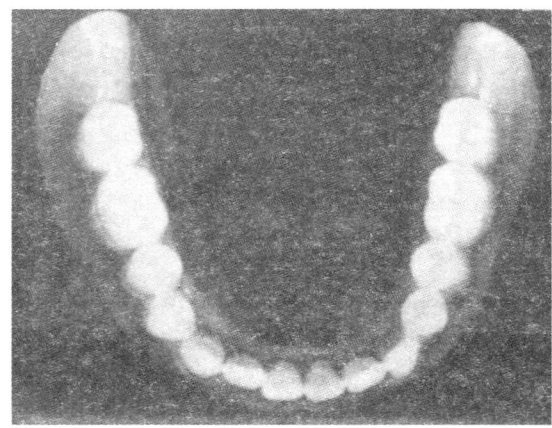

Fig. 2.15.78

# Insertion of Finished Denture and Patient Education

## CHAPTER 16

This is the last step in the CD fabrication. Here you will be demonstrating the patient about the denture insertion and removal along with its care.
This chapter also outlines the post insertional problems.

### INSERTION OF FINISHED DENTURE

Examine the inside of both dentures carefully, both visually and manually, and remove any small bubbles or sharp projections.

Insert the mandibular denture first. The soft tissues of the ridge will be deformed by the old dentures and the new dentures require at least 15 min. for tissue accommodation. If the maxillary denture is placed first, it may up lying on the patient's tongue -not a very good beginning for this visit! This occurs as the soft ridge tissues are often distorted from the ill-fitting old dentures but will later adapt to the new dentures. Also, it is easier to insert the mandibular denture first as there will be more space without the opposing denture. Then insert the maxillary denture.

Ask the patient if there are any areas of discomfort. If reasonably satisfactory, place a cotton roll on each side at about the first molar area and instruct the patient to maintain a firm closure for 10 minutes. The patient should not be allowed to close with the new dentures as the occlusion has not yet been corrected. A malocclusion would result in uneven pressure and unwanted tissue displacement.

### INSTRUCTIONS TO THE PATIENT

1. Always insert the mandibular denture first and then the maxillary. This is especially necessary for well extended mandibular dentures.
2. Always comment on how well the dentures look and restate that the dentures will feel and function better in time. It is also necessary to make the patient aware that some future discomfort is to be expected and follow-up adjustments and maintenance are always required.
3. Discuss the fact that mastication is always a problem for new denture wearers and often for experienced ones. Recommend that chewing food simultaneously on both sides will greatly reduce tipping, and greater chewing forces are possible. Demonstrate this using cotton rolls.

4. Give the patient the handout, "How to keep Your Dentures Clean".
5. Appoint the patient in 24 hours for an examination and adjustment.

## ADJUSTMENT APPOINTMENT

1. Check for peripheral overextensions which will have a red line or even an ulcerated area if severe.
2. Check for pressure areas on the ridge.
3. Check the centric occlusion with the carbon paper.
4. Evaluate the thickness of the flanges and make corrections if indicated.
5. Polish the denture base and teeth well after any correction.
6. Make the second adjustment 48 hours later and repeat the above.
7. The next appointment (the third adjustment) should be about 1 week after the initial insertion but see the patient sooner if problems are anticipated or by patient request.

## POST INSERTION PROBLEMS

1. Looseness or instability—a very common complaint.
2. Lower rises when mouth is opened—very common complaint
3. Sore spots—a common complaint and are usually related to poor occlusion and inadequate fit
4. Gagging
5. Feeling of space in upper denture; due to a previous history of anterior traumatic occlusion with subsequent paresthesia of the nasopalatine nerves.
6. Phonetic problems: Some patients cannot speak clearly and probably never will, but dentures can interfere with speech, especially the "S" sound.
7. Cannot eat most foods
8. Loss of taste
9. Clicking while eating or talking
10. Tenderness when swallowing, over-extension of the distolingual flange
11. Food under dentures
12. Saliva under dentures, usually seen in new denture wearers
13. Dislodgement when drinking
14. Drooling at corners of mouth
15. Excessive bulk
16. Dull teeth
17. Cheek, lip, or tongue biting
18. Halitosis—usually poor hygiene or can be a medical problem
19. Dry mouth (xerostomia)
20. Excessive salivation: New dentures, possibly psychic tensions.
21. Peculiar tastes—bitter metallic taste sometimes seen in menopause, worry, etc.
22. TMJ problems
23. Burning sensation

# Miscellaneous

**CHAPTER 17**

This chapter briefly discusses the reshaping and repair of a fractured denture along with the other aspects of prosthodontics like immediate dentures, over dentures, etc.

## RELINING AND REBASING

### RELINING

Relining is adding new denture base material to the existing denture base, thereby refitting the denture. It reestablishes denture tissue relation, more particularly when other relations are not disturbed by changes in the basal seats for dentures.

### REBASING

Resurfacing of the filling surface of the denture, undertaken when the dentures need to be refitted and re-oriented as well.

#### Observed Clinical Changes Include

- Loss of retention and stability
- Loss of dimension of occlusion
- Loss of support for facial tissues
- Horizontal shift of dentures incorrect occlusal relationship
- Reorientation of occlusal plane

### INDICATIONS

1. Immediate dentures at 3–6 months after their original construction
2. When residual alveolar ridge have resorbed and adaptation of the denture base to ridge is poor
3. When construction of new denture with the accompanying series of appointments can cause physical and (or) mental stress, such as for geriatric or chronically ill patients.

### GENERAL CONSIDERATIONS

1. The occlusal vertical dimensions should be satisfactory
2. The centric occlusion should coincide with centric relation

3. Patient's appearance should be acceptable to the patient and dental
4. Oral tissue should be in optimum health
5. The posterior limit of the maxillary denture is correct
6. The denture bases extensions are adequate
7. The denture base extensions ensure distribution of masticatory forces over as large an area possible.
8. The interocclusal distance is correct
9. Speech is satisfactory with the existing tooth arrangement.
10. There are no existing hard or soft tissue conditions, that would preclude the technique such as redundant tissue or severe osseous undercuts.

## CONTRAINDICATIONS

1. When an excessive amount of resorption has taken place.
2. When abused soft tissue are present. The refining is not indicated until the tissue recover and return as closely as possible to normal form
3. When patient complains of temporomandibular joint problems, until accurate diagnosis and treatment of the problem has been accomplished, relining or rebasing is contraindicated.
4. If the denture have poor aesthetics or unsatisfactory law relationships
5. If the denture creates a major speech problem.
6. When severe osseous undercuts exist, until surgical removal and healing takes place.

## METHODS OF RELINING TECHNIQUES

### Three Types

I. Static
   A. Open Mouth
   B. Closed Mouth
II. Functional
III. Chair side

### I. Static Technique

There are two major variations on the static impression techniques. In one variations, the dentures used are impression trays and either this existing centric occlusion, is used as means to seat the dentures with the lining impression material or the centric relation is recorded.

A. Open Mouth Reline Technique

The open mouth technique was described by Boucher (1973) and implies the following:

a. It is a method for relining both maxillary and mandibular dentures at the same appointment
b. The dentures are essentially being used as trays for making this new impression
c. The existing centric occlusion is not utilized and new centric relation record is accomplished after the impressions are made.

1. **Centric Relation:** Jaw relation recorded using both denture as recording bases, after making secondary maxillary and mandibular impression.
2. **Denture Preparation:** Posterior palatal seal formed on maxillary denture, 1mm space is provided inside denture for new impression material and borders shortened for the new impression material.
3. **Border Molding:** Using low fusing modeling compound
4. **Impression:** By zinc oxide eugenol for secondary impression.
5. **Occlusal Refinement**
6. **Follow Up Advantages**
   i. Loss of vertical dimension compensated during relining procedures.
   ii. Error in centric occlusion reduced during lab stages.
7. **Disadvantages**
   i. Time consuming
   ii. Procedure for establishment of occlusal vertical dimension highly questionable.

B. Closed Mouth Reline Technique

Each denture is used as an impression tray and the dentures occlusion is used to stabilize the tray when the impression material sets.

1. **Centric Relation**
   i. Existing intercuspation used to stabilize dentures
   ii. Interocclusal record made by use of wax of compound
2. **Denture Preparation**
   i. Large undercuts relieved
   ii. Hard resin surfaces relieved 1.5 to 2 mm
   iii. Tissue conditioner removed or relieved.
   iv. Escape holes drilled, particularly in maxillary bases. This will also assist during packing and processing.
   v. Dentures periphery shortened to create flat border.
3. **Impression Procedure**
   i. Border moulding achieved with low fusing compound material
   ii. Posterior palatal seal achieved with low fusing compound
   iii. Final impression achieved by choosing impression material that is soft and yet viscous

enough to support and register peripheral detail (polyether impression materials)

**4. Occlusal Refinement**

Permanent interocclusal record helps to position the dentures during the impression making and to orient the denture on articulator.

**5. Follow Up**

**6. Disadvantages**
   i. Possibility of moving maxillary denture forward is a problem
   ii. Wax interocclusal record is not accurate and safe record, that patient can close on several times without possibility of damaging the record.
   iii. This technique does not suggest any solution for difficulties of refining both dentures at the same time.

## II. Functional Impression Technique

It is a simple and practical tissue conditioner used as functional impression material.

### Procedure

The denture is checked intraorally and the posterior palatal seal is developed with compound (modeling) on the maxillary dentures.

Tissue conditioner is placed inside the denture and should flow evenly to cover the whole impression surface and the borders of the dentures with a thin layer. It voids evident should be filled with a fresh mix of liner material. Unsupported parts of liner indicate that localized border molding with stick modeling compound is needed before the placement of fresh mix of liner. Too low or narrow border indicates inadequate peripheral extension of the denture.

The patients mandible is guided in its most retruded position in maximum intercuspation to help stabilize the denture while the lining material is setting.

The excess material is trimmed away with a hot scalpel. Most of the material used for this purpose progress through plastic and then elastic stages before hardening which can take several days.

| | |
|---|---|
| PLASTIC STAGE (Tissue Conditioner) | Tissue conditioner in denture(s) denture base respond to functional/para functional stresses fit is improved few hours to few days. |
| ELASTIC STAGE (Tissue Conditioner) | Stress is cushioned; tissue recovery takes place (1 to 2 weeks) |
| FIRM STAGE (Reline Impression) | Surface is similar to polymerized resin surface except it is vulnerable to deterioration |

### The physical changes of tissue conditioners treatment liners

Simple rinsing of temporarily lined dentures and gentle brushing with a soft tooth brush are good measures to minimize the damage to the lining. 10–14 days should elapse before the material is firm enough to proceed with the clinical reline sequences.

At the next appointment the temporarily relined denture will be well retained, with well rounded peripheral borders and healthy appearing mucosa.

The cast should be poured when the material has reached the firm stages, otherwise, leads to recovery of compressed material when load is removed.

If the surfaces or peripheral deterioration is slight these areas can be trimmed with carbide but and denture prepared for wash/secondary impression with light bodied material.

The stone cast must be poured immediately after removal of the refined denture base from the mouth. The material should not be plastic or "self flow" because material's own weight may deform the impression. Also weight of the stone poured into the impression surfaces will cause distortion of the impression.

Maxillary casts may have to be scored in the selected posterior palatal seal area. Since the long period of plasticity of the material may not create sufficient displacement action in this area, a thin bead of compound material is used to augment posterior palatal seat. Making of a new centric relations record and remount procedure are, always necessary to ensure an optimal prosthodontics occlusion.

The recently introduced visible light cured (VLC) resin systems are non toxic and biocompatible, have imposed strength, ability to polymerise without residual components, ease of fabrication and manipulation, patient acceptance, ability to bond with other denture base resins and low bacterial adherence. VLC resin is used in chair side technique.

## III. Chairside Reline Technique

Several attempts have been made to produce an acrylic or other plastic material that could be added to the denture and allowed to set in the mouth to produce an instant chair side reliner/rebase. These have met with failure for several reasons;

A. The material have often produced a chemical burn on the mucosa

B. The result was often porous and subsequently developed a bad odor

C. The colour stability was poor

D. If the denture was not positioned correctly, the material could not be removed easily to start again.

# REPAIR OF DENTURE BASES

## FRACTURE OF DENTURE BASE

- A number of dentures which are brought by patients having cracked in the mouth have in fact been dropped. The crack passes unobserved and the stresses of mastication complete the fractures.
- Often the first thing to be noted by the patient is the sensation of a hair in the dentures and a very close inspection is often required to see the small crack at this stage.

### Factors

1. **Poor fit:** This is more readily described under separate headings
   
   i. *Alveolar resorption:* This causes the denture to be unevenly supported and is a common cause of fracture
   
   This will cause breakage in denture which have been worn for some consideration time or were made shortly after extraction of teeth.
   
   ii. *Warpage:* Dimensional change of acrylic is a cause of further fractures of denture which has already been replaced.
   
   iii. *Relief areas:*
   
   a. Failure to relieve the cast in prominent bony areas (torus palate) lead to excess flexure of denture.
   
   b. Excessive relief may make the denture plate so thin that its weakness causes fracture.

2. **Position of teeth:** If the upper teeth are set outside the ridges the force of mastication is also applied outside the ridge, the ridge itself becoming a fulcrum point, thus causing a large component force to be transmitted to the midline of the denture—the result is midline fractures.
   - However, if periphery is sufficiently wide to ensure a retentive force on the contralateral side as these shifts the fulcrum around which denture tilts and the load is more evenly distributed.
   - A balanced occlusion is also very important as a factor resisting midline fracture.

3. **Occasionally during deflasking procedures,** a maxillary denture will fracture at the labial frenum area. In the crack procedure a maxillary denture will fracture at the labial frenum area. The crack may continue through the palate, separating the denture in to two parts, or it may involve the labial flange and part of anterior ridge area.

Various denture base materials with greater impact and fatigue strength

1. Vinyl co-polymer and rubber acrylic graft copolymer
2. Incorporation of carbon fibers into the acrylics. This enhances mechanical properties but spoils aesthetics.
3. Incorporation of strengtheners like wire or mesh in to acrylic has the opposite effect and leads to areas of weakness.
4. In case of repeated fractures cobalt-chromium palate is carried up the lingual surfaces of the anterior teeth. This prevents initial fracture which invariably occurs between the upper incisor teeth.

## FRACTURE REPAIR

### Maxillary and Mandibular Fracture Repair

1. The broken edges of the dentures are cleaned of food and material debris and other interferences, so the two parts will fit together well.
2. The two halves are held together by means of an old bur or matchstick, which is luted to the denture teeth and the adjacent resin surface with sticky wax.
3. No wax is placed over the fracture. It prevents the halves from being examined for correct opposition.
4. Plaster is then gently vibrated onto the palatal surface of the denture, avoiding air bubble formation, and the remainder of the plaster is set on this to form the cast.

### Repair using Cold Curing Resin

After following the above 4 steps,

1. The cast is removed from the denture and the resin on the both sides of the break is cut away and beveled. A gap of minimum 1mm is created between the parts
2. Grooves are made along the break transversely (up to 2-3 mm) on both sides alternatively with the help of straight fissure bur No.585-560.
   
   The number of grooves made depend on the length of the fracture.
3. Then the cast is replaced, acrylic resin monomer is painted on the cut surfaces, and cold curing repair resin is placed in the break, by two methods
   
   i. Salt and pepper method (in this method monomer and polymer is added alternatively into the space)
   
   ii. Premixed monomer and polymer method.
   
   The premixed monomer and polymer are carefully flowed into the space until the area to be repaired is filled. The area should be slightly overfilled to allow for finishing.

### Curing under Air Pressure

1. Pressure can be maintained on the cold curing resin while it cures by immersing the denture in water in

a pressure cooker after the resin has been forced into place.
2. The water is preferably at 104°F and the pressure cooker is used according to manufacturer instruction (usually 20 to 25 Psi or 1.5 Kg/cm$^2$ is employed). This condenses the repair resin
3. Curing can be done when the repair resin is added in small increments of powder and liquid.
4. Without pressure, resin added in this manner will be less dense than that cured under pressure.

## IMMEDIATE DENTURE

### DEFINITION

Immediate denture is one that is fabricated before all the remaining teeth have been removed and inserted immediately after the removal of the teeth.

It can be complete denture or an over denture.

Immediate dentures may either be single or upper or lower immediate dentures.

An immediate denture is of 2 types:
1. **Conventional Immediate Denture (CID):** After heating is the immediate denture is either refitted or relined to serve as long term prosthesis
2. **Interim Immediate Denture (IID):** Worn by the patient only during the healing period. It is then replaced by a new prosthesis.

### CONTRAINDICATIONS

1. Patient's in poor general health and/or poor surgical risks
2. Patients who are uncooperative and do not understand limitations to the treatment
3. Patients with extensive bone loss adjacent to remaining teeth

### REQUIREMENTS

1. It should be compatible with the oral environment
2. Masticatory efficiency should be restored
3. It should be in harmony with functions like speech, mastication and deglutition
4. There should be good esthetics
5. Preservation of remaining tissues should take place

### ADVANTAGES

1. The patient does not have to suffer the embarrassment of being edentulous and can quickly resume most duties and social contacts.
2. The patient adapts to the denture more rapidly. Good speech and mastication are regained earlier.
3. The denture acts as a splint, controls bleeding and aids healing. There is usually less pain.
4. There is usually better ridge formation.
5. It is easier to obtain a more cosmetic denture.
6. Tooth position can be duplicated or modified.
7. Vertical dimension is usually duplicated or can be changed if indicated.

### DISADVANTAGES

1. Correction of the fit and occlusion is needed at frequent intervals, necessitating more visits and a higher fee.
2. The arrangement of the anterior teeth cannot be evaluated until the dentures are inserted, i.e., no trial denture visit.
3. More difficult to make impressions with correct extensions.
4. Existing teeth may not be in correct centric relation and/or vertical dimension
5. Recall, maintenance, and relines are mandatory so costs are higher.

## OVERDENTURE

### DEFINITION

It is a prosthesis that covers and is partially supported by natural tooth roots or dental implants.

### SYNONYMS

1. Biologic dentures
2. Hybrid dentures
3. Telescopic dentures
4. Onlay denture
5. Overlay denture
6. Root supported denture
7. Super imposed denture

### ADVANTAGES

1. The forces transmitted to the soft tissue are reduced.
2. Retained teeth provide physiologic stimulation to maintain the alveolar bone around the roots. This is probably the most important advantage.
3. When the teeth are drastically reduced and rounded, the potential for damaging horizontal forces is lessened considerably.
4. The cost is nominal, especially when compared to implants.

5. The vertical dimension is maintained by the retained supporting roots.
6. The patient is not rendered totally edentulous, an important psychological consideration for some patients.
7. Denture stability and retention as well as support are increased.
8. Proprioceptors in the periodontal ligaments are an aid for all functional jaw movements.
9. In the event of loss of supporting teeth, the denture alteration is simple and not expensive.
10. It is possible to obtain greatly improved retention with the use of an attachment.

## DISADVANTAGES

1. Quite expensive than conventional complete dentures
2. More bulkier
3. More patient acceptance of fixed denture. Hence they do not like overdenture as it is removable
4. If not kept clean, caries and periodontal diseases may occur
5. Greater effort for both patients and dentist.
6. Cannot be used in severe undercuts and reduction in interarch space.
7. Chances of failure due to acrylic are more
8. Cannot be used where teeth cannot be treated endodontically

## INDICATIONS

1. Patients with poor prognosis for complete denture
2. Patients having high palatal vault and sloping ridges
3. In patients, when the mandible has a poorly defined sublingual fold space, floor of mouth drapes, tongue falls back then positive retention and stability is hard to attain.
4. If pronounced vertical overlap of anterior teeth is required to produce a good aesthetic result.
5. When there is unfavorable crown foot ratio.
6. Extensive bone loss around the teeth to be retained
7. It increases stability and decreases residual ridge resorption when teeth with little bony support are taken for fabrication
8. Unilateral overdentures can be used if large amount of bone and soft tissues have been lost on one side of the arch.

## CONTRAINDICATIONS

1. Psychologically some patients cannot accept any type of removable denture
2. Uncooperative and under motivated patients
3. Patients with less interarch space and severe undercuts
4. In mentally and physically handicapped patients.

# SINGLE COMPLETE DENTURE OPPOSING NATURAL TEETH

A single complete denture opposed by a residual natural dentition, such as a maxillary complete denture opposing all or some of the mandibular natural dentition, or vice versa.

## OBJECTIVES

1. An acceptable interocclusal distance
2. A stable jaw relationship with bilateral tooth contacts in retruded closure
3. Stable tooth quadrant relationship, providing axially directed forces
4. Multidimensional freedom of tooth contacts throughout a small range of mandibular movement.

## INDICATIONS

A single complete denture may be desirable when it is to oppose any one of the following:
1. Natural teeth that are sufficient in number not to necessities a fixed or removable partial denture
2. A partially edentulous arch in which the missing teeth have been or will be replaced by a fixed partial denture
3. A partially edentulous arch in which the missing teeth have been or will be replaced by a removable partial denture
4. An existing complete denture.

# Section 3
# Removable Partial Denture

# Removable Partial Denture

**CHAPTER 1**

The removable partial denture is a prosthesis that is designed and fabricated to be removed by the patient. A removable partial denture is the treatment option for a partially edentulous dental patient who desires to have replacement teeth for functional or esthetic reasons and who cannot have a fixed partial denture (bridge) for any number of reasons, such as lack of required teeth to serve as support for a bridge (e.g. distal abutments) or due to finanical limitations. There are several types of removable partial dentures. All of them use standard denture teeth as replacement for the missing natural teeth. The differences between them are the materials that are used to support the denture teeth and retain the removable partial denture in the mouth.

### DEFINITION

- Any prosthesis that replaces some teeth in a partially dentate arch. It can be removed from the mouth and replaced at will.

### OBJECTIVES

1. To maintain or improve phonetics.
2. To establish or increase masticatory efficiency.
3. To stabilize the individual arch and prevent migration or drifting of remaining natural teeth.
4. To organize interarch function by control of interarch contacts and to prevent supraeruption of opposing teeth into edentulous spaces.
5. To develop required esthetics.

### INDICATION

1. In cases of long span edentulous areas.
2. When there is no tooth posterior to the edentulous space to act as an abutment and when placement of implant is not possible.
3. In cases where there is reduced periodontal and bony support for remaining teeth.
4. In cases of periodontally weakened teeth, where there is necessity for cross arch stabilization.
5. In cases where there is excessive bone loss within the residual ridge and regenerative therapy is not possible.
6. To replace teeth immediately after recent extractions.
7. If prognosis of abutment tooth is questionable or unfavourable for FPD, then RPD is indicated.
8. The lengthy preparation and construction procedures for fixed partial dentures can be tyring, especially for patients with physical or emotional problems. In such cases RPD is indicated.
9. When patients primary concern is esthetics.

10. In cases of unfavourable maxillomandibular relationships which include disharmonics in arch size, shape and position.
11. When patient desires removable partial denture in place of fixed partial denture (a) to avoid operative procedures on sound, healthy teeth. (b) to avoid the placement of one or more implants; and (c) for economic reasons.

## REQUIREMENTS OF CLASSIFICATION

1. It should permit immediate visualization of the type of partially edentulous arch that is being considered.
2. It should permit immediate differentiation between the tooth—supported and the tooth and tissue-supported removable partial denture.
3. It should serve as a guide to the type of design to be used.
4. It should be universally acceptable.

## CLASSIFICATION

Many classifications of partial dentures and their designs have been proposed by different clinicians. The confusion is not yet resolved and there is no universally accepted classification. But, the Kennedy's classification is widely followed.

### Kennedy Classification

- The Kennedy method of classification was originally proposed by Dr. Edward Kennedy in 1925. Kennedy divided all partially edentulous arches into four basic classes. Edentulous areas other than those determining the basic classes were designated as modification spaces (Figs 3.1.1 to 3.1.13).
  **Class I:** Bilateral edentulous areas located posterior to the natural teeth.

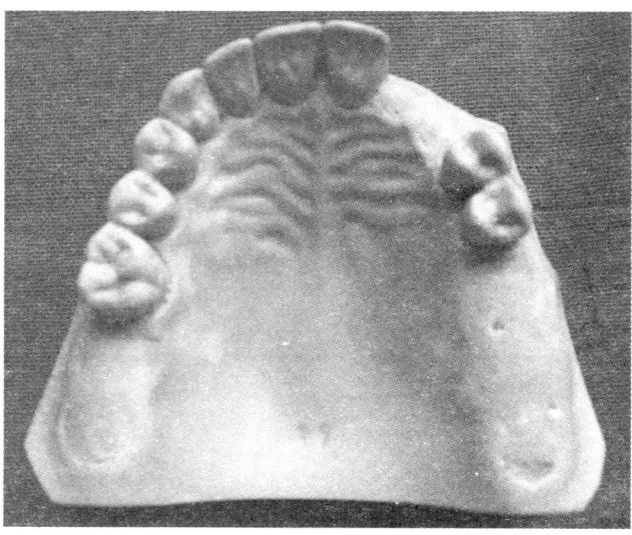

**Fig. 3.1.2:** Class I, Mod-1

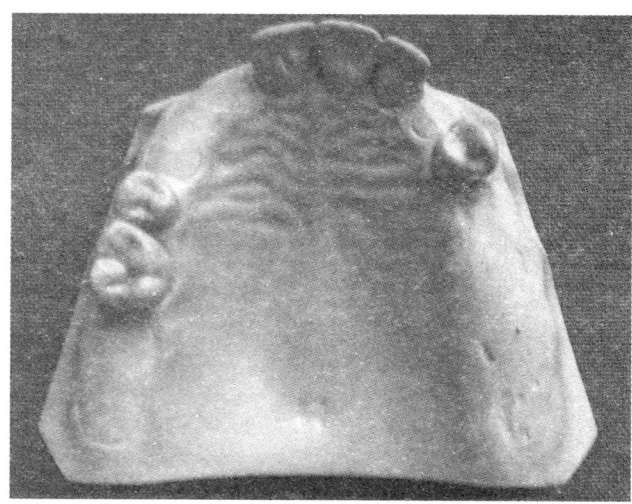

**Fig. 3.1.3:** Class I, Mod-2

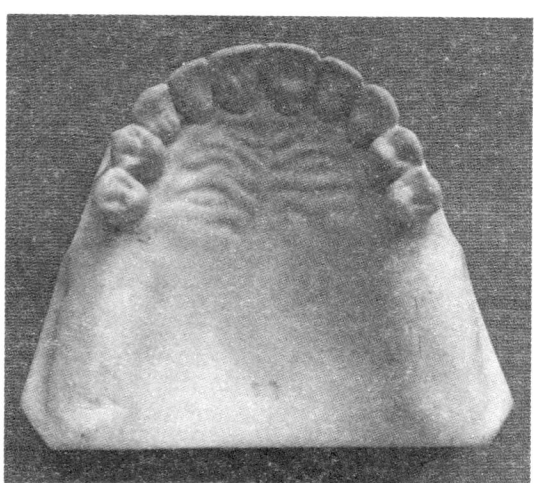

**Fig. 3.1.1:** Class I

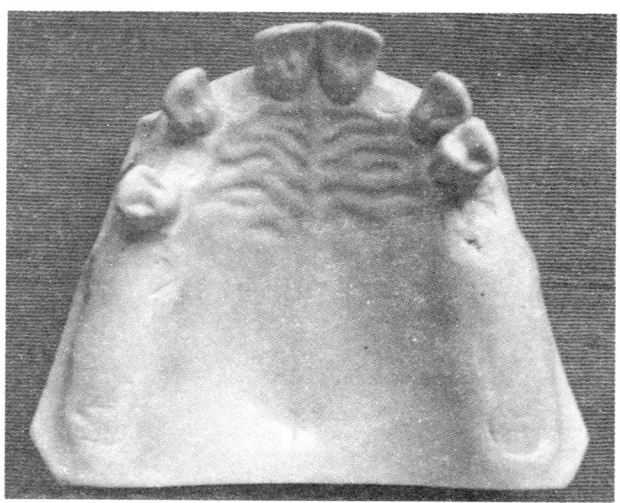

**Fig. 3.1.4:** Class I, Mod-3

**Class II:** A unilateral edentulous area located posterior to the remaining natural teeth.

**Class III:** A unilateral edentulous area with natural teeth remaining both anterior and posterior to it.

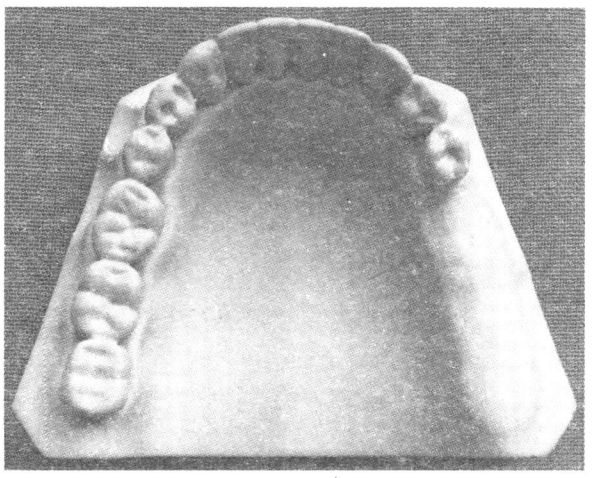
**Fig. 3.1.5:** Class II

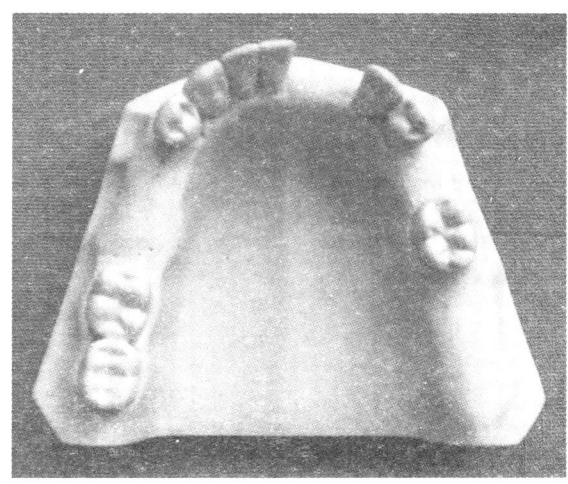
**Fig. 3.1.8:** Class II, Mod-3

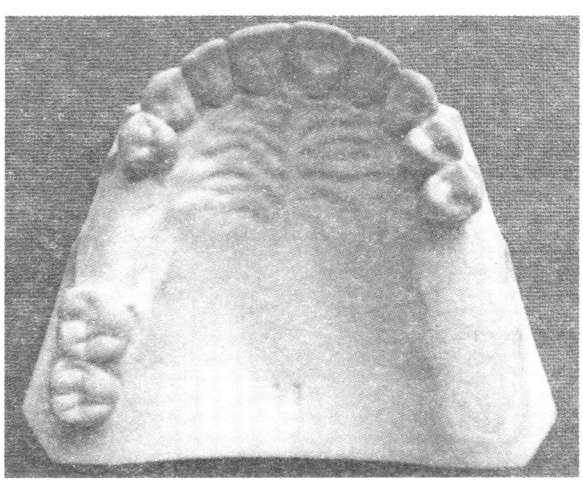
**Fig. 3.1.6:** Class-II Mod-1

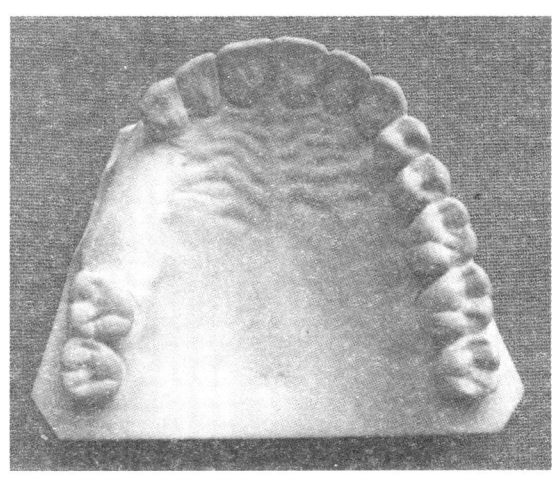
**Fig. 3.1.9:** Class III

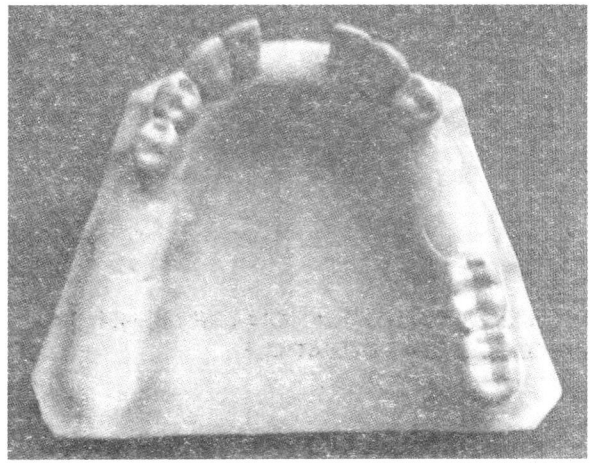
**Fig. 3.1.7:** Class II, Mod-2

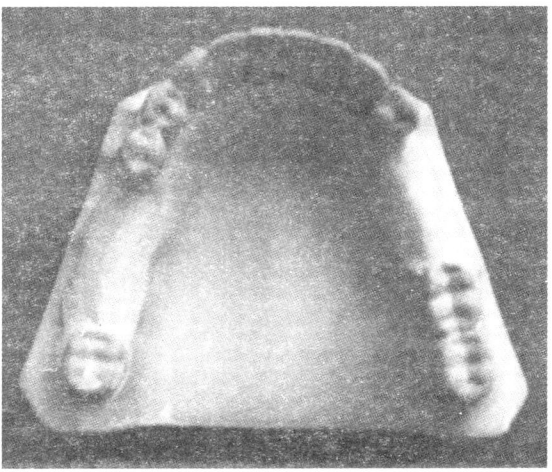
**Fig. 3.1.10:** Class III, Mod-1

**Class IV:** A single, but bilaterally crossing the midline, edentulous area located anterior to the remaining natural teeth.

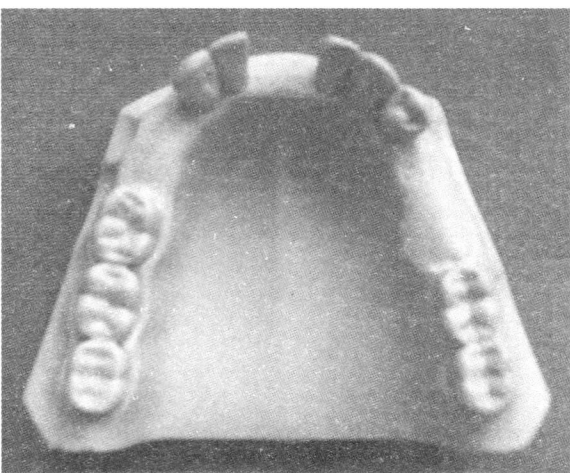

**Fig. 3.1.11:** Class II Mod-2

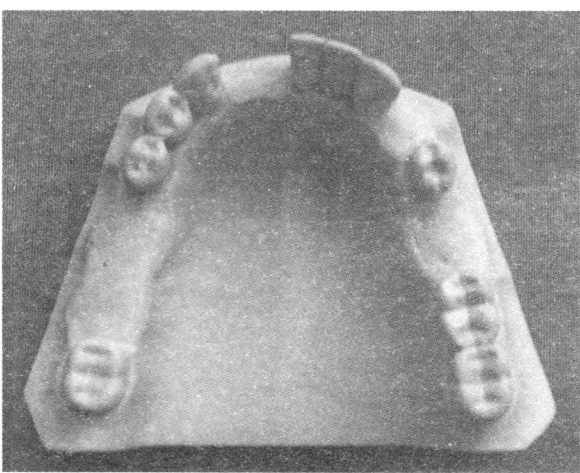

**Fig. 3.1.12:** Class III, Mod-3

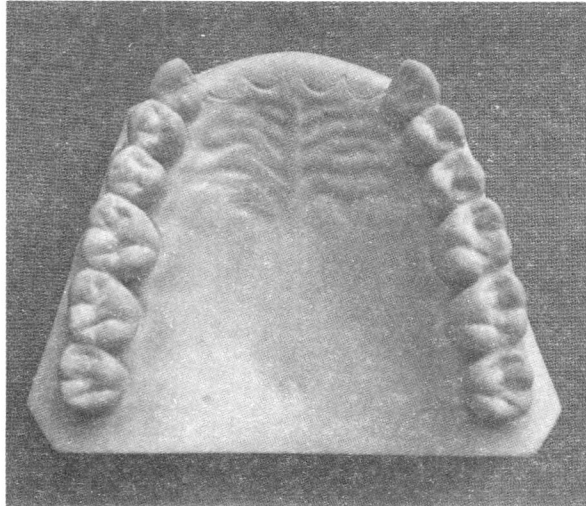

**Fig. 3.1.13:** Class IV

*Advantages of Kennedy Classification*

1. It permits immediate visualization of partially edentulous arch.
2. It allows easy distinction between tooth—supported versus tooth and tissue—supported prosthesis.
3. It can readily relate the arch configuration design to be used in the basic partial denture.
4. It permits a logical approach to problems of design.
5. It makes possible the application of sound principles of partial denture design and is therefore a logical method of classification.

*Drawbacks of Kennedy Classification*

1. It does not take into account the available support upon which the success or failure of any partial denture or bridge ultimately depends.

### APPLEGATE'S RULES FOR APPLYING THE KENNEDY CLASSIFICATION

The Kennedy classification would be difficult to apply to every situation without certain rules for application. Applegate provided eight rules governing the application of the Kennedy method of classification.

**Rule 1:** Classification should follow rather than precede any extractions of teeth that might alter the original classification.

**Rule 2:** If a third molar is missing and not to be replaced, it is not considered in the classification.

**Rule 3:** If a third molar is present and is to be used as an abutment, it is considered in the classification.

**Rule 4:** If a second molar is missing and is not to be replaced, it is not considered in the classification (e.g. if the opposing second molar is like wise missing and is not to be replaced).

**Rule 5:** The most posterior edentulous area (or areas) always determines the classification.

**Rule 6:** Edentulous areas other than those determining the classification area referred to as modifications and are designated by their number.

**Rule 7:** The extent of the modification is not considered, only the number of edentulous areas is considered.

**Rule 8:** There can be no modification areas in class IV arches. Other edentulous areas lying posterior to the single bilateral areas crossing the midline would instead determine the classification.

### APPLEGATE'S CLASSIFICATION (OR) KENNEDY-APPLEGATE'S CLASSIFICATION

Applegate modified Kennedy's classification in 1960 and enumerated the following six classes:

**Class I:** All remaining teeth anterior to the bilateral edentulous areas.

**Class II:** Remaining teeth of either right or left side anterior to the unilateral edentulous area (unilateral free end).

**Class III:** The edentulous space bounded by teeth both anteriorly and posteriorly.

**Class IV:** The edentulous space anterior to the remaining teeth, which bound it both to the right and left of the median line.

**Class V:** A space bounded by remaining teeth at its posterior and anterior terminals (there was an essential difference between class V and class III. In class V the space was long and the anterior tooth very weak).

**Class VI:** Same as class III and class V, but in class VI conditions were such that restoration could be made entirely tooth-borne.

## TYPES OF REMOVABLE PARTIAL DENTURES

### A. Based on Support

1. *Tooth supported removable partial denture*
   The tooth supported removable partial denture receives support from natural teeth at each end of the edentulous areas. In this type of partial denture the forces in function are borne primarily by the remaining natural teeth, which in turn transmit these forces to the periodontal ligament and to the bone structure for support.
   
   The Kennedy's class III and class IV partially edentulous arches fall into this category.

2. *Tooth and tissue—supported removable partial denture (or) distal extension removable partial denture*
   The distal extension removable partial denture are supported by the distal abutment teeth which are teeth at the anterior aspect of distal extension and by tissues of the distal extension areas.
   
   According to Glossary of prosthodontic terms, distal extension removable partial denture is defined as the removable partial denture that is supported and retained by natural teeth only at one end of the denture base segment and in which a portion of the functional load is carried by the residual ridge.
   
   The Kennedy's class I and class II partially edentulous arches fall into this category.

### B. Based on Term of Usage

1. *Short term removable partial dentures/temporary partial denture/treatment removable partial denture/ immediate removable partial dentures/ flippers:*
   They are made of acrylic denture bases and acrylic teeth which are generally used to make standard complete dentures. The advantage of this type of RPD is that new teeth and new denture base can easily be added to an existing treatment RPD. These are frequently fabricated even if the remaining teeth have existing decay or periodontal disease and their prognosis is doubtful. If later in the course of treatment some of the existing natural teeth are extracted for any reason, new artificial teeth can be added quickly to the partial denture, maintaining the patients appearance. In spite of the fact that they are considered a temporary solution, many people keep this type of appliance for many, many years, because as long as they are properly maintained, they look outwardly as good as the more expensive permanent removable partial dentures (Figs 3.1.14A and B).

2. *Long term removable partial dentures/permanent removable partial dentures/definitive removable partial denture:*
   a. *Cast metal removable partial dentures*
      Removable partial dentures with metal frame works are probably one of the oldest forms of

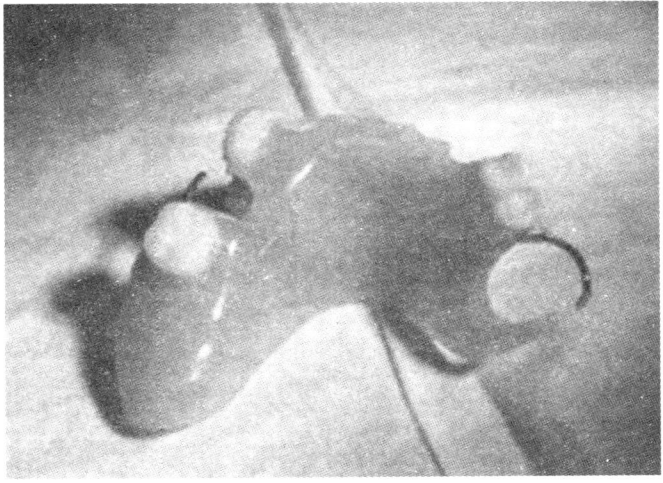

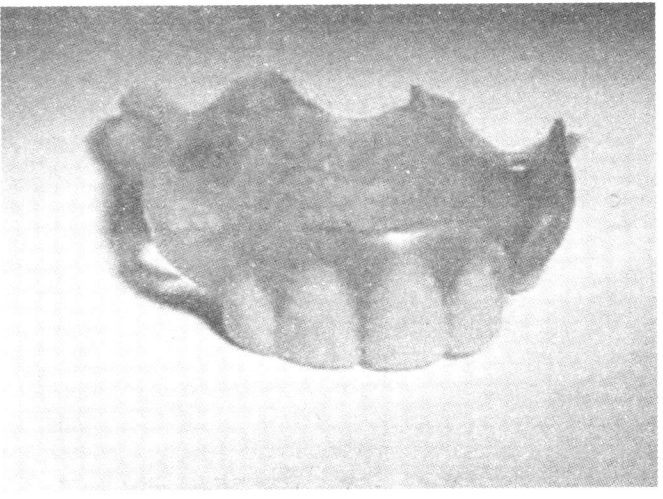

**Figs 3.1.14A and B**

dentistry. The materials used for fabrication of metal framework are type IV yellow gold alloy, silver-palladium alloys (white gold) or cobalt—chromium alloys. This type of partial denture offers numerous advantages over the treatment removable partial dentures. Since they sit on the teeth, as well as being attached to them, they are extremely stable and retentive. The metal framework does not contact the gums. Thus, as the gums resorb, this type of partial denture does not sink with them and rarely requires relining. They are extremely strong and thin when compared to temporary removable partial dentures made with acrylic. They do not impinge on surrounding tissues hence does not irritate or injure the tissues. They are also much less noticeable to the tongue (Figs 3.1.15A and B).

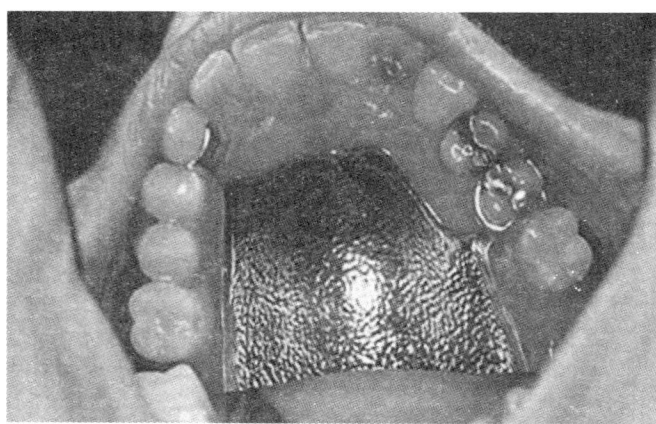

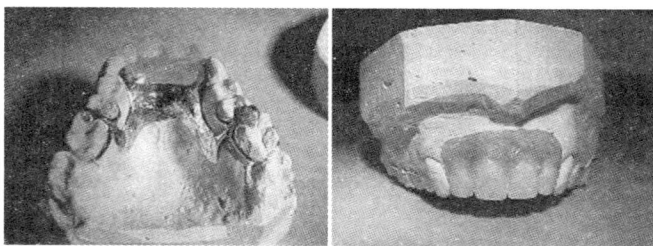

**Figs 3.1.15A and B**

b. *The flexible framework RPD's*
The most recent advance in dental materials has been the application of nylon-like materials to the fabrication of dental appliances. This material (the most common brand is valplast) generally replaces the metal and the pink acrylic denture material used to build the framework for standard removable partial dentures. Valplast is similar to the material used to build those flourescent orange traffic cones you see sometimes on highways. It is nearly unbreakable, is coloured pink like the gums, can be built quite thin and can form not only the denture base, but the clasps as well (Fig. 3.1.16).

c. *The cusil denture*
This type of denture is constructed when one or two teeth are remaining the arch. Even the presence of single remaining in tooth in an arch can make the denture much more stable and retentive. A cusil denture is essentially a full denture with holes allowing the remaining teeth to protrude through. The cusil denture is unique because the holes that surround the natural teeth are lined with a rubber gasket which snugly holds the teeth while allowing a natural suction to form under the denture (Figs 3.1.17A and B).

## Components of RPD

- To provide a systematic approach to partial denture treatment, it is important to identify the parts of a partial denture and their functions. Each part is

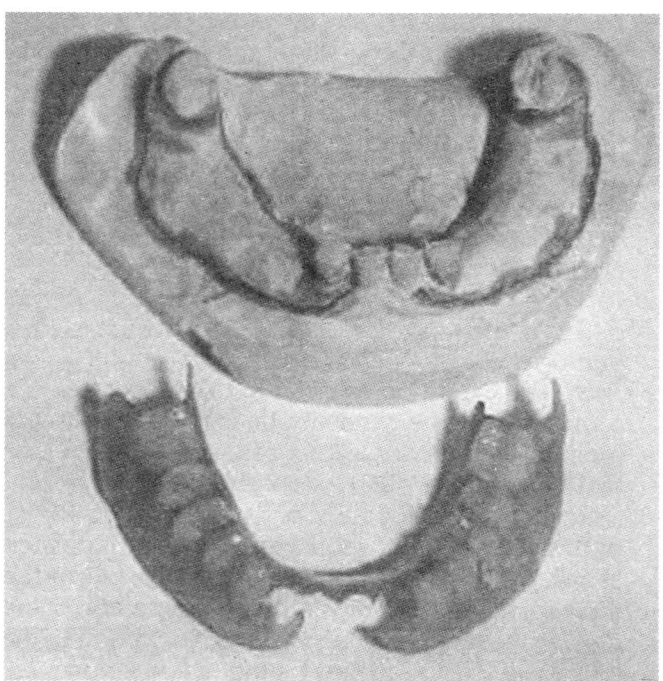

**Fig. 3.1.16**

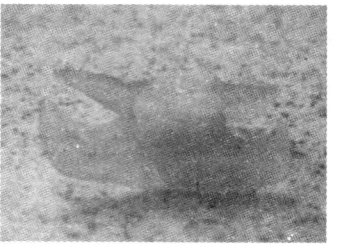 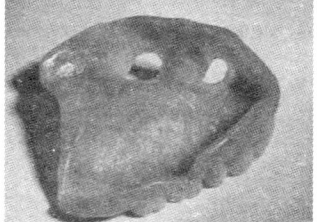

**Figs 3.1.17A and B**

presented individually in the sequence in which it is designed. The parts that receive major forces are considered first (Fig. 3.1.18).

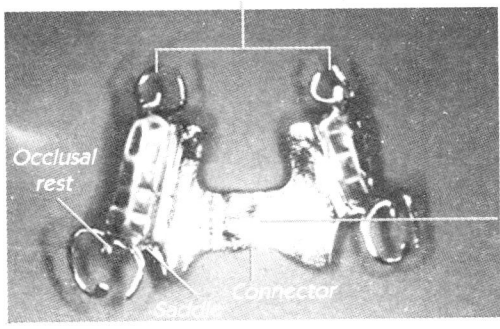

Fig. 3.1.18

### 1. Rests

A rest is the part of a removable partial denture that contacts a tooth and provides vertical support to the removable partial denture.

*Functions*
- They direct functional forces along the long axis of the tooth.
- They preserve the supporting oral structures by controlling the position of prosthesis in relation to teeth and the position of prosthesis in relation to periodontium and other supporting tissues.
- The types of rests are: - Occlusal rests
  - Cingulum rests
  - Incisal rests

### 2. Major Connectors

- It is defined as "a part of a removable partial denture which connects the components on one side of the arch to the components on the opposite side of the arch"—GPT.
- Major connectors can be classified as:
  1. Palatal plates and palatal bars.
  2. Lingual plates and lingual bars
  3. Labial plates and labial bars.

*Functions*
- It provides cross arch stabilization.
- It unites all remaining teeth and distribute occlusal forces to all the teeth equally.

### 3. Minor Connectors

- It is defined as the connecting link between the major connector or base of a removable partial denture and the other units of the prosthesis, such as the clasp assembly, indirect retainers, occlusal rests or cingulum rests—GPT.

- *Types of minor connectors*
  1. Minor connectors that connect the direct retainer to the major connector.
  2. Minor connectors that connect auxillary rests to major connectors.
  3. Minor connectors that connect denture base to the major connectors.
  4. Minor connectors that extend as the approach arm of a bar clasp.

  *Functions*
  1. Minor connectors transfer functional stress to the abutment teeth. This is a prosthesis-to-abutment function of the minor connector.
  2. Minor connectors transfer the effect of the retainers, rests and stabilizing components throughout the prosthesis. This is an abutment-to-prosthesis function of the minor connector.

### 4. Direct Retainers (clasps) (Fig. 3.1.19)

- It is defined as, "a clasp or attachment placed on an abutment tooth for the purpose of holding a removable denture in position"—GPT.

  *Classification*
  - Intracoronal direct retainer resides within the normal contours of an abutment and functions to retain and stabilize a removable partial denture. The first intracoronal direct retainder was introduced by Herman E.S. Chayes in 1906. The first component or matrix, is a metal receptacle contained within the normal contours of abutment teeth and the second component or patrix, is attached to the associated removable partial denture.
  - If components of intracoronal retainers are fabricated using high. precision manufacturing techniques, they are called as precision attachments. These attachments usually exhibit long, parallel walls and exceptional surface adaptation.
  - If components of intracoronal retainers originate as wax or plastic patterns, which are subsequently cast in metal, they are called as semi precision attachments. These attachments have less surface adaptation and often display gently tapering walls.
  - Extracoronal direct retainers consist of components that reside entirely outside the normal clinical contours of abutment teeth. They are of two types—extracoronal attachments and retentive clasp assemblies.
  - Extracoronal attachments derive their retention from closely fitting components termed matrices and patrices. Many of these attachments permit vertical movement of prosthesis during occlusal loading and act as stress breakers.

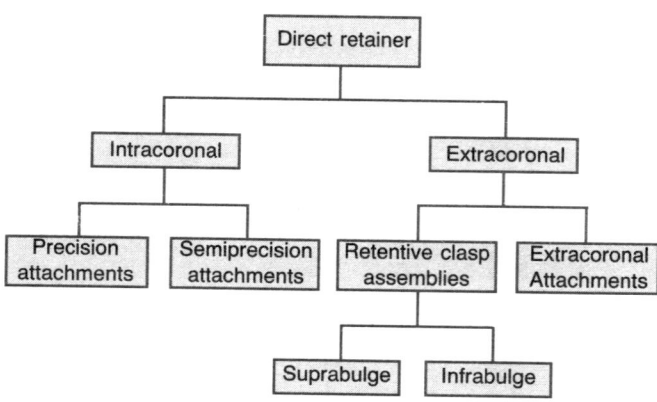

Fig. 3.1.19: Classification of direct retainers

- Retentive clasp assemblies represent the most common method for extracoronal direct retention. The retentive element of an individual clasp arm that displays a limited amount of flexibility. This flexibility allows the tip of the retentive clasp to pass over the greatest diameter of an abutment and contact the surface of the tooth as it converges apically.

*Functions*

1. Direct retainers ensure effective prosthesis retention.
2. Direct retainers minimize the transmission of detrimental forces to the associated abutments and supporting tissues.

### 5. Indirect Retainers

- It is defined as, "a part of a removable partial denture which assists the direct retainers in preventing displacement of distal extension denture bases by functioning through lever action on the opposite side of the fulcrum line"—GPT.
- Types of indirect retainers—Auxillary occlusal rests

*Functions*

- An indirect retainer is so called because it retains in position some part of a denture remote from itself. It works on the principle of counter balance.
- It tends to reduce anteroposterior—tilting leverages on the principal abutments.
- Anterior teeth supporting indirect retainers are stabilized against lingual movement.
- It may act as a auxillary rest to support a portion of the major connector facilitating stress distribution.
- It may provide the first visual indication for the need to reline an extension base partial denture.

### 6. Denture Bases

- Denture base is defined as the part of a denture that rests on the foundation tissues and to which teeth are attached—GPT.
- Materials used to fabricate denture bases
  1. Acrylic resins   - Heat activated
                      - Chemically activated
  2. Cast metal alloys - Cobalt-chromium alloys
                       - Nickel-chromium alloys
                       - Type IV gold alloys
                       - Titanium-aluminium-vanadium alloys
                       - Commercially pure titanium

*Advantages of Acrylic Resins*

1. Simulates the appearance of natural mucosa and gingiva.
2. Technique is reasonably simple and requires little special apparatus.
3. Can be used for whole denture including the teeth.
4. Forms a chemical union with acrylic teeth thus giving a very strong attachment.
5. Repairs and additions can easily be made.
6. Light in weight.
7. Easy to keep clean.
8. Insoluble and inert in oral fluids.

*Disadvantages of Acrylic Resin*

1. It has less strength.
2. Its resistance to fatigue is low, it frequently fractures after a few months in the mouth.
3. Has a tendency to warp during deflasking.
4. Its abrasion resistance is low and leads to rapid wear when used for posterior teeth; it is also easily abraded by cleaning with a stiff brush.
5. Residual monomer present in processed denture, weakens acrylic and also irritates oral mucosa.
6. Subject to porosity which affects strength, surface polish and water absorption and lead to dimensional changes.
7. Radiolucent, a problem if part of an acrylic denture is inhaled or swallowed detection by radiograph is impossible.
8. Subject to crazing which weakens the material.

*Advantages of Metals*

1. Increased strength.
2. Improved adaptation to underlying tissues.
3. Improved hygiene.
4. Enhanced thermal conductivity.

*Disadvantages of Metals*

1. Inability to reline or rebase poorly fitting areas.
2. The techniques of their fabrication are time consuming, require a high degree of skill and need special apparatus.

3. Their appearance does not simulate the natural mucosa.
4. They may cause electrolytic action if the denture is in contact with a dissimilar metal fitting.

*Ideal Requirements of Denture Base Material*

1. Accuracy of adaptation to the tissue, with minimal volume change.
2. Dense, non irritating surface capable of receiving and maintaining a good finish.
3. Thermal conductivity.
4. Low specific gravity, light weight in the mouth.
5. Sufficient strength; resistance to fracture or distortion.
6. Easily kept clean.
7. Esthetic acceptability.
8. Potential for future relining.
9. Low initial cost.

## 7. Tooth Replacements

- The prosthetic teeth of choice for removable partial dentures are commercially available acrylic resin denture teeth on most instances. The restoration of edentulous areas is accomplished by attaching such teeth to an acrylic resin denture base.
- Alternative methods of replacement include tube teeth, braided posts, reinforced acrylic pontics and metal pontics.

## ADVANTAGES OF REMOVABLE PARTIAL DENTURES OVER FIXED PARTIAL DENTURES (BRIDGES)

1. They can be constructed for any case, while bridges are confined to relatively short span bounded by healthy teeth and with a fairly normal occlusion.
2. They can be constructed of polymeric materials and therefore are cheaper.
3. They are more easily cleaned as are the natural teeth in contact with them.
4. They are more easily repaired and in many cases can have additions made to them.
5. They do not normally involve much preparation of the natural teeth.

## DISADVANTAGES OF REMOVABLE PARTIAL DENTURES

1. By harbouring food debris in close contact with the natural teeth a partial denture may promote caries and gingivitis.
2. They can damage the supporting tissues of the teeth.
3. They may loosen the natural teeth by leverage, clasps wrongly designed or carelessly constructed or indirect retainers badly placed, may cause excessive stresses on the natural teeth.
4. They can cause traumatic damage to the mucosa. Various types of damage which can be inflicted by a partial denture are hyperemia, hyperplasia and ulceration.

# Section 4
# Fixed Partial Denture

# Fixed Partial Denture

**CHAPTER 1**

A fixed partial denture (FPD) is a restoration designed to replace more than one missing natural tooth. In contrast to a removable partial denture, the dentist attaches an FPD to natural teeth (abutments) or roots by cementation. An FPD consists of two types of units: retainers and pontics. The unit castings are joined together by connectors. The overall size of the FPD is measured in units. Each pontic or retainer counts as one unit. For example, an FPD with three retainers and two pontics has a total of five units. The units of an FPD may be made entirely from metal, combination of metal or resin, or from a combination of metal and porcelain. This chapter will discuss the retainers, pontics, connectors, and abutments that make up the FPD in brief.

## INTRODUCTION

- Fixed prosthodontics is the art and science of restoration of damaged teeth with cast metal, metal-ceramic or all-ceramic restorations and of replacing missing teeth with fixed prosthesis. Successfully treating a patient by means of fixed prosthodontics requires a thoughtful combination of many aspects of dental treatment: patient education and the prevention of further dental disease, sound diagnosis, periodontal therapy, operative skills, occlusal considerations and sometimes, placement of removable complete or partial prostheses and endodontic treatment.
- Restoration by fixed prostheses depends on one's knowledge of sound biological and mechanical principles, the growth of manipulative skills to implement the treatment plan and the development of a critical eye and judgement for assessing detail.

## DEFINITIONS

*Fixed Prosthodontics*

- The branch of prosthodontics concerned with the replacement and/or restoration of teeth by artificial substitutes that are not readily removed from the mouth.

*Fixed Bridge/Fixed Partial Denture*

- A partial denture that is luted or otherwise securely retained to natural teeth, tooth roots and / or dental implant abutments that furnish the primary support for the prosthesis.

*Crown*

- An artificial replacement that restores missing tooth structure by surrounding part or all of the remaining structure with a material such as cast metal, porcelain or a combination of materials such as metals and porcelain.

*Types*

1. Full veneer crown
2. Partial veneer crown

## FULL VENEER CROWN/COMPLETE CROWN

### Definition

- A restoration that covers all the coronal tooth surfaces (mesial, distal, facial, lingual and occlusal / incisal).

### Types

*Complete Cast Crown Preparation*

– All-metal restoration often used on single posterior teeth as a retainer for a fixed partial denture, provides greater retention and resistance than any other type of restoration.

*Metal-Ceramic Crown Preparation*

- A fixed restoration that uses a metal sub-structure on which a ceramic veneer is fused.
- Collarless metal ceramic crown: A metal ceramic restoration whose cervical metal collar, has been eliminated. Porcelain is placed directly in contact with the prepared finish line.

*All-Ceramic Crown Preparation*

- Most esthetically pleasing prosthodontic restorations, because there is no metal to block light transmission, they can resemble natural tooth structure better in terms of color and transluency than any other restorative option can.

*Porcelain Laminate Veneers*

Laminate veneering is a conservative method of restoring the appearance of discolored, pitted or fractured anterior teeth. It consists of bonding thin ceramic laminates onto the labial surface of affected teeth.

## PARTIAL VENEER CROWN

A restoration that restores all but one crown surface of a tooth, usually not covering the facial surface.

### Types

*Anterior teeth:* Three quarter crown variations of three quarter crown; selberg crown.

*Posterior teeth:* Mesial one-half crown three quarter crown 7/8 crown

## BRIDGE/FIXED PARTIAL DENTURE

### Parts of Bridge (Fig. 4.1.1)

**1. Retainer**

"Any type of device used for the stabilization or retention of a prosthesis".

Retainer is that component of a fixed partial denture which supports and connects the body of the FPD to the abutment and restores the form, function and aesthetic of the abutment.

### Classification

*Class I: Extracoronal Restoration*

a. Complete crowns
   i. All metal
   ii. Metal + porcelain
   iii. All acrylic
   iv. Acrylic facing on metal
b. Partial crowns

*Division I: Anterior*

i. *Three quarter crown:* Covers 3/4 of the gingival circumference of tooth, leaving one surface intact. Facial surface commonly remains untouched.

*Division II: Posterior*

i. *Mesial one-half crown:* A 3/4 crown rotated 90°, preserving the distal surface of the tooth while veneering the remaining surfaces.
   *Indication:* Distal retainer of a mandibular FPD, with tilted molar abutment.
ii. Three quarter crown
iii. *Reverse three quarter crown:* Lingual surface of a mandibular posterior tooth is preserved.
   *Indicated:* Mandibular molar with severe lingual inclination used as FPD abutments.

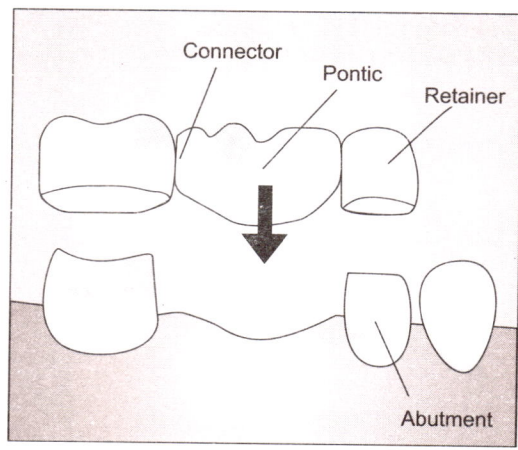

Fig. 4.1.1

iv. *Seven eighth crown:* Encompasser 7/8 of the gingival circumference of the tooth. Extends distal finish line to the midfacial surface avoiding unnecessary display of metal on mesial surface.
*Indicated:* Maxillary molars
Mandibular premolars

*Class II: Intracoronal Restorations*
i. Inlays
ii. Onlays
iii. Pinledges
iv. Combinations

*Class III: Radicular Retainers*
i. Cast core
ii. Blue island posts
iii. Parapost techniques
iv. Kurer techniques

2. **Connector**
That part of the dental bridge which unites the retainer with pontic.

*Types*
i. *Internal connector:* A non rigid connector of varying geometrical designs using a matrix to unite the members of a fixed partial denture.
ii. *Non-rigid connector:* Any connector that permits limited movement between otherwise independent members of a fixed partial denture.
iii. *Rigid connector:* A cast, soldered or fused union between the retainer(s) and pontic(s).
iv. *Subocclusal connector:* An interproximal nonrigid connector positioned apical to and not in communication with the occlusal plane.

3. **Pontic**
An artificial tooth on a fixed partial denture that replaces a missing natural tooth, restores its function and usually fills the space previously occupied by the clinical crown.

*Types*
i. *According to Designing of the Gingival Surface of Pontic*
 a. Conical/avoid pontic
 b. Saddle
 c. Ridge lap
 d. Modified ridge lap
 e. Spheroid pontic/bullet shaped
 f. Sanitary pontic/hygiene pontic
 g. Bar type
ii. *Based on Similarity to Natural Tooth*
 a. *Anatomic:* Resembles natural teeth.
    E.g. Saddle, ridge lap, modified ridge lap.
 b. *Non anatomic:* Except occlusal surface the remaining part does not resemble natural tooth. E.g. Sanitary, bar type.
iii. *Based on Fabrication*
 a. Prefabricated, e.g. porcelain teeth
 b. Custom made, Metal
    Metal-ceramic
    Ceramic
    Acrylic
    Metal-acrylic

4. **Abutment**
A tooth, a portion of a tooth or that portion of a dental implant that serves to support and / or retain a prosthesis.
**Pier abutment:** Any abutment other than the terminal abutment is called as peir abutment.
*Bridges may be classified as,*
i. Fixed-fixed: anterior, posterior
All component are rigidly joined together either by soldering the individual units together or one piece casting.
ii. Fixed-movable: anterior, posterior
iii. Cantilever bridge
iv. Spring cantilever
v. Compound bridge
vi. Conservative bridge: Resin bonded FPdor acid etched bridge.

# Section 5
# Prosthodontic Materials

# Prosthodontic Materials

**CHAPTER 1**

Many dental materials are unique to prosthodontic procedures. The improper use of any of these materials could cause a delay in the treatment and an inconvenience to the patient. You should be familiar with the use, handling, reaction time, and storing procedures for these materials. This knowledge is necessary for your successful performance as a prosthodontist.

## DENTAL ALLOYS

Although you do not make dental prostheses as a basic dental assistant, you must know enough about the materials used in their construction to document properly the treatment patients receive. When a patient's prosthesis is given to a dental lab for repair or change, they need to know its history to do the work properly, or a tragic result may follow. You should document all laboratory requests and patient dental records with information, such as alloy type used, solder type, and tooth shade if applicable. Dental alloys can be classified as precious, semiprecious, and nonprecious. For the purpose of training and clarification, we will classify them as **noble metal** or **base metal** alloys. **Noble Metal Alloys** Noble metals resist oxidation and corrosion. The four noble metals used primarily in dentistry are silver, platinum, palladium, and gold. Gold is very useful for dental purposes. Although too soft for use alone, it can be combined with other metals in varying proportions to produce alloys of almost any desired properties. Other noble metals are used in most dental labs to fabricate crowns and FPDs because of the high cost of gold. **Base Metal Alloys** Since base metal alloys do not contain noble metals, they are much stiffer and harder. Thus, they are useful for constructing RPDs and certain types of FPDs.

## IMPRESSION MATERIALS

Many types of impression materials are used in the dental clinic. However, no one material fulfills all requirements for making a perfect negative reproduction of the oral structures. The dentist will determine which material will best meet the requirements for each case. The two commonly used impression materials are alginate hydrocolloids and synthetic rubbers.

### Alginate Hydrocolloids

Hydrocolloids that change state because of thermal changes are known as *reversible* hydrocolloids because the process can be changed back and forth by altering the temperature. Those that are altered through a chemical change are known as *irreversible* hydrocolloids. Once the chemical change has taken place, it cannot be reversed or turned back to the previous state. Irreversible hydrocolloids, more commonly known as **alginates,** were developed from seaweed during World War II. Alginate impression material has largely replaced the reversible type for impressions. The advantages of alginate material are that it is easy to prepare and handle, it does not require excess equipment and advanced preparation, it is comfortable for the patient, and it is inexpensive. Alginate is used in making preliminary impressions for all study casts and most final impressions for RPD working casts. According to the American Dental Association (ADA) specifications, alginate materials are divided into two types based on gelling time: Type I—Fast set material, must gel in 1 to 2 minutes. Type II—Regular set material, must gel in 2 to 4.5 minutes after the beginning of the mix.

### Synthetic Rubber Materials

Rubber impression materials are supplied as pastes in collapsible metal tubes that require mixing. One tube contains the **base,** while the other contains an **accelerator** or a **catalyst.** When mixed in appropriate amounts, the mixture hardens to a synthetic rubber. Other types of materials come in the form of double-barreled injector cartridges that do not require mixing.

### Consistency Types

Rubber impression materials can be used for almost any impression. They come in three consistencies and are discussed in the paragraphs that follow.

*Light Bodied:* Light bodied impression materials are injected with a syringe onto preparations for inlays, crowns, and FPDs. It is also used as a "wash" impression for full dentures, relinings, and RPDs. Its high degree of flow registers the fine detail.

*Regular Bodied:* Regular bodied impression materials are used in an impression tray for inlays, crowns, and FPDs.

*Heavy Bodied:* Heavy bodied impression materials are used in a tray to force light bodied impression material onto the cavity preparation or with a copper band for impressions of single teeth.

### Material Types

Rubber impression materials can be grouped into three types depending on their composition: polysulfides, silicones, and polyethers.

### Polysulfides

The polysulfides (rubber base) can be identified by the usually dark color of one of the two pastes and their resulting opaque mix and sulfur smell. If the materials are improperly mixed, the impression will have streaks in it, thereby affecting dimensional stability. Mixing time is between 45 and 60 seconds with a 5-minute working time. The impression must not begin setting before placement in the mouth. If the 5-minute working time is exceeded, the resulting impression will have inadequate expansion, producing a smaller cast. The impression must set completely before removal from the mouth and poured no later than 1 hour after removal.

*Silicones:* Silicone (vinyl polysiloxanes) materials are generally lighter in color, translucent when set, and have a slight odor. Silicone types come in the form of a heavy putty, light, regular, and heavy bodied viscosities. The silicone material is used with a stock tray to make up the bulk of the impression and minimize distortion. Manufacturers have been able to control shrinkage resulting in impressions with greater accuracy when compared to all other rubber products. Impressions made from silicone do not have to be poured immediately. The material will remain accurate for several days so they can be repoured as necessary.

*Polyethers:* Polyethers have lighter colors than polysulfides, but are darker than silicones. The working and setting times are much shorter than the other two rubber impression materials. Polyether is just as good to use as polysulfides to control shrinkage. Unlike polysulfide, polyether will absorb water. This type of impression material is very stiff, making it difficult to remove from the mouth and a cast. The dentist must take care when removing the tray with the material from the mouth, because the polyether tears easily in thin areas like the subgingival sulcus. For best results, use this material with a custom tray.

## GYPSUM PRODUCTS

Gypsum products are supplied in powder form. When mixed with water in the correct proportions, a paste forms that will eventually harden. This setting process takes place over several minutes, during which time the mixture is soft and pliable, and can be formed into the desired shape. During the setting process, gypsum gives off heat, which is characteristic of all its products. Each material in the gypsum group is carefully compounded to give it the particular combination of physical properties needed for a particular work order. Dental plaster, stone, and die stone are the most frequently used gypsum products.

### Dental Plaster

The plaster must set within a definite time limit. Plasters made for dental use are specially processed to provide high purity and suitable working properties. One of the most important requirements is plaster has many uses. It can be used to form casts, construct matrices, and attach mount casts to an articulator. The initial setting time for most dental plaster is from 7 to 13 minutes. The final set is completed within approximately 45 minutes.

### Dental Stone

Compared to plaster, dental stone requires less water in mixing and sets more slowly. When it is set, it is harder, denser, and has a higher crushing strength. These differences make stone the choice to use over dental plaster when using it as a master cast for complete dentures and partial denture construction. Stone is more resistant to scratching and damage and can withstand more pressure in acrylic processing. Stone has many uses, including pouring, mounting casts, and flasking dentures for processing. The initial setting time of a typical stone mixture varies from 8 to 15 minutes. The final set occurs within approximately 45 minutes. **Die Stone** Historically, die stone was only used for making the first pour of a working cast for fixed prosthodontics. Improved die stone now is being used for working casts in removable prosthodontics.

## DENTAL WAXES

Dental waxes are important in the construction of dental prosthetic appliances. The waxes are supplied in different types, with each designed for specific purposes. Next we describe the waxes with which a chairside prosthetic technician needs to be familiar and be able to use.

### Baseplate Wax

Baseplate wax is used to create a spacer over the cast before custom trays can be made. Another use is as a block-out wax for undercuts on casts. It is available in sheet and ribbon form and is pink in color.

### Bite Registration Wax

Bite registration wax is a metal-impregnated wax in sheet form. It is used to record the occlusal relationships between a patient's opposing arches and to later transfer this relationship to the cast for articulation. Often without this record, it is impossible for the dentist or the laboratory technician to properly occlude the patient's cast.

### Indicator Wax

Indicator wax is usually green in color and is coated with a water soluble adhesive on one side. It is used for registering occlusal contacts on natural teeth, individual restorations, FPDs, RPDs, and CDs. It is sometimes used by the dentist to evaluate high spots on restorations.

### Sticky Wax

Sticky wax is made of beeswax, paraffin, and resin. Its colors are orange and the darker shades of blue, red, and violet. The resin gives the wax its adhesiveness and hardness. An important requirement of sticky wax is that it must break under pressure rather than bend or distort. This property makes it useful for holding the parts of a broken denture together so that it can be repaired.

### Utility Wax

Utility wax is a red or colorless wax that comes in rope form. It is extremely pliable and tacky at room temperature, making it usable without heating. Its main use is in beading (curbing) impressions before boxing and pouring. It can also be used on the impressions trays to avoid the flow of impression material to the back of the throat and to avoid injury to the soft tissue.

## ACRYLIC RESINS

There are a number of acrylic resins that you will use and need to be familiar with in prosthetic assisting. *Polymerization* is the term used to describe the processing or curing of acrylic resins. Acrylic resins can be classified by its method of curing. Some of the more common acrylic resins include the heat-cured, self-cured, and light-activated types. When handling acrylic resins, you should be sure to read the manufacturer's instructions and safety precautions before using.

### Methyl Methacrylate

Methyl methacrylate is the most widely used synthetic resin used in dentistry. The resin is usually supplied in a fine powder (polymer) and liquid (monomer). They are mixed to form a gel or dough and processed into a rigid solid.

### Clear Acrylic

Clear heat-cured acrylic resin is used to construct night guards and surgical templates. As a surgical template (band-aid) it is used after extraction of remaining teeth to show the possible interferences between the alveolar bone and the immediate denture.

## Crown and Bridge Resin

These tooth-shaded acrylic resins are used in fixed prosthodontics to make temporary and permanent restorations. The self-curing type is used as an interim restoration while the permanent one is being fabricated. This resin is normally used with a vacuum or pressure-formed matrix to sculpt the contours of the interim crown or bridge.

## Orthodontic Resin

Self-curing orthodontic resin is used to fabricate nightguards and orthodontic retainers. It is normally supplied in the clear and pink types and can be used with several tinted liquids to produce different shades.

## Repair Resins

These resins are used to fabricate interim RPDs and to repair any acrylic prosthesis. They are normally only stocked by the dental clinic in self-curing pink and light-pink fibered shades, oral tissues, head, and neck. Custom fluoride trays also are made out of this material for prescribed home treatment with fluoride gels.

## Separating Media

Separating media prevents one material from bonding to another material. The medium coats the cast and seals off the pores so acrylic resins can now be fabricated on a dental cast and removed. One type of separating media is tinfoil substitute that when used, forms a film on the cast. To use, paint it on the cast with a soft bristle brush. The film is fragile and can easily be scuffed off. If this occurs, remove the entire film and repaint. Place the acrylic resin to the cast within 1 hour of painting the film on the cast to avoid deterioration. Do not allow gypsum particles to contaminate the bottle of tinfoil substitute when applying to a cast. Many other commercially prepared separators are available to prevent bonding.

## Tray Adhesive Tray Acrylic

Self-curing tray acrylic is used to make customized impression trays. Tray acrylic is usually light blue or white in color. You can lengthen the working time of this material by submersing the dough in cold water before it is ready to use.

## OTHER PROSTHODONTIC MATERIALS

Along with the prosthodontic materials previously explained in the above categories, you need to become familar with other miscellaneous materials such as alcohols, mouthguard materials, separating media, tray adhesive, and treatment liners.

## Alcohols

Isopropyl, methanol, and denatured ethanol are examples of fuels used in an alcohol torch for softening plastic or melting wax. Of the three, denatured ethanol is preferred since it is safer to use and burns cleaner.

## Mouthguard Materials

Mouthguards are made from polyvinyl materials. This thermoplastic resin is molded over a cast by means of a vacuum-forming machine. The use of mouth protectors in sports is to reduce injuries to the custom impression trays are coated with this adhesive before they are filled with rubber impression material. This ensures that the impression material stays in the tray when it is removed from the mouth. Tray adhesive in spray form is also available for use with alginate impression materials and stock impression trays.

## Treatment Liners

Treatment liners, also known as tissue conditioners, allow oral tissues to recover, improving tone and health, before making a new denture or relining an existing one. The dentist changes the tissue conditioner at 3- to 4-day intervals since liners stiffen rapidly.

# INDEX

## A

Abutment  6, 209
Anatomic teeth  11, 131
Anatomic landmarks  26
Anterior teeth selection  131
Anterior vibrating line  34, 114
Anteroposterior curves  144
Applegate's classification  198
Applegate's modification  199
Applegate's rules  198
Appliance  5
Arbitrary face-bow  116
Arcon  149

## B

Balanced occlusion  142
Base plate  97
Beading  93
Bench curing  181
Border molding  89
Boxing  6, 93
Buccal shelf area  36

## C

Camper's line  123
Centric jaw relation  120
Compensating curves  144
Condylar guidance  143
Curve of Spee  7, 144

## D

Denture base  58
Diagnostic cast  53

## E

Eccentric jaw relation  121

## F

Face-bow  8, 116

## H

Hamular notch  8, 27
Hanau's quint  143

## I

Incisal guidance  152
Incisal guide pin  152
Incisal guide table  152
Indexing/Keying  54
Interpupillary line  123

## J

Jaw relation  115

## K

Kennedy's classification  196
Key of occlusion  154

## M

Modiolus  23
Mucocompressive impression  68

## N

Neutral zone  9, 146

## O

Occlusion rim  108
Orientation jaw relation  115

## P

Pontic  10, 209
Posterior teeth selection  135
Preliminary impression  74
Primary impression  74
Primary stress bearing area  29, 35, 36

## R

Rebasing  187
Record base  97
Relining  187
Removable partial denture  195
Rest  201
Retainer  201
Reverse curve  145

## S

Secondary impression  91
Secondary stress bearing area  29, 30, 32, 35
Semianatomic teeth  136, 137
Special tray  70

## V

Vertical jaw relation  119
Vibrating line  27, 34

## Z

0° teeth  11

# Reader's Notes